护理学研究方法

Nursing Research Methods

主　编　刘燕群

副主编　孟宪梅　邹智杰

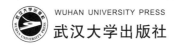

WUHAN UNIVERSITY PRESS

武汉大学出版社

图书在版编目(CIP)数据

护理学研究方法/刘燕群主编. —武汉:武汉大学出版社,2023.12
ISBN 978-7-307-24192-3

Ⅰ.护…　Ⅱ.刘…　Ⅲ.护理学—双语教学—医学院校—教材
Ⅳ.R47

中国国家版本馆 CIP 数据核字(2023)第 237287 号

责任编辑:李　玚　　　责任校对:李孟潇　　　版式设计:马　佳

出版发行:**武汉大学出版社**　　(430072　武昌　珞珈山)
　　　　　(电子邮箱:cbs22@ whu.edu.cn 网址:www.wdp.com.cn)
印刷:武汉科源印刷设计有限公司
开本:787×1092　　1/16　　印张:36　　字数:698 千字　　插页:2
版次:2023 年 12 月第 1 版　　　2023 年 12 月第 1 次印刷
ISBN 978-7-307-24192-3　　　定价:99.00 元

编　委　会

主　编

刘燕群　武汉大学护理学院

副主编

孟宪梅　武汉大学护理学院

邹智杰　武汉大学护理学院

编　委

陈永凤　广西壮族自治区人民医院

曹琼雅　湖北医药学院

林育敏　厦门大学附属妇女儿童医院

顾耀华　武汉大学护理学院

白锦兵　Emory University

孔令磷　湖北科技学院

鲜于云艳　武汉大学人民医院

王雪芬　武汉大学人民医院

冯毕龙　武汉大学中南医院

阮　景　广东省妇幼保健院

王　莉　武汉大学口腔医院

胡健薇　西安医学院

秘　书

臧恬滋　武汉大学护理学院

Contents

目 录

Contents
目 录

PART 2：Conceptualizing and Planning a Study to Generate Evidence for Nursing
第二部分　概念化及制订研究计划，为护理实践提供证据

Chapter 4：Research Questions and Hypotheses
第四章　确定研究问题、提出研究假设 / 79

PART 3: Designing and Conducting Quantitative Studies to Generate Evidence for Nursing
第三部分　设计及开展量性研究，为护理实践提供证据

Chapter 8: Quantitative Research Design
第八章　量性研究设计　／167

Chapter 9：Rigor and Validity in Quantitative Research

第九章　量性研究的严谨性和有效性　

Section Ⅰ Validity and Inference

第一节　有效性及推论　

Section Ⅱ Statistical Conclusion Validity

第二节　统计结论的有效性　

Section Ⅲ Internal Validity

第三节　内部效度　

Section Ⅳ Construct Validity

第四节　结构效度

PART 4：Designing and Conducting Qualitative Studies to Generate Evidence for Nursing

第四部分 设计及开展质性研究，为护理实践提供证据

Chapter 17：Qualitative Research Design and Approaches

第十七章 质性研究设计与方法 ／387

PART 5：Designing and Conducting Mixed Methods Studies to Generate Evidence for Nursing

第五部分　设计及开展混合方法研究，为护理实践提供证据

Chapter 25：Reporting Research Findings

第二十五章　报告研究结果　／520

PART 1：Foundations of Nursing Research

第一部分　护理研究的基础

Chapter 1：Introduction to Nursing Research
第一章　护理研究概述

Nursing is a comprehensive applied science based on the theories of natural science and social science. Science is a branch of knowledge system reflecting the objective laws of nature, society and thinking. The development of science corresponds to the process of human exploration of the world and the road of seeking truth constantly.

护理学是以自然科学和社会科学理论为基础的综合性应用科学。科学是反映自然、社会、思维等客观规律的分科的知识体系。科学的发展对应着人类探索世界的过程和不断地寻求真理的道路。

Section Ⅰ　Overview of Nursing Research
第一节　护理研究概述

Nursing is an applied science that combines theory and practice, finds and solves problems from practice, and improves existing nursing theories. Nursing research is to use scientific research methods to solve the problems in the nursing process. The concept, importance, development history and future prospects of nursing research will be described in detail below.

护理学是理论和实践相结合，从实践中发现和解决问题，完善现有的护理理论的应用型科学。护理研究是采用科学的研究方法解决护理过程中的问题。下面将详细描述护理研究的概念、重要性、发展历史及未来展望。

1. The Definition of Nursing Research(护理研究的概念)

Research is a systematic initiative to explore and find the source of problems and solutions, and to seek more supportive and reliable theoretical support. Nursing research is the systematic exploration of nursing problems through scientific methods, directly or indirectly applied to clinical nursing practice.

研究是系统性地主动探究和寻找问题的来源和解决方法，寻求更有支持性、更可靠的理论支持。护理研究是通过科学的方法，系统性地探究护理问题，直接或间接运用于临床护理实践。

In the past development of nursing, nursing researchers used appropriate research methods to make nursing research develop and solve many problems in nursing practice, but there are still many new problems that need to be explored and solved.

在过去护理学的发展过程中，护理研究者们运用合适的研究方法使得护理研究有了一定的发展，解决了许多护理实践中的问题，但如今仍有许多新的问题需要探索和解决。

2. The Importance of Research in Nursing(护理研究的重要性)

The development of nursing research contributes to the development of the nursing profession, and rigorous research results help clinical nurses make more appropriate nursing decisions. Nursing research can have a huge impact on current and future professional nursing practice.

护理研究的发展有助于护理专业发展，严谨的研究结果有助于临床护士做出更合适的决策。护理研究可以对当前和未来的专业护理实践产生具有巨大影响。

Since the 21st century, the role of the nurse has changed markedly. Nurses who work in hospitals, community health centers, nursing homes, etc., have different roles, but the main goal of professional nurses is to provide the best care for their patients through evidence from research results (Tingen MS, 2009).

进入21世纪以来，护士的角色发生了明显的变化。在医院、社区卫生服务中心、养老院等任职的护士虽然担任着不同的角色，但专业护士的主要目标都是通过研究结果获得的证据为患者提供最佳护理(Tingen MS, 2009)。

Nursing scientists are good at translating research findings into usable and effective interventions. With the development of nursing, modern nursing tends to be more evidence-based nursing and combined with basic medicine, psychology, computer science and other disciplines to conduct diversified research.

护理学家擅长将研究结果转化为可用的有效的干预措施。随着护理专业的发展，现代护理学更趋向于循证护理和与基础医学、心理学、计算机学及其他不同学科结合进行多样化研究。

3. Nursing Research in Historical Perspective(护理研究发展史)

In the 1850s, the cause of nursing research began with Mrs. Florence Nightingale (1820-1910). Around the time of the Crimean War in 1854, Nightingale improved the living conditions of patients in terms of their physical comfort and psychological comfort, made the wards ventilated, clean and bright, and increased the rounds of patients, so that the sick and wounded were better cared for and the mortality rate was greatly reduced. At that time, Nightingale mainly observed and recorded the phenomena she saw as the basis for improving nursing care, which was the beginning of nursing research. Her most famous research contribution was her analysis of the factors that influenced the mortality and morbidity of soldiers during the Crimean War. Based on skilled analysis, she transformed nursing and public health.

在 19 世纪 50 年代，护理研究事业始于弗洛伦斯-南丁格尔女士(1820—1910)。约在 1854 年克里米亚战争时，南丁格尔从病人的身体舒适和心理安慰等方面着手，改善病人的居住条件，使病房通风、清洁明亮，并增加对病人的巡视，使伤病员得到较好的护理，死亡率大大降低。当时南丁格尔主要通过观察和记录所看到的现象作为改善护理工作的依据，这就是护理研究的开始。她最著名的研究贡献就是对影响克里米亚战争期间士兵死亡率和发病率的因素进行了分析。基于科学分析，她改变了护理工作和公共卫生事业。

After Nightingale, most of the early research was on the education of nurses rather than clinical issues. In 1860, the first Nightingale Nursing School was established at ST. Thomas Hospital, London, which began systematic nursing education and played an important role in the development of nursing.

在南丁格尔之后，大多数早期研究是关于护士的教育而非针对临床问题。1860 年在伦敦圣汤姆院(ST. Thomas Hospital)建立了第一所南丁格尔护士学校，开始有系统地进行护理教育，对护理事业的发展起到重要作用。

The development of nursing research began primarily with the leaders in nursing education in the United States in the early 20th century, and the 1906 survey of nursing education was one of the earliest sources of nursing research. Many medical experts and nursing scholars have carried out research work in nursing since then and achieved great success.

护理研究的发展主要是从 20 世纪初美国护理教育的领导者开始。1906 年的护理教育调查报告是最早的一份护理研究资料。日后，相继有许多医学专家和护理学者进行护理方面研究工作，取得了很大成绩。

4. Current and Future Directions for Nursing Research(护理研究现状及展望)

Nursing research is a cognitive activity of repeated exploration, systematic observation, purposeful data collection, and rigorous scientific analysis of the unknown in the field of nursing by using scientific methods. The characteristics of nursing research include the specificity of the research object, the specificity of clinical research, and the difficulty of research methods. The focus of future nursing research will be on promoting the science of nursing. Nurse researchers and nurse practitioners will strengthen their research competencies and use them to address issues of importance to the profession and the populations it provides.

护理研究是运用科学的方法对护理学领域的未知事物进行反复地探索、系统地观察、有目的地收集资料、严谨地科学分析的一种认知活动。护理研究的特点包括研究对象的特殊性、临床研究的特殊性和研究方法的困难。未来护理研究的重点将是促进护理科学性。护理研究者和执业护士将加强他们的研究能力，并利用这些能力来解决对该专业及所护理人群非常重要的问题。

The current status of nursing research includes the expanding scope of nursing research, the gradual specialization of nursing research topics, the increasing investment in nursing research funds, the more rational application of nursing researchers, and the increased use of qualitative research methods in nursing research.

护理研究的现状包括：护理研究的范围不断扩大、护理研究的选题逐渐专业化、护理研究基金投入日益增多、护理研究人员的应用更加合理，以及护理研究中定性研究的方法增多。

Future directions for nursing research include the following:

护理研究未来发展的方向包括以下几个方面：

Firstly, the development of evidence-based nursing practice. For the nursing discipline, evidence-based nursing practice organically combines nursing research and nursing practice, making nursing truly a research-based profession and changing the habits and behaviors of clinical nurses based on experience and intuition. For society, the concept of evidence-based nursing practice combines science and technology, which is conducive to saving medical resources and controlling the excessive growth of medical costs, and has a health economics value that cannot be ignored.

首先，循证护理实践的发展。对护理学科而言，循证护理实践将护理研究和护理实践有机地结合起来，使护理真正成为一门以研究为基础的专业，改变了临床护士以经验和直觉为主的习惯和行为。对社会而言，循证护理实践的理念将科学与技术结合起来，有利于节约医疗资源，控制医疗费用的过快增长，具有不可忽视的卫生经济学价值。

Secondly, innovation in nursing research. The development of creative and innovative solutions to practice problems in nursing research. Innovative interventions and new ways of studying nursing problems will be part of the future field of nursing research.

其次，护理研究的创新。在护理研究中对于实践问题的创造性和创新性解决方案的发展。创新的干预措施和研究护理问题的新方法，会成为未来护理研究领域的一部分。

In addition, interdisciplinary collaborations have developed. In the 20th century, many difficult problems at the frontiers of science have achieved new developments in multidisciplinary integration and mutual transformation of results, and interdisciplinary cooperation has emerged in this context. The development of teaching aspects, research aspects, and practice aspects through interdisciplinary cooperation will further foster the development of interdisciplinary cooperation to promote nursing research toward internationalization in the new situation in the future.

此外，跨学科的合作发展。在 20 世纪，许多科学前沿的难题在多学科融合和成果的相互转化中取得了新的发展，跨学科合作也在此背景下产生。通过跨学科合作实现教学方面、科研方面、实践方面的发展，将进一步培养新形势下跨学科合作，从而推动护理研究未来向国际化方向发展。

Finally, increased attention to cultural differences in health. The issue of health disparities has become central to nursing and other health disciplines, along with increased awareness of the cultural sensitivity of health interventions and health care professionals in terms of cultural competence. Future research will continue to enhance the exploration of health literacy, behaviors, and values of culturally and linguistically diverse populations.

最后，加强对健康文化差异的关注。健康差异问题已经成为护理和其他健康学科的核心问题，同时也提高了人们对健康干预措施的文化敏感性和医护人员在文化胜任力方面的认识。未来的研究会不断加强对不同文化和语言人群的健康素养、行为和价值观的探讨。

Section Ⅱ Sources of Evidence for Nursing Research
第二节 护理研究的证据来源

1. Classification of Evidence in Nursing Research(护理研究的证据分类)

Evidence for nursing research can come from a variety of sources, from nurses' daily nursing practice，from expert advice，from published articles or guidelines.

护理研究的证据来源多样，可以来源于护士们日常的护理实践，也可以来源于专家意见，也可以来源于已经发表的文章或者指南。

According to different characteristics and needs of research and application，there can be the following classification：

根据研究和应用的不同特点和需求，可以有以下的几种分类：

（1）According to different research methods，it can be divided into primary research evidence and secondary research evidence.

按研究方法不同可以分为原始研究证据和二次研究证据两种。

Primary research refers to the research on causes，prevention，treatment，prognosis and other aspects directly carried out in animals or people. Direct data are usually used for analysis and statistics，and the final conclusion is drawn.

原始研究是指直接在动物或者人群中进行的有关病因、预防、治疗、预后等方面的研究，通常使用直接的数据进行分析统计，最终得出结论。

Secondary research usually needs to collect and use the original research data of relevant issues comprehensively，conduct integrated processing，analysis and statistics，and finally draw a comprehensive conclusion. Secondary study data are higher-level evidence.

二次研究通常是尽量全面收集并使用相关问题的原始研究数据，进行整合处理、分析统计，最终得出一个综合的结论。二次研究数据是更加高层次的证据。

While secondary research summarizes available studies in the form of reviews and meta-analyses，the actual studies are performed in primary research. See Figure 1. 2. 1 for a more detailed breakdown.

二次研究以综述和荟萃分析的形式总结现有研究，而实际研究是在原始研究中进行的。更详细的分类见图 1.2.1。

（2）According to different research problems，it can be divided into etiology research evidence，diagnosis research evidence，prevention research evidence，treatment research evidence and prognostic research evidence.

按研究问题不同可以分为病因研究证据、诊断研究证据、预防研究证据、治疗研究证据和预后研究证据。

（3）According to different needs of users，there are also different classifications，such as the evidence used by clinicians and nurses can be systematic evaluation，clinical practice guidelines，clinical decision analysis and clinical evidence manual，etc. Health education materials are available to the public.

根据用户不同的需要，也同样有不同的分类，如临床医师和护士使用的证据可以为系统评价、临床实践指南、临床决策分析和临床证据手册等。大众可以使用健康教育资料等。

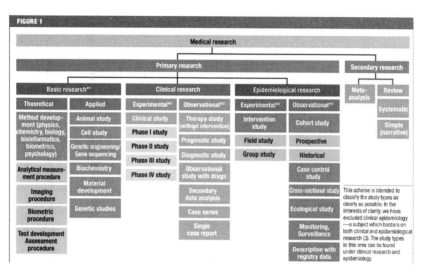

Figure 1.2.1　Classification of different study types（Röhrig B et al.，2009）

（不同研究类型的分类（Röhrig B 等，2009））

NOTE：＊1，sometimes known as experimental research；＊2，analogous term：interventional；＊3，analogous term：noninterventional or nonexperimental.

（4）According to different access channels，it can be divided into publicly published research evidence，gray literature（conference papers and internal data），research evidence under research and online information.

根据获取途径不同可以分为公开发表的研究证据、灰色文献（会议论文和内部资料）、在研的研究证据和网上信息。

2. Grading of Evidence in Nursing Research（护理研究的证据分级）

Evidence grading is based on the source，scientific nature and reliability of evidence. There are various evidence grading methods，such as OCEBM standard of EBM Center of Oxford University，internationally recognized GRADE standard，etc.

证据的分级是依据证据的来源、科学性和可靠性进行的等级划分，现在有多种证据分级方式，如英国牛津大学 EBM 中心的标准 OCEBM，国际公认的 GRADE 标准等。

GRADE（GRADE 标准）

With the development of evidence-based medicine, the quality of evidence has undergone a variety of grading methods, and finally formed the "GRADE". GRADE was released in 2000 by the "GRADE" Working Group, which was co-founded by 19 countries and international organizations, including WHO, and launched in 2004. "GRADE" focuses on transformation quality and integrates classification, grading and transformation standards from the perspective of evidence grading.

随着循证医学的发展，其证据质量先后经历了多种分级方式，最终形成了 GRADE 标准。"GRADE"在 2000 年由包括 WHO 在内的 19 个国家和国际组织共同创立的"推荐分级的评价、制定与评估"工作组发行，于 2004 年正式推行。GRADE 关注转化质量，从证据分级出发，整合了分类、分级和转化标准。

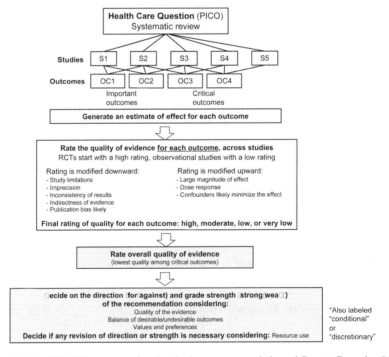

Figure 1.2.2　GRADE's process for developing recommendations（Guyatt G et al., 2011）

（GRADE 制定建议过程的示意图（Guyatt G 等, 2011））

GRADE offers a system for rating quality of evidence in systematic reviews and guidelines and grading strength of recommendations in guidelines, the system is designed for reviews and guidelines that examine alternative management strategies or interventions, which may include no intervention or current best management (Guyatt G et al., 2011).

GRADE 提供了一个在系统审查和指南中对证据质量进行评级的系统，以及对指南中建议的强度进行评级的系统，该系统是为审查替代管理战略或干预措施而设计的审查和准则，其中可能包括不干预措施或目前的最佳管理（Guyatt G 等，2011）。

In developing GRADE, researchers have considered a wide range of clinical questions, including diagnosis, screening, prevention, and therapy. Most of the examples in this series are clinical examples. The GRADE system can use in clinical problems and also can use in public health and health systems questions.

在发展 GRADE 的过程中，研究人员考虑了广泛的临床问题，包括诊断、筛查、预防和治疗。本系列中的大多数示例是临床示例。GRADE 系统可以用于临床问题，也可以用于公共卫生和卫生系统问题。

Section Ⅲ　Paradigms and Methods for Nursing Research
第三节　护理研究的范式及方法

A paradigm is a concept and theory proposed by Thomas Kuhn, a famous American philosopher of science, and described systematically in *The Structure of Scientific Revolutions* (1962). Kuhn points out that "In established usage, a paradigm is an accepted model or pattern". For Kuhn, paradigm is a fundamental commitment to ontology, epistemology, and methodology. A paradigm is a theoretical framework. Within the framework of the system, the paradigm's theories and laws are generally accepted by people.

范式的概念和理论是美国著名科学哲学家托马斯·库恩提出并在《科学革命的结构》(1962)中系统阐述的。库恩指出："按既定的用法，范式就是一种公认的模型或模式。"在库恩看来，范式是一种对本体论、认识论和方法论的基本承诺。范式是一种理论框架。在该体系框架之内的该范式的理论和定律都被人们普遍接受。

1. The Positivist Paradigm(实证主义范式)

The positivist paradigm is the mainstream of modern social science research paradigm, which is the research paradigm of natural science in a broad sense. Its purpose is to construct some new management theories by means of prediction, verification and falsification. The positivist paradigm has been applied to many fields such as management, education and so on.

实证主义范式是现代社会科学研究范式的主流，其广义上是自然科学的研究范式，其目的侧重于用预测、证实、证伪的方法来构建一些新的管理理论。实证主义范式已经被运用到了管理学、教育学等很多个领域中。

Positivism originates from "naive realism". The research methods of the positivist paradigm mainly include the method of verification and the method of falsification, both of which are methods of verification based on objective facts and things.

实证主义源于"朴素的现实主义"，实证主义范式的研究方法主要有证实法和证伪法两种，都是基于客观事实和事物进行验证的方法。

Table 1.3.1　**Understanding the positivist paradigm from ontology, epistemology and methodology** (从本体论、认识论、方法论的角度认识实证主义范式)

Angle(角度)	Contents(内容)
Ontology(本体论)	The positivist paradigm holds that the truths and laws of nature exist objectively and are not affected by subjective will. These phenomena and laws can be used in research. 实证主义范式认为自然的真理和规律是客观存在的，不受主观意志的影响。这些现象和规律是可以被使用于研究中的。
Epistemology(认识论)	The positivist paradigm emphasizes that objective facts are independent of individuals. When researchers maintain a neutral attitude to conduct research, the research results obtained will be true and can reflect objective phenomena and experiences. 实证主义范式强调客观事实独立于个体。当研究者保持中立的态度进行研究时，得到的研究结果将是真实的，可以反映客观的现象和经验。
Methodology(方法论)	The positivist paradigm believes that research methods are independent of individuals and have universal applicability. It emphasizes the use of quantitative methods to put forward hypotheses, deductively verify hypotheses with questionnaires and other methods, and study the nature of objective facts, and is mostly used in cross-sectional research. 实证主义范式认为研究方法独立于个体，具有普遍适用性。它强调通过量化的方法，提出假设，以问卷调查等方法演绎验证假设，研究客观事实的本质，多用于横断面研究。

2. The Constructivist Paradigm(建构主义范式)

The constructivist paradigm is one of the research paradigms of social science. It emphasizes that knowledge is actively constructed by individuals rather than objectively existing, and its purpose is to construct new theories with explanatory and dialectical methods. Constructivism paradigm is also widely used.

建构主义范式是社会科学研究范式的一种, 其强调知识是由个体主动建构的, 而不是客观存在的, 其目的侧重于用阐释、辩证的方法来构建新的理论。建构主义范式同样应用广泛。

The constructivist theory says that individuals eventually achieve their own balance through self-adaptation after being assimilated by the environment. The constructivist paradigm is also very similar. It emphasizes that objective facts do not exist, and subjective factors will affect the conduct of research, including concept description and research methods.

建构主义理论提出个体在受到环境的同化通过自我的顺应最终达到自身的平衡。建构主义范式也非常类似, 其强调客观的事实是不存在的, 主观因素会影响研究的进行, 包括概念描述、研究方法等。

Table 1.3.2 **Understanding the constructivist paradigm of positivism from ontology, epistemology and methodology**(从本体论、认识论、方法论的角度认识建构主义范式)

Angle(角度)	Contents(内容)
Ontology (本体论)	The constructivist paradigm holds that things are controlled by individuals and influenced by subjective factors, so there is no absolutely objective truth and law. Real things are unique, and there are differences between things in different regions. 建构主义范式认为事物都受到个体的支配, 有主观因素的影响, 所以不存在绝对客观的真理和规律。现实事物具有独特性, 不同区域的事物存在差异。
Epistemology (认识论)	The constructivist paradigm emphasizes that objective facts and research subjects are difficult to separate, there is no independent objective facts and laws. Research results are mixed with researchers' opinions. The same research in different regions, different populations and carried out by different researchers will produce different research results, which are regional and unique. 建构主义范式强调客观事实与研究主体难以分离, 不存在独立的客观事实和规律。研究结果掺杂着研究者的见解, 同一研究在不同区域、不同人群通过不同研究者的开展, 会产生不同的研究结果, 具有区域性和独特性。

续表

Angle(角度)	Contents(内容)
Methodology (方法论)	The constructivist paradigm holds that effective information can be obtained from objective facts through induction and understanding of the facts themselves, emphasizing that researchers have a deep understanding of the life of the participants. Constructivist paradigm emphasizes qualitative research methods, but does not oppose the use of quantitative research. 建构主义范式认为从客观事实出发，通过归纳和理解事实本身来得到有效的信息，强调研究者深入了解研究参与者的生活。建构主义范式强调质的研究方法，但并不反对采用量化研究。

3. Paradigms and Methods: Quantitative and Qualitative Research（定量和定性研究中的范式和方法）

Research method is the methods used by researchers to construct research, collect and analyze information relevant to research questions. Constructivist paradigm and positivist paradigm can be applied to quantitative and qualitative research respectively.

研究方法是研究人员用来构建研究、收集和分析与研究问题相关的信息的方法。建构主义范式和实证主义范式可以分别被运用到定量和定性研究中。

3.1　Paradigms and Methods in Quantitative Research（定量研究中的范式和方法）

The positivism paradigm focuses on the use of predictive, confirmatory, and falsified methods. When conducting quantitative research, researchers are more inclined to use positivism paradigm. The research methods of the positivist paradigm mainly include the method of verification and the method of falsification, both of which are methods of verification based on objective facts and things.

实证主义范式侧重于使用预测、证实、证伪的方法。在进行定量研究时，研究人员更加倾向于使用实证主义范式。实证主义范式的研究方法主要有证实法和证伪法两种，都是基于客观事实和事物进行验证的方法。

Quantitative research usually explores the influence of a specific factor on outcome variables by controlling confounding factors that may affect outcome variables. Positivist paradigm is also used to explore objective phenomena and experience, deducting and verifying hypotheses with structured methods.

定量研究通常是通过控制一些可能会影响结局变量的混杂因素，探究某一特定因素对结局变量的影响。实证主义范式也是用来探究客观现象和经验的，使用结构化的方法演绎验证假设是否成立。

3.2 Paradigms and Methods in Qualitative Research(定性研究中的范式和方法)

Both constructivist paradigm and positivist paradigm can be applied to qualitative research, which is mainly determined by the nature of qualitative research. Qualitative research can be to explore "what is this phenomenon", or to explore the opinions of different groups of people on a certain phenomenon, so both paradigms can be used.

建构主义范式和实证主义范式均可以被运用到定性研究中，这主要是由定性研究的性质决定的。定性研究可以是探究"这个现象是什么"，也可以探究不同人群对某一现象的见解，所以两种范式均可以运用。

4. Multiple Paradigms and Nursing Research(多重范式与护理研究)

Nursing research can not only rely on the two paradigms of constructivism and positivism to complete all the research, and the paradigm should be the motivation for us to further explore the nature of phenomena, rather than the shackles of research. A paradigm will always have its strengths and weaknesses, but they all share some common characteristics.

护理研究并不是单单仅依靠建构主义范式和实证主义范式这两种范式就可以完成所有的研究，范式应该是我们去更深入探究现象本质的动力，而不是禁锢研究的枷锁。一个范式总有它的优势和劣势，但是他们都有一些共同的特征。

4.1 Ultimate Goals(最终目标)

No matter what paradigm is used in research, the ultimate goal of research is to obtain the explanation of phenomena, no matter quantitative or qualitative research.

不管研究使用的范式是什么，无论是定量研究还是定性研究，研究的最终目的都是获得对现象的解释。

4.2 External Evidence(外部证据)

The research itself is not conducted through the researchers' own experience and experience, but through the exploration of objective phenomena to get answers, focusing on the collection and analysis of objective data.

　　研究本身不是通过研究人员的自身经历和经验而进行的，而是通过对客观现象的探索从而得到答案，侧重于收集和分析客观数据。

4.3　Reliance on Human Cooperation(依靠人类的合作)

Most nursing studies require the participation of the population, which needs to understand the research content and sign informed consent.

　　护理研究多数需要人群参与，需要研究人群了解研究内容并签署知情同意书。

4.4　Ethical Constraints(道德约束)

All research is subject to certain ethical principles, which we will discuss in detail in Chapter 7.

　　所有研究均需要遵循一定的道德伦理原则，我们将在第七章进行详细讲解。

4.5　Study Limitations(研究的局限性)

Virtually all studies have some limitations. Every research question can be addressed in many ways, and inevitably.

　　几乎所有的研究都有一些局限性。每个研究问题都可以以多种方式解决，这是不可避免的。

Section Ⅳ　The Purposes of Nursing Research
第四节　护理研究的目的

The purpose of nursing research is to find and solve the existing problems in the field of nursing and provide theoretical basis for the development of related fields and nursing intervention in the future. The purpose and role of nursing research include identification, description, exploration, explanation, prediction and control.

　　护理研究的目的是发现并解决目前在护理领域存在的相关问题，为今后相关领域的发展以及护理干预提供理论基础。护理研究的目的和作用包括识别、描述、探索、解释、预测和控制。

1. Identification and Description(识别和描述)

In the process of nursing research, the first step should be "identification". In qualitative research, we can usually get clear questions from some existing phenomena and describe them, which can solve problems such as "What is the name of this phenomenon?" and "What is this phenomenon?" In quantitative research, we usually have identified the problem to be studied.

在护理研究的过程中，首先要明确研究问题。在定性研究中，我们通常可以从现有的一些现象中明确得出问题并对其进行描述，可以解决像"这个现象叫什么?"和"这个现象是什么?"等问题。在定量研究中，我们通常已经明确了所要研究的问题。

2. Exploration(探索)

Exploratory research is usually a clinical phenomenon that attracts the attention of researchers, so as to further explore the causes, manifestations, results and influencing factors of this phenomenon. Exploratory research is more in-depth than descriptive research.

探索性研究往往是某种临床的现象引起了研究者的注意，从而去更深入地探索这种现象产生的原因、表现、造成的结果以及其影响因素等。探索性研究相比于描述性研究来说更加深入。

【 **Example 1** 】 Roshan et al. explores the effects of green coffee extract supplementation on anthropometric indices, glycemic control, blood pressure, lipid profile, insulin resistance and appetite in patients with the metabolic syndrome (Roshan et al., 2018).

【例1】Roshan 等人探索了青咖啡提取物补充对代谢综合征患者的人体测量指数、血糖控制、血压、脂质谱、胰岛素抵抗和食欲的影响 (Roshan 等, 2018)。

3. Explanation(解释)

Explanatory research is concerned with understanding natural phenomena and explaining their relationships (causality, opposition, etc.). Explanatory research is usually associated with theory. In quantitative research, theories are applied to research, hypotheses are made, and then verified. In qualitative research, explanatory research is to find out how this phenomenon exists, what it means and how to explain it.

解释性研究主要是了解自然现象并解释它们之间的关系(因果关系、对立关系等)。解释性研究通常与理论联系在一起。在定量研究中,将理论运用到研究中,做出假设,然后进行验证。在定性研究中,解释性研究就是去寻找这种现象如何存在的,它意味着什么以及如何去解释它。

4. Prediction and Control(预测和控制)

Prediction mainly refers to the ability to use scientific methods to make relatively reliable predictions after mastering the laws of the development of things. For example, in a specific situation, a researcher has measured a certain outcome variable in the early stage, and the probability of a specific outcome can be predicted based on these data.

预测主要是指掌握了事物发展的规律,就能够利用科学的方法做出比较可靠性的预测。如在特定情形下,在前期研究者测量了某一结果变量,可以根据这些数据去预测某一特定结果出现的可能性。

Control is usually the manipulation or manipulation of a phenomenon to produce a desired outcome, such as verifying whether a specific set of interventions designed by a nurse can help a patient achieve health goals.

控制通常是控制或操纵某种现象以产生想要的结果,比如验证护士设计的一组特定的干预措施是否能够帮助病人达到健康目标。

📖 Studies Cited in Chapter 1(第一章参考文献)

[1]Tingen, M. S., Burnett, A. H., Murchison, R. B., et al. The importance of nursing research[J]. The Journal of nursing education, 2009, 48(3): 167-170.

[2]Röhrig, B., Du Prel, J. B., Wachtlin, D., et al. Types of study in medical research: part 3 of a series on evaluation of scientific publications[J]. Deutsches Arzteblatt international, 2009, 106(15): 262-268.

[3]Guyatt, G., Oxman, A. D., Akl, E. A., et al. GRADE guidelines: 1. Introduction-GRADE evidence profiles and summary of findings tables [J]. Journal of clinical

epidemiology, 2011, 64(4): 383-394.

[4] Roshan, H., Nikpayam, O., Sedaghat, M., et al. Effects of green coffee extract supplementation on anthropometric indices, glycaemic control, blood pressure, lipid profile, insulin resistance and appetite in patients with the metabolic syndrome: a randomised clinical trial[J]. British Journal of Nutrition, 2018, 119(3): 250-258.

Chapter 2：Evidence-Based Nursing：Translating Research Evidence into Practice
第二章 循证护理：将研究证据转化为实践

Evidence-based practice as a concept and working method has a profound influence on the development of clinical medicine and nursing. Evidence-based nursing, as a branch of evidence-based practice, is a hot spot of concern for the development of nursing disciplines at home and abroad, and plays an important role in enhancing the scientific and professional level of nursing practice.

循证实践作为一种观念和工作方法，对当今临床医学和护理学的发展具有深远影响。循证护理作为循证实践的分支，是国内外护理学科发展的关注热点，对提升护理实践的科学性和专业化水平起到重要作用。

Section Ⅰ Background of Evidence-Based Nursing
第一节 循证护理的背景

1. Definition of Evidence-Based Nursing（循证护理的概念）

Evidence-based nursing（EBN）is the process by which nursing staff discreetly, explicitly, and judiciously integrate scientific findings with their clinical experience and patient desires in the planning of nursing activities, and making clinical nursing decisions based on obtained evidence. EBN is a philosophy and approach to guide scientific and effective clinical nursing decision-making. It's based on the clinical practice and emphasis specific problems as a starting point, and including four core elements.

循证护理是指护理人员在计划护理活动过程中，审慎地、明确地、明智地将科研结论与其临床经验以及病人愿望相结合，并根据获得的证据做出临床护理决策的过程。循证护理是引导科学、有效地开展临床护理决策的理念和方法，构建在临床实践基础上，强调以临床实践中特定、具体的问题为出发点，包括四个核心要素。

1.1 The Best Available External Evidence from Systematic Research
（所有可获得的来自研究的最佳证据）

Evidence refers to the practice and methods that have been proven to be credible, effective, and powerful in promoting positive changes in medical or nursing outcomes as a result of research and clinical application.

证据是指经过研究及临床应用后，证明可信、有效、能够有力促进医疗或护理结局向积极方向改变的措施、方法。

1.2 Clinical Professional Judgment（护理人员的专业判断）

Professional judgment refers to making professional decisions based on the nursing staff's sensitivity to clinical issues and extensive clinical knowledge and experience, as well as proficient clinical skills. Professional judgment requires nursing staff have systematic clinical knowledge, rich practical experience, sensitivity to identify problems, rigorous thinking, and proficient practical skills.

专业判断是指护理人员对临床问题的敏感性，以及应用其丰富的临床知识和经验、熟练的临床技能做出专业决策。专业判断要求护理人员具有系统的临床知识、丰富的实践经验、敏感的发现问题的能力、缜密的思维以及熟练的实践技能。

1.3 Patient Preference（患者的需求和偏好）

Patient preferences are the core of evidence-based decision-making. Advanced treatment methods require patients' acceptance and cooperation in order to achieve the best outcomes. Nursing staff must be patient-centered and focus on assessing and meeting patients' individual needs.

患者的需求和愿望是开展循证决策的核心。任何先进的诊治手段必须得到患者的接受和配合才能取得最好的效果，护理人员必须秉持以患者为中心，注重对患者个体需求的评估和满足。

1.4 Context（应用证据的场景）

The findings achieved significant results in a particular context may not be applicable to all clinical settings. In implementing evidence-based nursing, the application context (e.g., resource distribution, hospital conditions, patient affordability, culture, and beliefs) should be fully considered to evaluate the feasibility, appropriateness, and clinical significance of evidence.

在某一特定情境获得明显效果的研究结论不一定适用所有的临床情景，在开展循证护理的过程中，应充分考虑证据的应用情景，如资源分布、医院条件、患者的经济承受能力、文化习俗和信仰等，充分评估证据应用的可行性、适宜性和临床意义。

2. The Origin, Current Status and Future of Evidence-based Nursing（循证护理的起源、现状及展望）

EBN is rooted in evidence-based medicine. Considering increasing numbers of research papers in health care, and varying quality of research, not all treatment decisions were based on the latest and optimal evidence, British clinical epidemiologist Archie Cochrane first raised the issue of efficacy and efficiency in medical decision making in his 1972 book, *Efficacy & Efficiency: Random Reflections on Health Services*, calling for systematic reviews of published randomized controlled trials. In 1992, Professor David Sackett, a leading physician and clinical epidemiologist at McMaster University in Canada, formally developed the concept of EBM. In 1992, The Cochrane Centre was established in the UK, and then the Cochrane International Collaboration Network was developed in 1993.

循证护理的发展源于循证医学。英国临床流行病学家 Archie Cochrane 最早根据医疗卫生保健领域研究论文数量日益增多，信息传播迅速，但研究质量参差不齐，不是所有治疗决策都依据最新最佳研究证据的现象，在其 1972 年的著作《疗效与效益：卫生保健服务的随机反思》中提出了医疗决策的疗效和效益问题，呼吁要对公开发表的随机对照试验进行系统评价。1992 年加拿大麦克马斯特大学的著名内科医生和临床流行病学家 David Sackett 教授正式提出"循证医学"的概念。1992 年，英国成立 Cochrane 中心；1993 年，成立 Cochrane 国际协作网。

With the influence of evidence-based medicine, York University School of Nursing established the world's first Evidence-Based Nursing Centre in 1995, and primarily developed the concept of EBN. In 2005, the JBI Evidence-Based Health Care Model was proposed. Based on the model, a nursing-focused global collaborative network was built for the integration, dissemination, and application of healthcare evidence in areas of nursing, midwifery, geriatric care, psychotherapy, infection control, physical therapy, and cancer patient support. Since 2008,

JBI collaborated with the Cochrane Collaboration Network, and take responsibility for the 17th professional group in Cochrane—Cochrane Nursing Care Field（CNCF）. In 2012, the International Council of Nursing（ICN）released a white paper entitled "Evidence-Based Nursing Practice—Closing the Gap: From evidence to action" that sparked a boom of evidence-based practice in nursing throughout the world.

随着循证医学的影响不断深入，1995 年，英国 York 大学护理学院成立了全球第一个"循证护理中心"，首次提出"循证护理"的概念。2005 年，提出 JBI 循证卫生保健模式，以该模式为指导，建立以护理为核心的循证卫生保健相关证据的整合、传播和应用的全球协作网，包括护理、助产、老年照护、心理治疗、感染控制、物理治疗、癌症患者支持等领域。2008 年起，JBI 与 Cochrane 协作网合作，负责 Cochrane 下的第 17 专业组——护理组的工作。2012 年，国际护士理事会发布了题为"循证护理实践——缩短证据与实践之间的差距"的白皮书在全球护理领域引发了循证实践的热潮。

After becoming a Chinese Cochrane Center in 1999, the West China Hospital of Sichuan University became the first institution in mainland of China that provided evidence-based practice training to nursing staff and helped them develop evidence-based practice in the clinical setting. Starting from 2004, the JBI Evidence-Based Care Global Collaborative Network（JBC）has established sub-centers in mainland of China. These institutes aim to promote evidence-based practice adopted in clinical nursing, nursing research, and nursing education.

1999 年四川大学华西医院成为中国 Cochrane 中心后，对护理人员进行循证实践相关培训，并将循证实践的方法应用于临床护理实践，是大陆地区首次将循证实践引入护理学科的机构。自 2004 年至今，JBI 循证护理全球协作网(JBC)先后在中国大陆设立分中心。这些循证护理研究机构旨在运用循证实践的观念开展临床护理、护理研究和护理教育，促进研究成果在护理实践中的应用。

3. The Role of Nurses in Evidence-based Practice(护理人员在循证实践中的角色)

Nursing staff are the main body for implementing evidence-based care. They can fully use their own duties to cultivate a supportive environment for implementing and facilitating evidence-based practice.

护理人员是实施循证护理的主体。他们可以充分利用自己的职责，为实施和促进循证实践营造一个支持性的环境。

Firstly, working as an information promoter. Nursing administrators, nursing educators, and clinical nurses should spread the importance and benefits of evidence-based nursing to foster awareness and promote behavior change in practice.

第一，信息传播的倡导者。护理管理者、护理教育者、临床护士大力宣传循证护理实践的重要性和益处，培养开展循证实践的意识并促进其行为改变。

Secondly, working as partnership facilitator. Effective partnerships help organizations collaborate with each other, decrease duplication inputs and negative resource competition, and facilitate strategy and resource mobilization for evidence-to-practice translation.

第二，伙伴关系的推动者。有效的伙伴关系有助于相互合作和学习，减少重复投入及资源竞争，促进证据向实践转化的信息分享、策略发展和资源调动。

Thirdly, working as a performer of competence enhancement to promote nursing professional and evidence-based practice. These include improving the availability of evidence-based resources, spreading the experience of evidence-based nursing practice, arousing interest in nursing research, providing training opportunities, establishing feedback mechanisms, and changing management practices.

第三，提升能力的执行者。促进护理专业能力及循证实践能力的提升，包括提高循证资源的可及性、传播循证护理的实践经验、激发护理科研的兴趣、提供培训机会、建立反馈机制、改变管理方式等。

Fourthly, working as a summarizer of practice experience. In clinical work, nurses provide care to patients from a variety of social backgrounds, which allows nurses to fully understand how environmental factors affect patients and their families and how they respond to various health policies and services. Summarizing clinical experiences and conveying them to policymakers will benefit to clarify existing problems and designing policy support for evidence-based practice.

第四，实践经验的总结者。在临床工作中，护士为各种社会背景的患者提供护理，这使护士可以全面理解各种环境因素如何影响患者及其家庭，以及他们对于各种卫生政策和服务有何反应，及时将临床护理工作中的心得、体会、意见经验进行总结，传递给卫生政策制定者，使其明确护理实践存在问题及需要的支持，为循证实践争取政策倾斜和支持。

4. The Importance of Evidence-Based Nursing(循证护理的重要性)

EBN is a concept and working method. It is clinically important to carry out evidence-based practice to promote the scientific and effectiveness to save health resources.

循证护理是一种观念和工作方法，开展循证护理对促进临床护理的科学性和有效性以此来节约卫生资源具有重要的临床意义。

Firstly，EBN helps nursing staff update the professional vision and improve working methods. Secondly，EBN promotes the transfer of nursing knowledge to clinical practice. Thirdly，EBN follows the trend of effective use of resources in healthcare. Fourthly，EBN promotes the scientificity and effectiveness of clinical nursing practice. Fifthly，EBN contributes to the scientific and effective decision-making of clinical nursing. Sixthly，the implementation of evidence-based practice pushes our nursing staff to integrate with the multidisciplinary and international platforms.

第一，循证护理帮助护理人员更新专业观，改进工作方法；第二，循证护理促进护理知识向临床实践转化；第三，循证护理顺应了医疗卫生领域有效利用资源的趋势；第四，循证护理可促进临床护理实践的科学性和有效性；第五，循证护理有利于科学、有效地制定临床护理决策；第六，开展循证实践是将我国护理人员推向多学科合作和国际化平台的契机。

5. Evidence-based Practice Challenges(循证实践挑战)

EBN carried forward the merit of practices and rationality in natural science and reflected the emphasis on patients' personal values and expectations of modern nursing. It has important practical significance for improving the quality of clinical nursing and promoting the professional development. However，in the process of understanding and implementing evidence-based care，some misconceptions about its concept and methods have emerged. For example，simply equating evidence-based care with the application of results from a literature review to clinical practice，equating systematic reviews with general reviews，equating evidence-based care with systematic evaluation or Meta-analysis，equating evidence-based care with conducting original research，and equating evidence with results of randomized controlled trial（RCT）. These misconceptions affect the proper implementation of evidence-based nursing practice.

循证护理发扬了自然科学实践与理性的传统，又体现了现代护理对病人个人价值观和期待的重视，对于提高临床护理工作质量、促进护理学科发展有重要现实意义。然而，在认识和推广循证护理过程中，出现了一些对循证护理概念和方法理解的误区，如简单地将循证护理等同于将文献综述后的结果应用于临床实践、将系统评价等同于一般综述、将循证护理等同于系统评价或 Meta 分析、将循证护理等同于开展原始研究、将证据等同于随机对照试验(RCT)结果，影响了循证护理实践的正确实施和推广。

Section Ⅱ Evidence-Based Practice in Nursing
第二节 循证护理实践

1. Models for Evidence-based Practice(循证护理实践的相关模式)

Evidence-based nursing practice is a multidimensional and multistage process. With related concepts interacting with each other, it requires guidance from theoretical models. Commonly used models are described in the followings.

循证护理实践涉及多层面、多环节，相关概念相互影响，需要理论模式的指导，下面介绍常用的模式。

1.1 The JBI model for evidence-based healthcare(JBI 循证卫生保健模式)

The "JBI model of evidence-based healthcare" was proposed by Professor Alan Pearson, et al. in 2005. The model describes the nature, process, and logical relationship between related concepts of evidence-based healthcare. It provides a clear conceptual framework and methodological guidance for researchers and practitioners to implement evidence-based practice, which has been widely used and updated in 2016 (See Figure 2.2.1 the JBI model for evidence-based healthcare).

Alan Pearson 教授等人于 2005 年提出的"JBI 循证卫生保健模式"，阐述了循证卫生保健的本质、过程和相关概念之间的逻辑关系，为研究者和实践者开展循证实践提供了清晰的概念框架和方法学指导，在循证实践领域被广泛应用，并于 2016 年进一步更新(见图 2.2.1 JBI 循证卫生保健模式)。

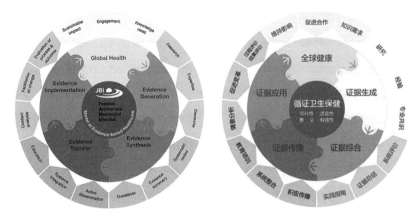

Figure 2.2.1 The JBI model for evidence-based healthcare(JBI 循证卫生保健模式)

The model conceptualizes evidence-based healthcare as a clinical decision-making process that considers the best available external evidence from systematic research，the judgment of the health professional，patient preference，and the context in which the care is delivered. The process of promoting healthcare involves a comprehensive and systematic assessment of the evidence，focus on its feasibility，appropriateness，meaningfulness，and effectiveness. These four elements consist of the FAME structure of evidence-based healthcare and inner circle of the model.

该模式认为循证卫生保健是综合可获得的最佳证据、临床情景、患者的需求和偏好，以及卫生保健人员的专业判断进行临床决策的过程。推动卫生保健的过程中，要对证据的可行性、适宜性、临床意义以及有效性进行全面系统的评估、分析和判断，该四个属性是循证卫生保健的 FAME 结构，构成了该模式图的内圈。

The middle circle is four components of evidence-based health healthcare，i. e.，evidence generation，evidence synthesis，evidence transfer，and evidence application to promote global health，which forms a proactive，healthy，dynamic，two-way cycle.

中圈是循证卫生保健的四个环节，即卫生保健是一个从证据生成、证据综合、证据传播、证据应用到促进全球健康的主动、健康、动态、双向的循环过程。

The outer circle is a concrete step of evidence-based health care，driven by global health. Based on the assessment of practice needs，practitioners uphold a pluralist philosophy，acquiring knowledge from research，experience，and professional consensus. Then，focus on a specific topic，summarizing evidence in the form of systematic evaluation，evidence summaries，and clinical practice guidelines，and promoting active evidence utilization in the clinical setting through training and system integration at al. Furthermore，based on scenario analysis，practitioners promote evidence into practice，and keep it continuous application via process and outcome evaluation to unit collaboration among stakeholders to achieve the goal of global health，and which will become the driving force for the next round of evidence-based practice.

外圈是循证卫生保健的具体步骤，由全球健康所驱动。在评估实践需求的基础上，秉持多元主义的哲学观，获取包括研究、经验、专业共识在内的知识，以系统评价、证据总结及临床实践指南的形式评价、汇总某一特定主题相关证据，借助教育培训、系统整合等方式推动证据在临床中的积极传播。在情景分析的基础上促进证据向实践转化的积极变革，通过过程及结果评价推动证据持续应用，维持变革的影响及促进利益相关者的密切合作，以达到全球健康这一目标，并成为下一轮循证实践的驱动力。

1.2　Johns Hopkins Nursing Evidence-based Practice Model

（Johns Hopkins 循证实践概念模式）

The model was proposed by Newhouse, et al. at Johns Hopkins University School of Nursing in 2007 (See Figure 2.2.2 Johns Hopkins Nursing Evidence-Based Practice Model).

该模式由约翰斯·霍普金斯大学护理学院 Newhouse 等学者于 2007 年提出（见图 2.2.2 Johns Hopkins 循证实践模式）。

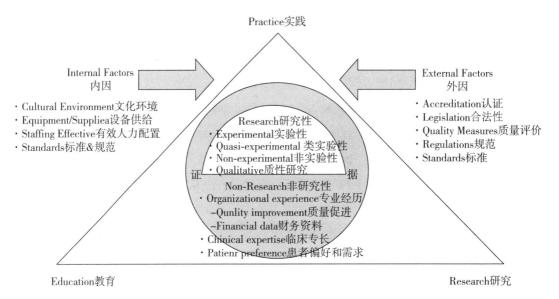

Figure 2.2.2　Johns Hopkins Nursing Evidence-Based Practice Model

（Johns Hopkins 循证实践模式）

The model considers the evidence to be central to the triangle of professional practice, education, and research, and that evidence includes those from research and from non-research evidence. Their balanced relationship is influenced by internal organizational factors and external environmental factors, which may enhance or limit the implementation of evidence.

该模式认为专业实践、教育、研究的三角关系中，核心是证据，证据包括来自研究的证据和非研究的证据。该平衡关系受内部组织因素、外部环境因素的影响，这些因素可能提高或限制证据的实施。

The model considers that evidence-based practice consists of three components: practical problem, evidence, and translation. It includes 16 steps: defining the problem, defining the scope, assigning responsibilities, conducting a team meeting, searching for internal and external evidence, evaluating the evidence, summarizing the evidence, classifying the quality level, forming a recommendation, analyzing the suitability and feasibility of evidence translation, constructing an action plan, implementing transformation, evaluating the effectiveness, internal decision support, clarifying the follow-up plan, and publishing the results.

该模式认为循证实践包括三个环节：实践问题、证据、转化。其中包括 16 个步骤：明确问题、界定范畴、分配职责、召开团队会、检索内外证据、评估证据、总结证据、划分质量等级、形成推荐意见、证据转化适宜性和可行性分析、构建行动方案、实施变革、评价效果、内部决策支持、明确后续方案、发布结果。

2. The Basic Steps of Evidence-based Nursing Practice（循证护理实践的基本步骤）

Evidence-based nursing practice includes evidence generation, evidence synthesis, evidence transfer, and evidence utilization. It includes eight steps：defining the problem, systematically searching the evidence, critically evaluating the evidence, synthesizing the evidence through systematic evaluation, disseminating the evidence, introducing the evidence, applying the evidence, and evaluating the effectiveness of the evidence after application.

循证护理实践包括证据生成、证据综合、证据传播和证据应用。具体包括 8 个步骤：明确问题、系统检索文献、严格评价证据、通过系统评价汇总证据、传播证据、引入证据、应用证据、评价证据应用后的效果。

2.1 Evidence Generation（证据生成）

That is the generation of evidence. The evidence sources are diverse, including research results, expert consensus, expert clinical experience, mature expertise, logical deduction, and reasoning, etc. They need to have feasibility, appropriateness, clinical meaningfulness, and effectiveness, i. e., the FAME attributes of evidence.

即证据的产生。证据来源是多元化的，包括研究结果、专家共识、专家临床经验、成熟的专业知识、逻辑演绎和推理等，但需具备可行性、适宜性、临床意义和有效性，即证据的 FAME 属性。

2.2 Evidence Synthesis （证据综合）

The evidence is generated through systematic review. This phase includes four steps.

通过系统评价确立证据。该阶段包括四个步骤。

(1)Clarifying the problem in clinical practice, and structuring it in a specific way.

明确临床实践中的问题,并将其特定化、结构化。

(2)Based on the proposed question, systematically searching the literature to find evidence.

根据所提出的问题进行系统的文献检索以寻找证据。

(3)Critically evaluating the quality of retrieving literature to filter the appropriate studies, including the scientificity and rigor of design, feasibility and appropriateness of results, and clinical significance of the study.

严格评价检索到的文献质量,包括设计的科学性和严谨性、结果推广的可行性和适宜性,以及研究的临床意义,筛选合适的研究。

(4)Summarizing the included studies, i. e., to conduct Meta-analysis for similar studies with homogeneity and conduct qualitative summary for similar studies that cannot be Meta-analyzed.

对筛选后纳入的研究进行汇总,即对具有同质性的同类研究结果继续 Meta 分析,对不能进行 Meta 分析的同类研究进行定性总结和分析。

2.3 Evidence Transfer(证据传播)

It refers to the transmission of evidence to nursing systems, nursing managers, and nursing practitioners through the publication of Clinical Practice Guidelines, Best Practice Information Sheet, and other forms of media such as professional journals, professional websites, and education and training. It includes four steps.

证据的传播指通过发布临床实践指南、最佳实践信息册等形式,由专业期刊、专业网站、教育和培训等媒介将证据传递到护理系统、护理管理者、护理实践者中,包括四个步骤。

(1)Label the grade or recommendation of evidence, which is the fundamental characteristic of evidence-based practice.

标注证据的等级或推荐意见,是循证实践的基本特征。

(2)Organize the evidence resources into a form that can be easily disseminated and applied by professionals, such as clinical practice guidelines (CPG), care bundles, and evidence summary.

将证据资源组织成易于传播并利于专业人员理解、应用的形式,如临床实践指南、集束化照护方案、证据总结。

(3) Understand the specific needs of the target population for evidence.

详细了解目标人群对证据的需求。

(4) Deliver evidence and information in the most cost-effective way.

以最经济的方式传递证据和信息。

2.4 Evidence Utilization(证据应用)

It refers to utilizing evidence to reform nursing practice, including:

证据应用即遵循证据改革护理实践活动，包括：

(1) Context analysis, understanding the gap between evidence and practice, and introducing evidence.

情景分析，了解证据与实践之间的差距，引入证据。

(2) Promoting change, formulating the adopted evidence into actionable workflows, quality standards, and incentive policies, and conduct staff training to reach consensus and improve performance.

促进变革，将采纳的证据制定成可操作的流程、质量标准、激励政策，通过全员培训达成共识，提高执行力。

(3) Evaluate the effectiveness of evidence application, dynamically monitor the process, and continuously improve quality until the change of the nursing system.

评价证据应用效果，动态监测证据应用过程，以护理系统发生整体变革为标志，持续质量改进。

3. Asking Well-worded Clinical Questions(如何提出一个好的循证问题)

Raising an evidence-based question is the first step in implementing a proper and effective literature search, and is the beginning of evidence-based nursing. Evidence-based nursing questions should be concise, precise, specific, and with the appropriate components. According to the different purposes, there are two categories: questions for evidence creation and questions for evidence utilization.

提出循证问题，是实施正确、有效文献检索的第一步，是循证护理的开端。循证护理问题应简明、准确和具体，具备相应的构成要素。根据不同的目的，分为两类：基于创证的循证问题和基于用证的循证问题。

3.1　Questions for Evidence Creation(基于创证的循证问题)

For quantitative studies, an ideal evidence-based question should include 5 elements, i. e., PICOS: P for population, I for intervention/exposure, C for control/comparator, O for outcome, and S for study design. With the development of evidence-based practice, extended models of PICO such as PECO, PEO, and PICOSST have been proposed. Furthermore, the evidence-based questions of qualitative research generally include 4 aspects of PICoS: P for participant, I for interest of phenomena, Co for context, and S for study design.

针对量性研究，一个理想的循证问题应包括5个要素，即 PICOS：特定的人群、干预或暴露因素、对照组或另一种可用于比较的干预措施、结局、研究设计。随着循证实践的发展，又提出了 PECO、PEO、PICOSST 等 PICO 扩展模式。质性研究的循证问题一般包括 PICOS 4 个方面：患者或服务对象、感兴趣的现象、具体情景、质性研究的类型。

3.2　Questions for Evidence Utilization(基于用证的循证问题)

In the process of conducting evidence-based practice, PIPOST can be used to structure the questions to accurately retrieve the related evidence, specifically:

在应用证据开展循证实践过程中，为准确检索到相应的证据，可采用 PIPOST 构建结构化的循证问题，具体为：

(1)P for the target population.

P 代表证据应用的目标人群。

(2)I for the intervention.

I 代表干预措施。

(3)P for the professional staff who use the evidence.

P 代表应用证据的专业人员。

(4)O for outcomes from the system, practitioner, and patient.

O 代表系统、实践者、患者相关的结局。

(5)S for setting.

S 代表证据应用场所。

(6)T for the type of evidence, such as clinic al practice guidelines, systematic reviews, and summaries of evidence.

T 代表证据类型，如临床实践指南、系统评价、证据总结。

4. Evidence Resources and the Retrieval of Evidence(证据资源及检索方法)

4.1　Evidence Resources(证据资源)

The widely acknowledged classification of evidence resources is the "6S" pyramid model proposed in 2009. Each "S" represents a type of evidence resource. From the top to the bottom of the pyramid, evidence includes：

国内外关于循证资源最经典的分类是 2009 年的"6S"证据资源金字塔模型，每个"S"代表一种证据资源类型，从塔顶自上而下具体为：

(1)System, such as computerized decision support systems.

系统，如计算机决策支持系统。

(2)Summaries, such as evidence-based clinical practice guidelines, and evidence-based textbooks.

专题证据汇总，来源如基于循证的临床实践指南、基于循证的教科书。

(3)Synopses of syntheses, such as the Database of Abstracts of Reviews of Effects.

系统评价摘要，来源如效果评价文摘数据库。

(4)Syntheses, such as The Cochrane Library, The Campbell Library.

系统评价/证据综合，来源如考克兰图书馆、坎贝尔图书馆。

(5)Synopses of studies, such as evidence-based abstraction journals.

研究摘要，来源如循证摘要杂志。

(6)Studies, such as original articles published in journal.

原始研究，如发表在期刊的原始研究论文。

4.2　Evidence Retrieval(证据检索)

There are two types of evidence retrieval：

循证护理的证据检索包括两种：

(1)Retrieval for the purpose of evidence translation. It emphasizes accuracy and enables nursing staff to retrieve the best evidence in a short period of time.

以"用证"为目的的检索强调查准率，便于临床护理人员在短时间内检索到最佳证据。

(2)Search for the purpose of evidence creation. It generates evidence through systematic evaluation/meta-analysis, which emphasizes the systematic, comprehensive, unbiased, and integrity of evidence retrieval.

以"创证"为目的的检索，即通过系统评价/meta 分析产生证据的过程，更强调检索的系统、全面和无偏移，应尽可能提高检索的查全率。

However, both have similar steps, except for the different focus on databases and search terms. The basic steps are as follows.

无论是"用证"还是"创证"的检索，检索基本步骤和基本检索方法大同小异，主要在数据库的选择和检索词的确定方面各具特点。基本步骤如下：

(1) Identify the clinical question. Structuring it in PICOS element to clarify population, intervention, comparator, outcome, and study design in the question.

明确临床护理问题。使用 PICOS 策略进行解析，明确研究对象特征、干预措施、对照措施、临床结局和研究类型。

(2) Select database. For evidence translation, evidence of 6S pyramid model should be searched in descending order. Only if the required evidence is still not available should the original research be searched. For evidence creation, the database of the original study is the priority. In order to find as much original research, conference paper databases, dissertation databases, gray literature data, and online registration databases are included.

选择数据库。以"用证"为目的的检索，按照"6S"证据金字塔模型，应从最高的资源等级开始依次往下检索，如果仍不能得到所需要的证据，才需要检索原始研究。以"创证"为目的的文献检索，直接从原始研究开始检索，为了保证查全率，还需检索会议论文数据库、学位论文数据库、灰色文献数据和在线注册数据库等。

(3) Determining appropriate search terms. It is necessary to use both subject term and keyword to search available evidence. As for evidence translation, if there are too many results of the initial search, the feature terms in Comparator and Outcome can be used to limit the results and improve their accuracy. As for evidence creation in systematic reviews or meta-analysis. If there are too many results of the initial search, the feature terms in study design can be used to narrow the results. However, terms of Comparator and Outcome cannot be used to search for evidence.

确定恰当的检索词。为了提高检索质量和效率，在检索时需要同时运用主题词检索和关键词检索。"用证"检索，若初次检索的结果数量较大，可以将对照措施项和结局指标中的重要特征词为检索词进行限定检索，提高查准率。若是"创证"检索制作系统评价或 meta 分析，在初步检索文献量较大时，可同时将研究类型(s)作为检索词进行限定。对照措施和结局指标不作为检索词使用。

（4）Develop and implement search strategies. If high sensitivity is required, OR operator can be used to expand the search scope and improve the detection rate of relevant documents. If high specificity is required, AND or NOT operator can be used to narrow the search scope and improve the detection rate.

制定检索策略并实施。对敏感性检索要求高时，可选择 OR 运算符来扩大检索范围，提高相关文献的检出率；对特异性检索要求高时，可选择 AND 或 NOT 运算符来缩小检索范围，提高查准率。

（5）Assess whether the available results answered the proposed questions. According to the inclusion criteria of the proposed questions, related literature was organized. Then, the scientific evaluation criteria of clinical epidemiology and evidence-based medicine were applied to evaluate the grade, truthfulness, and appropriateness of evidence to offer support for clinical nursing.

评估检索结果是否回答了提出的问题。根据循证护理问题的性质，制定文献纳入标准，将收集到的文献整理分析，应用临床流行病学/循证医学的科学评价标准，从证据的级别、真实性、适用性等方面评价研究证据，在此基础上选择最佳证据，为临床护理决策提供科学依据。

（6）Update regularly.

定期更新。

5. Appraising the Evidence(证据/文献的评价)

5.1 Significance of the Evidence/Literature Appraisal(证据/文献评价的意义)

Critical appraisal of the literature is required in systematic reviews. The reliability of systematic reviews depends on the truthfulness of the included original studies. Only the acceptable quality of original studies can guarantee the reliability of the systematic review and offer a solid basis for health policymakers.

文献严格评价是系统评价的必要步骤。对原始研究进行系统评价得出的结论是否可靠，取决于所纳入的原始研究的结果是否真实。只有纳入质量合格的研究，才能确保系统评价结果的可靠性，为卫生政策制定者提供可靠依据。

5.2 Contents of Evidence/Literature Appraisal(证据/文献评价的要素)

It includes internal truthfulness, clinical importance, and applicability of evidence/

literature.

文献严格评价的基本要素包括内部真实性、临床重要性和适用性 3 个方面。

5.2.1 Internal Truthfulness(内部真实性)

It is the degree to which the results of a given study are close to the true value, i. e., the degree to which the results are influenced by various biases. Biases are selection bias, implementation bias, measurement bias, reporting bias, etc.

内部真实性是指某个研究结果接近真值的程度，即研究结果受各种偏移的影响程度，偏倚来源主要有选择偏倚、实施偏倚、测量偏倚、报告偏倚等。

5.2.2 Clinical Significance(临床重要性)

It refers to the value of the clinical application. The focus of its appraisal should be on whether the clinical questions addressed by the evidence are clear and specific, and whether the measurements are correct.

重要性是指研究是否具有临床应用价值，评估证据的临床重要性应重点关注证据所涉及临床问题是否明确、具体，所选择的评价指标是否正确等问题。

5.2.3 Applicability(适用性)

It refers to the external validity of the study and whether the findings can be generalized to populations beyond the study population. Evaluation of the evidence applicability should take into account: whether the population served by the evidence matches the participant's inclusion criteria of the study; whether the health care environment in which the evidence is served has the necessary human resources, technical strength, facilities and equipment conditions, and socioeconomic factors to implement the evidence; evaluate the potential advantages and disadvantages of applying the evidence to the population served; and the willingness of the population served to use the evidence.

研究的外部真实性，指研究结果能否推广应用到研究对象以外的人群。评价证据的适用性应考虑：证据服务对象与证据中研究对象的纳入标准是否相符，证据服务对象所处的医疗环境是否具备应用该证据所需的人力、技术力量、设施和设备条件、社会经济因素等，应用证据可能对服务对象产生的利弊权衡，服务对象自身使用该证据的意愿。

5.3 Procedure for Evidence/Literature Appraisal(证据/文献评价的程序)

It includes the following steps：

进行证据/文献评价的程序为：

(1) Selecting the appropriate literature truthfulness appraisal tool based on the type of literature，and two appraisers independently evaluate the same literature according to the each item of appraisal tool and make separate judgments.

根据文献的类型选择相应的文献真实性评价工具，由 2 名评价者对同一篇文献对照评价工具中的每个条目独立评价，分别作出结果判定。

(2) Two appraisers discuss their appraisal results together，and negotiate when there are different opinions on the judgments，and asking a third person to discuss with them if they cannot reach agreement.

2 名评价者一起讨论各自的评价结果，在每个评价项目的结果判定出现意见分歧时，由 2 名评价者进行协商，不能达成一致时请第三人共同讨论。

(3) Making a decision on the inclusion，exclusion，or cautious inclusion of the literature.

对该文献做出纳入、排除或审慎纳入的决定。

5.4 Methods of Evidence/Literature Appraisal(证据/文献评价的方法)

Different methods are used for different types of literature appraisal. Detailed reference resources include the Cochrane Handbook for Systematic Reviews of Interventions version 6.3 (2022)，JBI Manual for Evidence Synthesis (2021)，and the Critical Appraisal Skills Program (CASP) Checklist (2022)，etc.

不同类型的文献采用不同的评价方法，具体可参考 Cochrane 协作网关于干预性研究系统评价的手册 6.3 部分(2022)、澳大利亚 JBI 循证卫生保健中心证据综合手册(2021)、文献严格评价项目清单(2022)等。

The JBI Manual for Evidence Synthesis (2021) contains critical appraisal checklist for different types of publications，such as randomized controlled trials，quasi-experimental studies，cohort studies，case-control studies，analytical cross-sectional studies，case series/case reports/ expert opinion，qualitative studies，systematic reviews，etc. The reviewers are required to give a "yes"，"no" "unclear" and "not applicable" for each appraisal item，and decide whether the study is included，excluded，or requires further information via a group discussion.

澳大利亚 JBI 循证卫生保健中心证据综合手册(2021)包含针对随机对照试验、类实验性研究、队列研究、病例对照研究、描述性研究、案例系列/个案报告/专家意见类、质性研究、系统评价等不同类型论文的评价工具，评价者需对每个评价项目做出"是""否""不清楚""不适用"的判断，经过小组讨论决定该研究是纳入、排除，还是需要获取进一步信息。

6. Types of Evidence and Evidence Hierarchies(证据类型及等级)

6.1　Type of Evidence(证据类型)

The widely acknowledged classification of evidence resources is the "6S" pyramid model proposed in 2009. Each "S" represents a type of evidence resource. From the top to the bottom of the pyramid，evidence include a computerized decision support system, summaries, synopses of syntheses, syntheses, synopses of studies, studies.

国内外关于循证资源最经典的分类是 2009 年的"6S"证据资源金字塔模型，每个"S"代表一种证据资源类型，从塔顶自上而下分别为：计算机决策支持系统，专题证据汇总，系统评价摘要，系统评价/证据综合，研究摘要，原始研究。

6.2　Grades of Evidence(证据等级)

It includes the quality level and recommendation grade of the evidence. Evidence quality refers to the truthfulness level of the predicted values in evidence, which is often distinguished by high-quality evidence, moderate-quality evidence, and low-quality evidence. Recommendation grade is the degree to follow a particular recommendation, often distinguished by a strong or weak recommendation. In combination with approach of the Grading of Recommendations, Assessment, Development and Evaluation (GRADE) Working Group, the JBI developed GRADE pre-rankings in 2014. It inherited the evidence grade by study design and separately graded quantitative and qualitative studies. It performs the recommendation grade based on the FAME attribute of the evidence, which is easy to understand and apply by users.

证据的等级性包括证据的质量等级和推荐级别。证据质量是指对预测值的真实性有多大把握，常用高质量证据、中等质量证据、低质量证据来区分。推荐强度是遵循某一特定推荐意见的强度，其程度常用强推荐或弱推荐区分。结合 GRADE 系统的推广，2014 年，JBI 循证卫生保健中心制定了证据预分级标准。它保留了按照研究设计分级的思路，将量性研究和质性研究分别划分等级，并根据证据的 FAME 属性执行了相应的推荐级别，便于使用者理解和应用。

6.2.1 GRADE Pre-rankings for Quantitative Studies(量性研究的证据预分级标准)

After a critical evaluation of the truthfulness of a single study, the evidence is graded into levels 1 to 5 by its study design. Experimental studies are defined as level 1 evidence, quasi-experimental studies are defined as level 2 evidence, observational studies are defined as level 3 evidence, descriptive studies are defined as level 4 evidence, and expert opinion and animal studies are defined as level 5 evidence. Within the same level of evidence, it was further divided into sublevels based on whether the evidence is integrated, defining the integrated level of evidence as higher than that of the single original study.

对单篇文献的真实性进行严格评价后，按照文献的研究设计，将证据分为1~5级。将实验性研究定义为1级证据，将类实验性研究定义为2级证据，观察性研究定义为3级证据，描述性研究定义为4级证据，专家意见和基础研究定义为5级证据。在同一级别的证据中，又根据证据是否被整合分为亚级，定义整合后的证据级别高于单项原始研究。

6.2.2 GRADE Pre-rankings for Qualitative Studies(质性研究的证据预分级标准)

After a critical evaluation of the truthfulness of a single study, the evidence was classified into levels 1 to 5 according to whether qualitative studies were integrated or not. Systematic reviews of mixed design studies are defined as level 1 evidence, Meta-integration of qualitative studies is defined as level 2 evidence, single qualitative study is defined as level 3 evidence, systematic evaluation of expert opinion is defined as level 4 evidence, and single expert opinion is defined as level 5 evidence.

对单篇文献的真实性进行严格评价后，按照质性研究整合与否，将证据分为1~5级。将混合设计研究的系统评价定义为1级证据，质性研究的 Meta 整合定义为2级证据，单项质性研究定义为3级证据，专家意见的系统评价定义为4级证据，单项专家意见定义为5级证据。

6.2.3 Recommendation Grade(推荐级别)

JBI grading the evidence into A-level recommendations (i.e., strong recommendations) and B-level recommendations (i.e., weak recommendations) based on the full consideration of FAME attributes of the evidence, i.e., its feasibility, appropriateness, clinical significance, and validity. Since the recommendation grade does not completely depend on the level of evidence, high-level evidence may not make a strong recommendation, and low-level evidence may not make a weak recommendation.

JBI 建议依据证据的 FAME 属性，即充分考虑证据的可行性、适宜性、临床意义和有效性，将推荐级别划分为 A 级推荐(即强推荐)和 B 级推荐(即弱推荐)。由于推荐级别的确定不完全取决于证据级别，所以高级别的证据未必做出强推荐，低级别的证据也未必做出弱推荐。

7. System Reviews(系统评价)

7.1　Concept of Systematic Review(系统评价的概念)

Systematic Review refers to the systematic and comprehensive collection of all published or unpublished studies for a specific clinical problem (such as disease etiology, diagnosis, treatment, prognosis, nursing care, etc.), and using rigorous principles and methods of epidemiology to screen out literature that meets quality standards, then perform qualitative or quantitative synthesis of results to draw comprehensive and reliable conclusions. Due to the strict organization and quality control system of the Cochrane Collaboration Network, system reviews from the Cochrane Collaboration Network have higher quality than other system reviews.

系统评价(Systematic Review, SR)是指针对某一具体临床问题(如疾病的病因、诊断、治疗、预后、护理等)，系统、全面地收集所有已发表或未发表的临床研究，采用临床流行病学严格评价文献的原则和方法，筛选出符合质量标准的文献，进行定性或定量合成，得出综合、可靠的结论。由于 Cochrane 协作网有严密的组织管理和质量控制系统，Cochrane 系统评价的质量通常比非 Cochrane 系统评价质量更高。

7.2　Procedures and Methods of Systematic Review(系统评价的基本步骤和方法)

The systematic review is a kind of scientific research. Similar to original research, it contains procedures of the design-implementation-result analysis-summary report, etc. Taking systematic reviews from the Cochrane Collaboration Network as an example, the following is a brief description of steps and methods of systematic review. It includes the followings:

系统评价是一种科学研究，同原始研究一样，都要经过设计—实施—结果分析—总结报告等阶段。下面以 Cochrane 系统评价为例，简述系统评价的基本步骤和方法。系统评价的步骤包括:

(1) Determine and register the title, and clarify its four elements, namely, the study

population, interventions and controls, outcome indicators, and type of study.

确立题目并注册，围绕研究问题明确四个要素，即研究对象类型、干预措施和对照措施、结局指标、研究类型。

（2）Develop a proposal for systematic review, including title, background, purpose, and methodology (e. g., strategy for literature retrieval, criteria for literature inclusion and exclusion, methods for literature quality appraisal, methods for collecting and analyzing data).

制定系统评价计划书，内容包括题目、背景资料、目的、方法（如文献检索的策略、文献纳入和排除标准、文献质量评价方法、收集和分析数据的方法）。

（3）Systematically and comprehensively search literature based on retrieval strategies.

根据检索策略进行系统、全面的检索。

（4）According to the inclusion and exclusion criteria, select literature that can answer the research questions.

根据纳入和排除标准，选择能够回答研究问题的文献资料。

（5）Two evaluators (at least) evaluate the quality of the literature independently and critically, contents include internal truthfulness, clinical importance, and applicability of evidence.

至少由 2 名评价人员独立、盲法地严格评价文献质量，评价内容包括内部真实性、外部真实性和临床适用性。

（6）Extract accurate data from original studies, and ensure the truthfulness and reliability of the systematic reviews.

从原始文献中准确提取数据，为保证系统评价的真实性和可靠性。

（7）Conduct data analysis and describe results. Data analysis includes qualitative and quantitative analysis. The description of the results should follow the general requirements of biomedical writing.

进行数据分析和结果描述，数据分析包括定性分析和定量分析，结果描述应遵循生物医学写作的一般要求。

（8）Interpret the results of the systematic reviews in five main dimensions, including a summary of the main findings, the applicability of the evidence, the quality of the evidence, possible biases or limitations, and similarities and differences with other studies or systematic reviews.

解释系统评价的结果，主要包括主要研究结果的总结、证据的可应用性、证据的质量、可能存在的偏移或局限性、与其他研究或系统评价的异同点等五个方面。

(9) Update the systematic reviews regularly.

定期更新系统评价。

7.3　Meta-analysis of Interventional Studies or Observational Studies

（干预性研究或观察性研究的 Meta 分析）

Meta-analysis is a quantitative and comprehensive analysis method that can statistically increase the sample size and improve the efficiency of the test, so as to draw more scientific, reasonable, and reliable conclusions. Its procedure is similar to that of the systematic reviews, and the followings focus on its statistical analysis process. It mainly includes:

Meta 分析是一种定量综合分析方法，能从统计学角度达到增加样本量、提高检验效率的作用，从而得出更为科学、合理和可信的结论。其步骤与系统评价类似，现重点介绍 Meta 的统计分析过程，主要包括：

(1) Clarify the types of data and their effect sizes. The five common types of data in Meta-analysis are dichotomous variables, continuous variables, hierarchical variables, categorical variables, and survival data.

明确数据的类型及效应量表达。Meta 分析中常见的数据类型有二分类变量、连续性变量、等级资料、计数变量和生存资料等 5 类。

(2) Extract relevant information from included studies for data aggregation.

提取纳入研究的相关信息，进行数据汇总。

(3) Heterogeneity tests. Only based on the clinical and methodological homogeneity, the test of statistical heterogeneity between studies can be performed.

进行异质性检验及处理。只有在临床和方法学同质性的基础上，方可进入研究间统计学异质性检验。

(4) Combined effect sizes and tests. It reflects the combined effect of multiple similar studies. if heterogeneity is not significant, a fixed-effects model can be used to estimate the combined effect size. When there is significant heterogeneity, a random-effects model can be used to estimate the combined effects size.

合并效应量及检验。用合并效应量反映多个同类研究的综合效应。当异质性不明显时，可采用固定效应模型估计合并效应量；当存在异质性，可选用随机效应模型估计合并效应量。

(5) Conduct sensitivity analysis to evaluate whether the Meta-analysis results are reliable and stable.

敏感性分析，用于评价 Meta 分析结果是否稳定可靠。

（6）Analyze publish bias，such as the method of funnel plot.

发表偏移分析，常用漏斗图法。

（7）Interpret the results of Meta-analysis. Forest plots are often used to present the results of statistical analysis. The combined effect size is evaluated for statistical significance based on whether the diamond intersects with the null line.

解释 Meta 分析结果。常使用森林图来展示统计分析结果，根据菱形是否与无效线相交来判断合并效应量有无统计学意义。

7.4　Meta-integration of Qualitative Studies（质性研究的 Meta 整合）

Meta-integration of qualitative studies refers to the understanding, interpretation, and inductive combination of multiple qualitative research findings. It aims to deepen the understanding and inquiry about the nature of phenomena, and promotes nursing knowledge accumulation and theoretical development. There are 7 steps：

质性研究的 Meta 整合是对多个质性研究结果进行理解、解释和归纳组合，从而深入理解和探究现象本质，促进护理知识积累和理论发展。包括 7 个步骤：

（1）Develop a rigorous proposal. Defines the evidence-based question through PICO, i. e., clarifies elements including participant, interest of phenomena, and contexts in which the study is conducted.

制订严谨的计划书。通过 PICO 界定循证问题，即明确研究对象、研究的现象、研究对象所处的情景。

（2）Develop a comprehensive search strategy, select appropriate databases, and conduct a systematic search of relevant qualitative literature.

制定系统的检索策略，选择合适的数据库，全面检索相关质性研究文献。

（3）Critically evaluate the truthfulness of qualitative research, e. g., the JBI appraisal checklist for qualitative research.

严格评价质性研究的真实性，如可采用 JBI 质性研究真实性评价工具。

（4）Read the full text carefully to extract information from the original qualitative study.

仔细阅读全文，提取质性研究中的资料。

（5）Summarize, analyze, interpret and synthesize the results of original research to form new concepts or interpretations.

概括、分析、解释和综合原始研究的结果，形成新的概念或解释。

(6) Use a structured way to systematically report integration results.

通过结构化的方式，系统地报告整合结果的方法。

(7) Evaluate the overall quality of Meta integration, mainly focusing on the credibility and dependability of the comprehensive body of evidence.

评价 Meta 整合的总体质量，主要评价综合性证据体的可信度和可靠性。

7.5 Systematic Review of Expert Consensus and Opinions

（专家共识、专家意见类研究的系统评价）

In the fields of nursing and psychology, evaluated expert consensus and opinion can temporarily serve as a basis for decision-making as fewer RCTs are available. Specific steps showed in the followings:

在护理学、心理学等领域，因 RCT 较少，经过评价的专家共识和专家意见可暂时成为决策依据。具体步骤包括：

(1) Raise and structure questions. Systematic reviews of expert consensus and opinion are more similar to qualitative research. The PICO (i.e., participant, interest of phenomena, and contexts) can be used to define the evidence-based question.

提出和构建问题。专业共识、专家意见类系统评价更接近质性研究的特点，可使用 PICO(即研究对象、感兴趣的现象、研究对象所处的情景)模型界定循证问题。

(2) Set inclusion/exclusion criteria based on the essential elements of the evidence-based question.

依据问题的基本要素，制订纳入/排除标准。

(3) Develop search terms according to the research question and determine the search strategy for a comprehensive search.

根据研究问题凝练检索词，确定检索策略进行全面检索。

(4) Two or more researchers independently screen literature following the inclusion/exclusion criteria.

由两名及以上研究员按照纳入/排除标准进行文献筛选。

(5) Conduct rigorous quality appraisal and establish a literature quality appraisal form.

进行文献严格质量评价，建立文献质量评价表。

(6) Two evaluators extract literature information against the data extraction instrument to maintain the integrity of the original data.

两名评价者根据文献提取工具进行资料提取，保持原始数据的完整性。

(7) Adopt method like the thematic synthesis to synthesize the content and mark the reliability of the synthesis results.

采取如主题综合的方式进行资料综合，并对综合的结果进行可信度标记。

(8) Present and discuss the results to provide an insightful interpretation and inference of the research questions.

报告及讨论结果，对研究问题进行深入阐释及推断。

7.6　Reviews of Systematic Reviews(系统评价的再评价)

It refers to summary of existing systematic reviews related to a given topic or question, such as treatment, etiology, diagnosis, and prognosis of the same disease or health problem. It aims to provide evidence for decision-making. It mainly includes the following circumstances: summary existing systematic reviews of multiple interventions related to the same clinical problem; summary of existing systematic reviews of a specific intervention conducted on different populations; summary of existing systematic reviews on different outcomes for the same intervention or phenomena of interest; Using a wider perspective to summarize relevant systematic reviews in a given area.

系统评价的再评价是指全面收集同一疾病或健康问题的治疗或病因、诊断、预后等方面的相关系统评价进行汇总分析，为决策者提供证据支撑。主要包含以下几种情况：对同一临床问题的多个干预措施相关系统评价进行汇总；对某一干预措施用于不同人群的多个系统评价进行汇总；对涉及同一干预或研究现象不同结局指标的多个相关系统评价进行汇总；从更广的范围对某一领域的相关系统评价进行汇总。

Procedures include(步骤包括):

(1) Identifying research questions with attributes of practicability and feasibility.

确定具有实用价值和可行性的研究问题。

(2) Setting literature inclusion and exclusion criteria based on the elements of the PICOS.

根据 PICOS 结构化问题的要素，确定文献纳入和排除标准。

(3) Developing a literature search strategy and conducting a comprehensive search using multiple databases.

制定文献检索策略，使用多个数据库进行全面、广泛的检索。

(4) Designing the information extraction form and have at least 2 evaluators independently screened the literature and extract information.

设计好资料提取表格，至少由 2 名评价者独立筛选文献和提取资料。

（5）Evaluating the literature quality via appraising the methodological quality and grading evidence level.

从方法学质量评价和证据质量分级两个方面进行文献质量评价。

（6）Using text, summaries table of results, graphics, or statistical methods to conduct data analysis.

采用文字、结果汇总表、图示或统计学方法进行资料分析。

（7）Analyzing and interpreting the results, reporting the results of the literature retrieval, the basic characteristics of the included studies, the quality appraisal results of the included studies, and the effect sizes of the interventions, etc.

分析和解释结果，分别报告文献检索结果、纳入研究的基本特征、纳入研究的质量评价结果、干预措施效应量描述等内容。

（8）Discussing the results, pointing out the significance of the study in guiding clinical practice and unresolved issues need to focus on, and presenting the reader with relevant information rather than providing recommendations.

以研究结果为依据进行讨论，指出研究对临床实践的指导意义和尚未解决的关键问题，向读者呈现相关信息而非提供建议。

7.7　Appraisal and Application of Clinical Practice Guidelines in Nursing
（护理临床实践指南的评价和应用）

In order to rigor the development process and improve the quality of the guide, a group of international guideline developers and researchers formed the Appraisal of Guidelines for Research & Evaluation (AGREE) Collaboration. In 2003, they developed AGREE instrument and updated it into AGREE Ⅱ in 2009.

为了规范指南制作过程，提高指南质量，全球的指南制定和研究人员成立了临床实践指南研究与评价国际工作组，并于 2003 年发布了指南研究与评价工具 AGREE，于 2009 年进行修订，并推出 AGREE Ⅱ。

The AGREE Ⅱ consists of 23 key items organized within 6 domains followed by 2 global rating items ("Overall Assessment"). Each of the AGREE Ⅱ items and the two global rating items is rated on a 7-point scale (1-strongly disagree to 7-strongly agree). Higher scores increase means more criteria are met and more considerations are addressed. The six AGREE Ⅱ domains are scored separately and should not be aggregated into a single quality score. AGREE Ⅱ is designed to assess guidelines developed by local, regional, national, or international groups or affiliated governmental organizations. These include original versions and updates of existing guidelines. The AGREE Ⅱ can be applied to guidelines in any disease area, including diagnosis, health promotion, treatment, interventions, and nursing etc. Each guideline is recommended to assessed by at least 2 appraisers and preferably 4 as this will increase the reliability of the assessment.

该工具包括6个维度23个条目及两个概述性的条目（总体评价），每个条目1—7分（1—强烈不同意，7—强烈同意），得分越高说明该条目符合程度越高。6个领域独立评分，不能合并为一个总分来评价一个指南的好坏。可用于评价地方、地区、国家、国际组织或联合政府发行的新指南、现有指南或更新版指南的方法学质量和指南报告质量，适用于任何疾病领域，包括诊断、健康促进、治疗、干预、护理等。为保证评价结果的可信度，AGREE Ⅱ推荐每个指南至少由2名、最好由4名评价人员进行评价。

8. Knowledge Translation and Evidence Implementation(知识转化和证据应用)

The Canadian Institutes of Health Research defines knowledge translation as "the exchange, synthesis and ethically sound application of knowledge—within a complex system of interactions among researchers and users— to accelerate the capture of the benefits of research for patients through improved health, more effective services and products, and a strengthened health care system". Although a large number of research findings are powerful enough to change clinical practice, there is a huge gap in its clinical application. Healthcare providers take responsibility to facilitate knowledge translation and evidence application in practice.

加拿大卫生研究所将知识转化定义为："有效地、及时地、符合伦理地将整合性知识应用于卫生保健实践，促进研究者和实践者的互动，从而保证最大限度地发挥卫生保健体系潜力，获得卫生保健的最佳效果。"尽管大量的研究结果足以改变临床实践，但在实践应用中存在巨大鸿沟。促进知识转化及临床实践中的证据应用，是卫生保健人员的职责。

Knowledge translation and evidence application is a continuous quality improvement process to identify problems, find evidence, and solve problems. Steps include:

知识转化和证据应用本质是一个发现问题、寻找证据、解决问题的持续质量改进过程。步骤如下：

（1）Identifying clinical problems and clarify PICO elements based on principles of importance, severity, resolvability, and disparities that exist between evidence and practice.

根据重要性、严重性、可解决性及证据和实践之间存在的差异等原则，确定临床问题，明确 PICO 要素。

（2）Searching for evidence, we first search for integrated evidence resources, beginning with the top of the evidence in the "6S" model, and then search for original studies if other integrated evidence resources are lacking or insufficient.

检索证据，首先检索经过整合的循证资源，根据"6S"模型，从证据顶端开始检索，在循证资源缺乏或不足的情况下，再检索原始研究。

（3）Appraising and integrate the evidence. Conduct a rigorous quality appraisal for the retrieved resources, including the integrated evidence resources and original studies, to ensure that the evidence is truthful, rigorous, and reliable. All included original studies should all be conducted systematic review first.

评价、整合证据，对检索到的资源，包括整合的循证资源和原始研究进行严谨的质量评价，确保证据真实、严谨、可靠，纳入的原始研究均应进行系统评价。

（4）Evidence application, including the three elements of context analysis, strategy building, and action-taking. Context analysis carries out the assessment of evidence, organizational context, and barrier factor. Based on the contextual analysis, develop effective and diversified intervention strategies, then establish an instrumental, process-oriented, and systematic action plan, and conduct a pilot application of the evidence.

应用证据，包括情景分析、构建策略、采取行动三个要素。情景分析进行证据评估、组织环境评估和障碍因素评估，基于情景分析结果构建策略，发展有效的多元化干预策略，制定工具化、流程化、系统化的行动方案，并进行证据应用试点。

（5）Evaluating outcomes, establish sensitivity outcome indicators, and comprehensively evaluate the impact of evidence application on systems, practitioners, and patients at the structural, process, and outcome levels. Feasible, appropriate, and effective evidence is embedded into the hospital system in the form of the flow path, norms, and tools to sustain evidence application.

评价结果，制订敏感性指标，从结构、过程及结果层面全面评价证据应用对系统、实践者及患者的影响。并将被证实可行、适宜、有效的证据，以流程、规范、工具等形式植入医院系统中，维持证据应用。

📖 Studies Cited in Chapter 2（第二章参考文献）

[1]胡雁，郝玉芳. 循证护理学：第 2 版[M]. 北京：人民卫生出版社，2018.

［2］胡雁. 循证护理学［M］. 北京：人民卫生出版社，2012.

［3］胡雁，周英凤. 循证护理——证据临床转化理论与实践［M］. 上海：复旦大学出版社，2021.

［4］李幼平. 循证医学（研究生）［M］. 北京：人民卫生出版社，2014.

［5］李峥，刘宇. 护理学研究方法［M］. 北京：人民卫生出版社，2012.

［6］Jordan，Z.，Lockwood，C.，Aromataris，E.，et al. The updated JBI model for evidence-based healthcare［M］. Melbourne：The Joanna Briggs Institute，2016.

［7］Higgins，J. P. T.，Thomas，J.，Chandler，J.，et al. Cochrane Handbook for Systematic Reviews of Interventions version 6. 3［EB/OL］.［2022-02］. www. training. cochrane. org/handbook，2022.

［8］Critical Appraisal Skills Programme. CASP Checklist［EB/OL］.［2002］https://casp-uk. net/referencing/.

［9］Aromataris，E.，Munn，Z. JBI Manual for Evidence Synthesis［EB/OL］.［2020］. https://synthesismanual.jbi.global.

［10］Porritt，K.，McArthur，A.，Lockwood，C.，et al. JBI Handbook for Evidence Implementation［EB/OL］.［2020］. https://implementationmanual.jbi.global.

［11］The Joanna Briggs Institute levels of Evidence and Grades of Recommendation Working party. Supporting Document for the Joanna Briggs Institute levels of Evidence and Grades of Recommendation［EB/OL］.［2014］. http://joannabriggs. org/jbi-approach. html # tabbed-nav＝levels-of-evidence.

［12］Phibrick V. Johns Hopkins Nursing EBP：Model and Guidelines［J］. Aorn Journal，2013，97（1）：157-158.

［13］Holger Schünemann，Jan Brozek，Gordon Guyatt，et al. Handbook for grading the quality of evidence and the strength of recommendations using the GRADE approach［EB/OL］.［2013］. https://gdt.gradepro.org/app/handbook/handbook.html#ftnt_ref1.

［14］International Council of Nurses. Closing the gap：from evidence to action. International Nurses Day Kit［EB/OL］.［2012］. http://www. icn. ch/publications/2012-closing-the-gap-from-evidence-to-action/.

［15］AGREE Next Steps Consortium. The AGREE Ⅱ Instrument［EB/OL］.［2009］. http://www.agreetrust.org.

Chapter 3: Key Concepts and Steps in Qualitative and Quantitative Research
第三章 质性研究和量性研究中的重要概念及步骤

Section I Fundamental Research Terms and Concepts
第一节 基本研究术语和概念

Nursing research has its own language—terms. Some terms are used by both quantitative researchers and qualitative researchers, some are used just by one group of researchers. This chapter provides a review of fundamental research terms and steps in the research process.

护理研究有自己的语言——术语。一些术语被量性研究人员和质性研究人员共同使用，一些术语仅由一类研究人员使用。本章回顾了研究过程中的基础研究术语和步骤。

1. Subjects/ Study Participants(研究对象/参与者)

In a quantitative study, the people being studied are called study participants, respondents, or subjects. In a qualitative study, those cooperating in the study are called participants, informants, or key informants.

在量性研究中，被研究的人称为研究对象、被调查者或受试者。在质性研究中，参与研究的人被称为参与者、信息提供者或关键信息提供者。

2. Researcher/Investigator(研究者/调查者)

The person who conducts a study is called the researcher or investigator. When a study is done by a team, the person directing the study is the principal investigator (PI).

开展研究的人称为研究者或调查者。当研究由一个团队共同完成时，负责指导该研究的人称为项目负责人或首席研究人员(PI)。

3. Theories，Models and Frameworks(理论、模型及框架)

3.1　Theory(理论)

Polit and Beck （2017） have defined a theory as " A theory is a systematic， abstract explanation of some aspect of reality". Grove and Gray （2018） described a theory as "a set of concepts and statements that present a view of a phenomenon". Concepts are the basic building blocks of a theory. Theories are composed of concepts and the relationships among these concepts，which is logical and holistic.

Polit 和 Beck(2017)将理论定义为"对现实某些方面的系统、抽象的解释"。Grove 和 Gray(2018)将理论描述为"一组呈现现象观点的概念和陈述"。概念是理论的基本组成部分。理论由概念和这些概念之间的关系组成，具有逻辑性和整体性。

Theories are developed to describe，explain，or predict a phenomenon or outcome. Many theories have been developed by nurses and are closely related to nursing practice；some theories come from other disciplines. Theories differ in their level of generality and abstraction. According to the theoretical level or scope，nursing theory is often classified as grand theory，middle-range theory，and micro or practice theory.

开发理论是为了描述、解释或预测现象或结果。很多理论由护理人员开发，并与护理实践紧密相关，部分理论则来自其他学科。理论的普遍性和抽象程度均不同。根据理论水平或范围，护理理论常划分为广域理论、中域理论、微观或实践理论。

Early nursing theorists developed conceptual models that helped to define the discipline of nursing. These conceptual models are broad in scope and are frequently referred to as grand theories，including Orem's Self-Care Model，Rogers's Science of Unitary Human Beings，Roy's Adaptation Model，and Neuman's Systems Model.

早期的护理理论家发展了有助于定义护理学科的概念模型。这些概念模型的范围很广，经常被称为广域理论。包括 Orem 的自我照顾模型、Rogers 的整体人科学、Roy 的适应模型和 Neuman 的系统模型。

Practice theory （micro theory or situation-specific theory），are highly specific，narrow in scope，and have an action orientation. While middle-range theories are more specific and applicable to nursing practice，it may not include guidance for specific nursing interventions.

Practice theories aim to propose specific approaches to particular nursing practice situations. The theory of heart failure self-care (Riegel, Dickson & Faulkner, 2016) is an example of practice theory that proposes specific nursing actions for a specific population. However, there is ongoing debate about whether they should be called "theory" (Peterson & Bredow, 2012).

　　实践理论(微观理论或情境理论)，具有高度的针对性，范围较窄且具有行动导向。虽然中等理论更具体，更适用于护理实践，但它可能不包括对特定护理干预的指导。实践理论旨在针对特定的护理实践情况提出具体的方法。心力衰竭自我护理理论（Riegel, Dickson & Faulkner, 2016）是实践理论的一个例子，它提出针对特定人群的特定护理行动。然而，关于它们是否应该被称为"理论"的争论一直存在(Peterson & Bredow, 2012)。

3.2　Models(模型)

Model is a graphic or symbolic representation of a phenomenon. Conceptual models, conceptual frameworks, made up of concepts and propositions that state the relationships among the concepts. Whereas a theory focuses on statements or explanations of the relationships among phenomena, a model focuses on the structure or composition of the phenomena. What is absent from conceptual models is the deductive system of propositions that specify and explain relationships among concepts, so the way it organizes and presents phenomena is considered less formal than theory.

　　模型是用图形或符号来表现某种现象。概念模型(也称概念框架)，由概念和陈述概念之间关系的命题组成。理论侧重于对现象之间关系的陈述或解释，而模型侧重于现象的结构或组成。概念模型中缺少明确和解释概念之间关系的命题演绎系统，故认为它组织和呈现现象的方式不如理论正式。

3.3　Frameworks(框架)

A framework for a research study helps organize the study and provides guidance for research or practice. The framework identifies the key concepts and describes their relationships to each other and to the phenomena (variables) of concern to nursing. Not every study is based on a formal theory or conceptual model, but every study has a framework. In a study based on a theory, the framework is a theoretical framework, and in conceptual model-based research, it is a conceptual framework. Theoretical framework and conceptual framework are often used interchangeably in the literature. The two types frameworks are similar in that both provide a background or foundation for a study. However, there are differences in these two types of frameworks.

研究框架有助于组织研究并为研究或实践提供指导。该框架确定了关键概念，描述它们之间的关系以及与护理相关的现象(变量)的关系。并非每项研究都基于正式的理论或概念模型，但每项研究都有一个框架。在基于理论的研究中，这个框架是理论框架，在基于概念模型的研究中是概念框架。理论框架和概念框架在文献中经常互换使用。这两种类型的框架相似，都为研究提供了背景或基础，但这两种类型的框架也存在差异。

A theoretical framework is based on the existing theories, and presents a broad, general explanation of the relationships between the concepts in a research study. When using a theoretical framework, each main study concept is related back to a concept from an existing theory. If none of the existing theories fit well with the concepts in the current study, the researcher may construct a conceptual framework to be used in the research study.

理论框架基于现有的理论，它为研究中所涉及概念的相互关系提供了广泛、综合的解释。在使用理论框架时，每个主要研究概念都与现有理论的概念相关联。如果现有理论均不太适合当前研究中的概念，研究人员可以构建一个概念框架以用于该研究。

A conceptual framework helps explain the relationship between concepts, but rather than being based on one theory, this type of framework may link concepts selected from several theories from previous research results or from the researcher's own experiences in a logical manner. A conceptual framework is a less well-developed structure than a theoretical framework, but it is the basis for the formulation of a theory.

概念框架有助于解释概念之间的关系，但这种类型的框架不是基于某个理论，而是以合乎逻辑的方式，将来自先前的研究结果或研究人员自身经验的多个理论中的概念联系起来。概念框架的结构不如理论框架完善，但它是理论形成的前期基础。

Theories and conceptual models guide researchers in understanding the phenomena and why they occur. Theories often provide a basis for predicting phenomena. In turn, prediction has implications for the control of those phenomena. Therefore, theory is an important basis for developing nursing interventions.

理论和概念模型能够指导研究人员了解现象及其发生的原因，且理论往往为预测现象提供依据。反过来，预测对这些现象的控制也会产生影响。因此，理论是制定护理干预措施的重要依据。

4. Variables(变量)

A variable is any quality of a person, group, or situation that varies or takes on different values. For example, weight is a variable when studying the relationship between weight and high blood pressure, but if everyone weighs 50kg, weight is not a variable. Variables can be divided into continuous, discrete and categorical variables.

变量是指不同的人、群体或者场景所具有的可变化的一种品质。例如：在研究体重和高血压的关系时，体重是一个变量，但如果每个人的体重都为 50kg，则此时体重就不是一个变量。变量可分为连续性、离散和等级变量。

5. Conceptual and Operational Definitions(概念定义和操作性定义)

In quantitative studies, principal concepts need to be defined at the outset so their meaning is clear to the researcher and to the reader of a research report. Concept can be concrete or abstract. Researchers operationalize the variables or concepts in a study by identifying conceptual and operational definitions.

在量性研究中，需要从一开始就定义研究的主要概念，以便研究人员和读者清楚地了解它们的含义。概念可以是具体的或抽象的。研究人员通过概念定义和操作性定义来明确研究中的变量或概念。

A conceptual definition provides a variable or concept with theoretical meaning (Gray et al., 2017), and it can be derived from a theorist's definition of a variable or concept, or developed through concept analysis. Alternatively, the conceptual definition also may be drawn from literature review, previous publications on the same topic, a medical dictionary, and even a standard dictionary, and then synthesized by the researcher so as to encompass the study's intended focus.

概念定义提供了具有理论意义的变量或概念(Gray et al., 2017)，它可以从理论家对变量或概念的定义中推导出来，也可以通过概念分析发展而来。或者，概念定义也可以从文献综述、之前发表的同一主题的研究、医学词典甚至标准词典中得出，然后由研究人员综合以涵盖研究的预期重点。

An operational definition indicates how a variable will be observed or measured. With an operational definition, a concept is converted into a variable and it becomes clear how it will be measured in that particular study. The researcher selects the operational definition that results in a measurement that is best for that study. Concepts in qualitative research are not measured during the research process, the key phenomena may be a major end product, so it makes little sense to define them operationally. However quantitative research does involve measurement, so each variable that will be measured must be operationally defined to reveal the way in which it will be measured.

操作性定义说明如何观察或测量变量。通过操作性定义，概念被转换为一个变量，并明确在该特定研究中将如何进行测量。研究人员选择产生最适合该研究的可测量的操作性定义。质性研究中的概念不是在研究过程中测量的，一些重要现象可能是研究的主要结果，因此对其进行操作性定义意义不大。然而，量性研究确实涉及测量，因此需测量的每个变量都要有操作性定义，以揭示它是如何被测量的。

6. Data(数据)

Data are the pieces of information obtained in a study. In quantitative studies, researchers identify and define their variables and then collect relevant data from study participants. In qualitative studies, researchers collect qualitative data, that is, narrative descriptions and reactions.

数据是指研究中获得的信息片段。在量性研究，数据指研究者根据他们所定义的变量所收集的研究对象相关资料；在质性研究中，研究者收集定性数据，数据指研究者所收集到的研究对象对于一个问题的回答及反应。

Section II　Major Types of Quantitative and Qualitative Research
第二节　量性研究和质性研究的主要类别

1. Major Types of Quantitative Research(量性研究的主要类别)

A variety of quantitative research designs are implemented in nursing studies. The four most common types are experimental research, quasi-experimental research, descriptive research and correlational research.

在护理研究中可实施多种量性研究设计。最常见的四类量性研究设计类型是实验性研究、类实验性研究、描述性研究和相关性研究。

1.1 Experimental Research(实验性研究)

The purpose of experimental research is to test the null hypothesis by means of applying an intervention to experimental subjects, and then measuring the effect on the dependent variable.

Experiments are characterized by manipulation, control, and randomization. The quality of experiments depends on the validity of their research design.

实验性研究的目的是通过对实验对象进行干预来检验原假设，然后测量其对因变量的影响。实验的特点是干预、对照和随机化。实验的质量取决于其研究设计的有效性。

Manipulation in interventional research means that the researcher enacts an intervention that alters the value of the independent variable, then measures the resultant effect on one or more dependent variables. The researcher decides what is to be manipulated (e. g., selected nursing interventions), to whom the manipulation applies, when the manipulation is to occur according to the specification of the research design, and how the manipulation is to be implemented.

实验性研究中的干预是指研究人员实施改变自变量值的操纵，然后测量对一个或多个因变量的结果影响。研究人员决定要干预什么(例如，所选择的护理干预措施)，干预适用的对象，根据研究设计何时进行干预，以及如何实施干预措施。

Control in research design means control for the effects of potentially extraneous variables, a serious issue for interventional research. Controlling the effects of extraneous variables through the research design is the most straightforward way of making sure they do not affect the researcher's conclusions related to the effect of the independent variable on the dependent variable. Use of random assignment is the most generically efficient way to control for the effects of extraneous variables. However, when it is not feasible to control for the effects of known extraneous variables through design, it is possible to measure them in the course of the study. After data collection is complete, the researcher analyzes the effects of one or more extraneous variables by measuring their relationships with the dependent variable.

研究设计中的对照意味着控制潜在的无关变量的影响，这是实验性研究的一个重要问题。最直接的方法是通过研究设计控制外来变量的影响，以确保不影响自变量对因变量影响的结论。采用随机分配是控制无关变量影响的最普遍有效的方法。但是，当无法通过研究设计控制已知的外来变量的影响时，可以在研究过程中对其进行测量。待数据收集完成后，研究人员通过测量它们与因变量的关系来分析一个或多个无关变量产生的影响。

Randomization entails two separate processes: random selection of study participants from the population and random assignment of participants to intervention or control groups. When researchers try to generalize findings to the entire target population, they need to randomly select the study sample. Samples can be selected from an accessible study population using random number tables, computer programs, coin toss or other methods. During the random selection process, every individual within the accessible study population has an equal chance of being selected. Random assignment occurs after study participants have been selected and have agreed to participate in a study. Random assignment is the process of assigning each member of the study participants to one of the groups, so that each of them has the equal chance of being in a certain group.

随机化需要两个独立的过程: 从人群中随机选择受试者以及将受试者随机分配到干预组或对照组。当研究人员试图将研究结果推广到整个目标人群时, 需随机选择研究样本。可使用随机数字表、计算机程序、抛硬币或其他方法从可及的研究总体中选择样本。在随机选择过程中, 可及研究总体的每个个体都有同等机会被选中。在选择研究对象并同意参加研究后进行随机分配。随机分配是将样本的每个成员(研究对象)分配到其中一个组的过程, 使每个对象都有同等机会进入某个组。

1.2 Quasi-Experimental Research(类实验性研究)

Experiments are characterized by manipulation, control, and randomization. However, when conducting research in a practical setting, it is not always possible to implement a research design that meets all these three criteria. As with experimental research, quasi-experimental research includes an independent variable and a dependent variable in a proposed cause-and-effect relationship. However, quasi-experimental research is lacking in one or more of the other attributes of experimental research: researcher-controlled manipulation of the independent variable, the control group, random selection and random assignment of study participants.

实验的特点是操纵、控制和随机化。然而, 在实践环境中开展研究时, 研究设计并不总是能够满足这三个标准。与实验性研究一样, 类实验性研究在所提出的因果关系中包括一个自变量和一个因变量。然而, 不同于实验性研究的是, 类实验性研究缺乏实验性研究的一个或多个其他属性: 研究人员控制自变量的干预, 对照组, 以及随机选择和分配研究对象。

Quasi-experimental research is a useful way to test causality in settings when it is impossible or unethical to randomly assign subjects to intervention and control groups or to withhold treatment from some research participants. The main disadvantage of quasi-experimental research is the increased threat to internal validity. Many quasi-experimental research designs exist. Some of these frequently used quasi-experimental research designs are the one-group pretest-posttest design, nonequivalent control group design and time series design.

当无法将研究对象随机分配到实验组和对照组, 或不给予某些研究对象治疗措施不符合伦理规范时, 类实验性研究是测试环境中因果关系的有效方法。类实验性研究的主要缺点是增加了对内部有效性的威胁。常用的类实验研究设计有自身前-后对照设计、不对等对照组设计、时间连续性设计等。

1.3　Descriptive Research(描述性研究)

The general purpose of descriptive research is to explore and describe phenomena in real-life situations. Descriptive research is performed when knowledge about a phenomenon is incomplete, for example, no relevant research has been conducted or existing knowledge of the research is limited. Descriptive researches are classified as cross-sectional or longitudinal. Quantitative descriptive methodologies include surveys, measurement tools, chart or record reviews, physiological measurements, meta-analyses, and secondary data analyses. There are many descriptive research designs, like the simple descriptive design, the comparative descriptive design, the longitudinal descriptive design, the cross-sectional descriptive design and so on.

描述性研究的一般目的是探索和描述现实生活中的现象。当关于某一现象的知识不完整时，例如尚未进行任何相关研究或现有的研究认知有限，则会进行描述性研究。描述性研究主要包括横断面研究和纵向研究。量性描述性研究方法包括调查、工具测量、图表或记录审查、生理测量、Meta 分析和二次数据分析等。描述性研究设计有很多种，如简单描述性研究设计、比较描述性研究设计、纵向描述性研究设计、横断面描述性研究设计等。

1.4　Correlational Research(相关性研究)

In a correlational study, the relationship between two or more variables is examined. The researchers test whether the variables covary, and quantify the strength of the relationship between variables or test a hypothesis or research question about a specific relationship.

在相关性研究中，研究人员检验两个或多个变量之间的关系，测试变量是否共同变化，并量化变量之间关系的强度或测试关于特定关系的假设或研究问题。

The magnitude and direction of the relationship between two variables is indicated by a correlation coefficient. Correlation coefficients may be positive (+) or negative (−) and range from − 1. 00 (perfect negative correlation) to 1. 00 (perfect positive correlation). If the correlation coefficient has no sign in front of it, a positive relationship is indicated, which means that as the value of one variable increases, the value of the other variable increases. A negative correlation coefficient is preceded by a negative sign, which means that as the value of one variable increases, the value of the other variable decreases. A correlation coefficient of 0.00 indicates there is no relationship between variables. There are three correlational research designs, the simple correlational design, the predictive correlational design, and the model testing design.

两个变量之间关系的大小和方向用相关系数表示。相关系数可以是正（+）或负（-），范围从-1.00（完全负相关）到 1.00（完全正相关）。如果相关系数前面没有符号，则表示正相关，即随着一个变量的值增加，另一个变量的值也增加。负相关系数前面有一个负号，则表明随着一个变量的值增加，另一个变量的值减小。0.00 的相关系数表明变量之间没有关系。相关性研究设计分为简单相关性设计、预测相关性设计和模型检验相关性设计三种。

A correlational design is a very useful design for clinical studies because many of the phenomena of clinical interest are beyond the researcher's ability to manipulate, control, and randomize. In terms of evidence for practice, the researchers based on the literature review and findings, frame the utility of the results in light of previous research and therefore help establish the "best available" evidence that, combined with clinical expertise, informs clinical decisions regarding the study's applicability to a specific patient population.

对于临床研究而言，相关性研究是一种非常有用的研究设计，因为许多临床感兴趣的现象超出了研究人员实施干预措施、设置对照和随机抽样和分配的能力。在实践证据方面，研究人员根据文献回顾和研究结果，从而帮助形成"最佳可用"证据，为临床决策提供依据。

2. Major Types of Qualitative Research(质性研究的主要类别)

Qualitative research focuses on gaining insight into a phenomenon or understanding about an individual's perception of events. It does not rely on manipulation and control, but focuses on observing and describing things as they naturally occur. Qualitative research is best suited for research aimed at rich description or in-depth understanding of a phenomenon, rather than determining causality. Qualitative approaches are most often chosen when little is known about a topic or when new perspectives are needed. Other functions of qualitative approaches include generating hypotheses, refining theory, providing illustrative examples, creating taxonomies, and generating items for instrument development.

质性研究侧重于深入了解一种现象或了解个体对事件的看法。它不依赖于干预和控制，而是专注于观察和描述事物的自然发生过程。它最适合于旨在对现象进行丰富描述或深入理解的研究，而非确定因果关系。当对某个主题知之甚少或需要新观点时，通常会选择质性研究方法。质性研究方法的功能还包括生成假设、完善理论、提供说明性示例、创建分类法以及研制测量工具时生成条目。

Although many qualitative research designs share some common features, they still vary widely in their approach and purpose. There is no agreed classification system for these research methods. One system is to categorize qualitative research according to disciplinary traditions. This section provides an overview of several most common qualitative designs, including phenomenology, ethnography, grounded theory, and more details will be described in later chapters.

尽管许多质性研究设计有一些共同的特征，但它们的方法和目的仍然存在很大差异。对于这些研究方法，尚未有一致的分类系统。其中一种分类系统是根据学科传统对质性研究进行分类。本节概述了几种最常见的质性研究设计，包括现象学、民族志、扎根理论。更多的内容将在后面的章节进行描述。

2.1　Phenomenology(现象学)

Phenomenology, rooted in a philosophical tradition developed by Husserl and Heidegger, is an approach to understanding people's everyday life experiences. The goal of phenomenological studies is to describe the meaning that experiences hold for each participant.

现象学植根于 Husserl 和 Heidegger 发展起来的哲学传统，是一种理解人们日常生活经验的方法。现象学研究的目标是描述经验对每个参与者的意义。

In phenomenologic studies, in-depth conversations are the main data source, with researchers and informants as co-participants. Researchers help informants to describe lived experiences without leading the discussion. Through in-depth conversations, researchers strive to gain entrance into the informants' world, to have full access to their experiences as lived. Multiple interviews or conversations are sometimes needed.

在现象学研究中，深入的对话是主要的数据来源，研究人员和信息提供者是共同参与者。研究人员在不引导讨论的情况下帮助信息提供者描述生活经历。通过深入的对话，研究人员努力进入信息提供者的世界，充分了解他们的生活经历。有时需要进行多次访谈或对话。

The phenomenologic approach is especially useful when a phenomenon has been poorly defined or conceptualized. The topics appropriate to phenomenology are ones that are fundamental to the life experiences of humans. An example of phenomenological study is shown in Box 3.2.1.

当一个现象的定义或概念化不明确时, 现象学方法特别有用。适用于现象学的是人类生活经验至关重要的主题。以下展示了一个现象学研究的例子(见方框 3.2.1)。

📝 Box 3.2.1 Phenomenological Study(现象学研究)

Loaring, Larkin, Shaw, and Flowers (2015) used the phenomenologic approach to study how breast cancer diagnosis and treatments may affect the relational context of women's coping and the impact upon their intimate partners. Their study focused on couples' experiences of breast cancer surgery, and its impact on body image and sexual intimacy. Using interpretative phenomenological analysis, the researchers conducted an in-depth analysis of the personal meaning of experiences. The researchers concluded that gendered coping styles and normative sexual scripts are an important part of the experience and that management of expectations regarding breast reconstruction may be helpful.

Loaring、Larkin、Shaw 和 Flowers (2015) 使用现象学方法来研究乳腺癌的诊断和治疗如何影响女性应对的关系情境以及对其亲密伴侣的影响。研究重点关注乳腺癌手术夫妻的经验, 及其对身体形象和性亲密的影响。使用解释性现象学分析, 研究人员对经验的个人意义进行了深入分析。研究人员得出结论, 性别化的应对方式和规范的性脚本是经验的重要组成部分, 对乳房重建的期望管理可能会对其有所帮助。

For nurses, phenomenology provides a systematic approach in understanding the way humans view themselves, their experiences, and their relationships with others. This is foundational to person-centered health care. Here, face-to-face interviews are used as a primary method to provide access to human being's lived experience (Willis et al., 2016). Investigational findings are requisite for the development of health interventions in promoting health, and in ameliorating suffering while meeting the human needs for humanistic care (Willis, Grace & Roy, 2008).

对于护士来说, 现象学提供了一种系统的方法来理解人类如何看待自己, 看待自己的经历以及与他人的关系。这是以人为本的医疗保健的基础。在这里，面对面访谈是一种提供人类生活体验的主要方法(Willis 等，2016)。调查结果对于发展健康干预措施以促进健康，及减轻痛苦以满足人类对人文关怀的需求都是必不可少的(Willis，Grace 和 Roy，2008)。

2.2 Ethnography(民族志)

Ethnography is a specific naturalistic written description of the "folk" and refers to both a specific naturalistic research method and the written product of that method. As a research process, ethnography investigates patterns of human behavior and cognition through observations and interactions in natural settings. As a written product, ethnography is a descriptive or interpretive analysis of the patterns of beliefs, behaviors, and norms of a culture.

民族志是对民间的特定文化的书面描述，既指特定文化研究方法，也指该方法的书面产物。作为一个研究过程，民族志通过在自然环境中的观察和互动来研究人类行为和认知模式。作为一种书面产物，民族志是对某种文化的信仰、行为和规范模式的描述性或解释性分析。

Ethnography does require spending considerable time in the setting, studying, observing, and gathering data. Participant observation is the primary method of ethnographers (Patton, 2015). The researcher frequently spends extended periods of time with the group, exploring their rituals and customs together and becomes part of their culture. During these interactions, the researcher maintains the etic perspective, noting aspects of shared culture, including behaviors, rules, power structures, customs, and expectations. An entire cultural group or just a subgroup may be studied.

民族志确实需要在设定、研究、观察和收集数据上花费大量时间。参与者观察是民族志学家的主要研究方法(Patton，2015)。研究人员经常与群体一起度过很长一段时间，一起探索他们的仪式和习俗，并成为他们文化的一部分。在这些互动过程中，研究人员保持理性的观点，注意共享文化的各个方面，包括行为、规则、权力结构、习俗和期望。可以研究整个文化群体或只是一个子群体。

Among health care researchers, ethnography provides access to the health beliefs and health practices of a culture or subculture. Ethnographic inquiry can thus help to facilitate understanding of behaviors affecting health and illness. The following is an example of an ethnographic study in a healthcare setting, is represented in Box 3.2.2.

在医疗保健研究人员中，人种学提供了一种文化或亚文化的健康信念和健康实践的途径。因此，民族志调查有助于促进对影响健康和疾病的行为的理解。以下是一个医疗保健环境中的民族志研究示例(见方框 3.2.2)。

> ### ✍ Box 3.2.2 Ethnographic Study(民族志研究)
>
> Saleem et al. (2015) conducted an ethnographic study of clinical end-users interacting with electronic medical records systems in Veterans Affairs Medical Centers. They analyzed data and identified barriers to effective adoption and optimization of electronic medical records systems. Identifying the barriers explained some of the challenges with the optimization of the electronic medical records systems across the Veterans Affairs Medical system. They were then able to make recommendations about how to improve adoption of systems for more effective use by Veterans Affairs healthcare providers.
>
> Saleem 等(2015) 对退伍军人事务医疗中心的电子病历系统临床终端用户进行了民族志研究。研究者分析了数据并确定了有效采用和优化电子病历系统的障碍。识别障碍解释了在整个退伍军人医疗系统中优化电子病历系统所面临的一些挑战。然后，研究者针对如何改进采用系统提出建议，以便退伍军人事务部医疗保健提供者更有效地使用系统。

2.3 Grounded Theory(扎根理论)

Grounded theory seeks to explain variations in social interactional and social structural problems and processes. Although the grounded theory approach was developed by sociologists, the approach is very appropriate for use by nurse researchers. When a researcher is interested in an area in which little research has been done or in which existing theories are not sufficient, grounded theory studies are a good choice. The goal is to generate theory from the data and resultant conceptual schema. Grounded theory, an important method for the study of nursing phenomena, has contributed to the development of many middle-range nursing theories.

扎根理论旨在解释社会互动的变化，及社会结构问题和过程的变化。尽管扎根理论方法是由社会学家开发的，但该方法非常适合护理研究人员使用。当研究人员对研究很少或现有理论不足的领域感兴趣时，扎根理论研究是一个不错的选择。扎根理论研究的目标是从数据和由数据产生的概念模式中发展理论。扎根理论是研究护理现象的重要方法，促进了许多中等护理理论的发展。

A fundamental feature of grounded theory research is that data collection，data analysis，and sampling of participants occur simultaneously. Grounded theories are focused on what may be unarticulated phenomena discovered through observation and interview data，and are particularly well suited to nursing studies conducted to uncover the nature of clinically relevant phenomena such as chronic illness，caregiving，and dying in real-world rather than laboratory conditions. The resulting theoretical formulation not only explains human experience and associated meanings but also can provide a basis for nursing intervention research and nursing practice. An example of Grounded Theory is shown in Box 3.2.3.

扎根理论研究的一个基本特征是数据收集、数据分析和参与者抽样同时发生。扎根理论侧重于通过观察和访谈数据发现的可能未阐明的现象，特别适用于为揭示临床相关现象的性质而进行的护理研究，例如现实世界而非实验室条件下的慢性病、护理和死亡。由此产生的理论表述不仅解释了人类经验和相关含义，而且还可以为护理干预研究和护理实践提供依据。方框3.2.3内展示了一个扎根理论的研究实例。

📝 Box 3.2.3　Grounded Theory Study（扎根理论研究）

Fritz（2015）used grounded theory method to examine the process by which low-income（mostly minority）women develop the skills to integrate diabetes self-management into daily life and the conditions that affect the process. The researcher used semi-structured interviews，photo elicitation，time geographic diaries，and a standardized assessment to collect data from ten low-income women with type 2 diabetes. The resulting theory，the Transactional Model of Diabetes Self-Management（DSM）Integration，depicts the theorized process whereby low-income women accept aspects of diabetes education and training as a part of their circumstances，act on them，and practice with them until they become integrated into daily life.

Fritz（2015）使用扎根理论方法来研究低收入（主要是少数族裔）女性将糖尿病自我管理融入日常生活技能的过程以及影响该过程的条件。研究人员使用半结构化访谈、照片引谈法、时间地理日记和标准化评估，收集来自10名患有Ⅱ型糖尿病的低收入女性的数据。由此产生的理论，糖尿病自我管理（DSM）整合模型，描述了低收入女性接受糖尿病教育和培训的各个方面作为其境遇的一部分、采取行动并与她们一起练习直到这些融入其日常生活。

Section Ⅲ Major Steps in a Quantitative Study
第三节 量性研究的主要步骤

Though different authors describe steps in quantitative research in different ways, the steps vary from study to study. But most quantitative studies follow some commonly accepted steps in the research process, and in general, the scientific research process proceeds in an orderly fashion.

尽管不同的作者以不同的方式描述量性研究的步骤，不同研究的步骤会有所不同。但大多数量性研究都遵循研究过程中一些普遍接受的步骤，总的来说，科学研究过程是有序进行的。

1. Identifying the research problem(确定研究问题)

Quantitative researchers begin by identifying an interesting, significant research problem and formulating research questions. In a nursing study, the research problem is an area where knowledge is needed to advance the practice of nursing. Generally, a broad topic area is identified, then the topic is narrowed down to a specific problem to be studied.

量性研究人员首先确定一个有趣的、重要的研究问题并确定研究问题。在护理研究中，研究问题是需要知识来推进护理实践的领域。通常，确定一个广泛的主题领域，然后将主题缩小到要研究的特定问题。

2. Determining the Purpose of the Study(确定研究目的)

The research problem addresses what will be studied, the purpose provides why the study is being done.

研究问题涉及将要研究的内容，目的则表明了开展某项研究的原因。

3. Formulating the Research Question(阐述研究问题)

A research question is the specific question that the researcher expects to be answered in a study. The research question should specify the variables and the population that are being studied. A variable is a characteristic or attribute that differs among the persons, objects, events, and so forth being studied (e. g., age, blood type).

研究问题是研究人员希望在研究中回答的具体问题。研究问题应具体说明正在研究的变量和人群。变量是在被研究的人、物体、事件等(例如年龄、血型)之间不同的特征或属性。

4. Reviewing the Literature(文献回顾)

Quantitative research is conducted in a context of previous knowledge. Besides determining the extent of the existing knowledge related to the study topic, the review of the literature also helps develop a theoretical or conceptual framework for a study. And review of the literature can also help the researcher clarify research methods, for example, instruments or tools may be discovered that can be used to measure the study variables. A comprehensive literature review lays the foundation for new evidence, which is usually conducted before collecting data.

量性研究是在先前知识的背景下进行的。除了确定与研究主题相关的现有知识的范围外，文献回顾还有助于建立研究的理论或概念框架。文献回顾也有助于研究人员明确研究方法，例如，可发现能用于测量研究变量的仪器或工具。全面的文献回顾为新证据奠定了基础，通常在收集数据之前进行。

5. Developing a Theoretical/Conceptual Framework(制定理论/概念框架)

Theoretical/conceptual frameworks are a valuable part of scientific research. Research and theory are closely intertwined. Research can test theories as well as help develop and refine theories. The theoretical/conceptual framework assists in the selection of the study variables and in defining them. The framework also directs the hypotheses and the interpretation of the findings. When quantitative research is performed within the context of a theoretical framework, the findings often have broader significance and utility.

理论/概念框架是科学研究的重要组成部分。研究和理论紧密相连。研究可以检验理论，也可以帮助发展和完善理论。理论或概念框架有助于研究变量的选择和定义，还可以指导假设和对研究结果的解释。当在理论框架的背景下进行量性研究时，研究结果通常具有更广泛的意义和效用。

6. Formulating Hypotheses(确定研究假设)

A researcher's expectation about the results of a study is expressed in a hypothesis. A hypothesis predicts the relationship between two or more variables. The hypothesis furnishes the predicted answer to the research question. In addition, the hypothesis proposes the relationship between the independent and the dependent variables. Each scientific investigation is based on hypotheses, and these hypotheses should be stated explicitly. But often studies are based on certain hypotheses that the researcher did not list these hypotheses. A hypothesis must be testable or verifiable empirically, and most quantitative studies involve testing hypotheses through statistical analysis.

研究人员对研究结果的期望以假设的形式表现。假设预测两个或多个变量之间的关系，提供了对研究问题的预测答案。此外，该假设提出了自变量和因变量之间的关系。每项科学研究都基于假设，应明确说明这些假设。但往往研究基于某些假设，研究人员却没有列出这些假设。假设必须在经验上是可检验或可验证的，大多数量性研究涉及通过统计分析来检验假设。

7. Defining the Study Variables/Terms(定义研究变量/术语)

Researchers should have a clear vision of the concepts in the study, including conceptual definition and operational definition. A conceptual definition is a dictionary definition or theoretical definition of an abstract idea that is being studied by the researcher. An operational definition indicates how a variable will be observed or measured. Operational definitions frequently include the instrument that will be used to measure the variables.

研究人员应该对所研究的概念有着清晰的认识，包括概念定义及操作性定义。概念定义是研究人员正在研究的抽象概念的字典定义或理论定义。操作性定义说明将如何观察或测量变量。操作定义通常包含将要用于测量变量的工具。

8. Selecting the Research Design(选择研究设计)

The research design is the plan for how the study will be conducted. It is concerned with the type of data that will be collected and the means used to obtain these data. For example, the researcher must decide if the study will examine cause-and-effect relationships or only describe existing situations, indicate how often data will be collected, what types of comparisons will be made, and where the study will take place. The researcher chooses the design that is most appropriate to test the study hypotheses or answer the research questions.

研究设计是研究如何开展的计划，它关注将收集的数据类型和用于获取这些数据的方法。例如，研究人员必须决定研究是检查因果关系还是只描述现有情况，表明数据收集的频率、将进行哪些类型的比较，以及研究将在何处开展。研究人员选择最适合检验研究假设或回答研究问题的设计。

9. Identifying the Population(确定研究总体)

The population is a complete set of individuals or objects that possess some common characteristic of interest to the researcher. Quantitative researchers need to clarify the group to whom study results can be generalized—that is, they must identify the population to be studied. There are two types of population, the target population and the accessible population. The target population is made up of the group of people or objects to which the researcher wishes to generalize the findings of a study. The accessible population is the group that is actually available for study by the researcher.

总体是一组完整的个体或对象，具有研究人员感兴趣的某些共同特征。量性研究人员需要明确研究结果可以推广到的人群，也就是说，他们必须确定要研究的人群。分为两类人群，目标人群和可达人群。目标人群由研究人员希望将研究结果推广到的一组人或对象组成。可访问人群是研究人员实际可用于研究的人群。

10. Designing the Sampling Plan(设计抽样计划)

Although researchers are always interested in populations, usually a subgroup of the population, called a sample, is studied. The sample is chosen to represent the population, and is used to make generalizations about the population. In a quantitative study, a sample's adequacy is assessed by its size and representativeness. The quality of a sample depends on how typical or representative it is in the population. The sampling plan specifies how the sample will be selected and recruited and how many research participants there will be.

尽管研究人员总是对研究总体感兴趣，但通常只会研究总体的一个子集，称为样本。

选择样本来代表总体，并用于对总体进行概括。在量性研究中，样本的充分性是通过其规模和代表性来评估的。样本的质量取决于样本在总体中的典型性或代表性。抽样计划规定了如何选择和招募样本，以及将有多少研究对象。

11. Specifying Methods to Measure Research Variables（明确测量研究变量的方法）

Quantitative researchers must be clear about how to measure research variables. The primary methods of data collection include self-reports, observations and biophysiologic measurements.

量性研究人员必须明确采用何种方法来衡量研究变量。数据收集的主要方法包括自我报告、观察和生物生理测量。

12. Developing Methods to Safeguard Human/Animal Rights（制定保障人/动物权利的方案）

Most nursing research involves humans, and so procedures need to be developed to ensure that the study adheres to ethical principles. A formal review by an ethics committee is usually required.

大多数护理研究涉及人类，因此需要制定程序以确保研究符合伦理原则。通常需要伦理委员会的正式审查。

13. Conducting a Pilot Study（进行试点研究）

It is advisable to conduct a pilot study before the study participants are approached and the actual study is carried out. People are selected for the pilot study with similar characteristics to those of the sample that will be used for the actual study. In a pilot study, researchers may evaluate the readability of written materials to assess if participants with low reading skills can comprehend them, or they may pretest their measuring instruments to see if they work well.

建议在接触研究参与者并进行实际研究之前进行试点研究。选择与将用于实际研究的样本具有相似特征的人进行试点研究。在试点研究中，研究者可能会评估书面材料的可读性，以评估阅读能力低的研究对象是否能够理解它们，或者可能会预先测试他们的测量工具，看看是否能正常使用。

14. Collecting the Data(收集数据)

Data are the pieces of information or facts that are collected in research. The actual collection of data in quantitative studies often proceeds according to a preestablished plan. The plan typically spells out procedures for training data collection staff, for actually collecting data (e. g., where and when the data will be gathered), and for recording information.

数据是在研究中收集的信息或事实。量性研究中数据的实际收集通常按照预先制定的计划进行。该计划通常会详细说明如何培训数据收集人员，如何收集数据(例如，收集数据的地点和时间)，以及记录信息的程序。

15. Preparing the Data for Analysis (数据分析准备)

Data collected in a quantitative study must be prepared for analysis. One preliminary step is coding, for example, coding gender information as "1" for females and "2" for males. Another step may involve transferring the data from written documents onto computer files for analysis. This step of the research process should have been carefully planned, ideally with a statistician, long before the data were collected.

在量性研究中，收集的数据必须为分析做好准备。一个初始步骤是编码，例如，将性别信息编码为女性"1"和男性"2"。另一个步骤可能涉及将数据从书面文件传输到计算机文件中进行分析。研究过程的这一步应该早在收集数据之前就已经仔细计划好，最好是由统计学家协助进行。

16. Analyzing the Data(分析数据)

Quantitative researchers analyze the data through statistical analyses, which include simple procedures (e. g., computing an average) as well as ones that are more complex. Some analytic methods are computationally formidable, but the underlying logic of statistical tests is fairly easy to grasp.

量性研究人员通过统计分析来分析数据，其中包括简单的程序(例如，计算平均值)和更为复杂的程序。一些分析方法的计算量很大，但统计检验的基本逻辑却很容易掌握。

17. Interpreting the Results(解释研究结果)

After the data are analyzed, the findings should be interpreted in light of the study hypotheses or research questions. If a hypothesis was tested, a determination is made as to whether the data support the research hypothesis. Researchers attempt to explain the findings in light of prior evidence, theory, their own clinical experience and the methods they used in the study. Interpretation also involves drawing conclusions about the clinical significance of the results, envisioning how the new evidence can be used in nursing practice, and clarifying what further research is needed.

分析数据后，应根据研究假设或研究问题解释研究结果。如果对假设进行了检验，则确定数据是否支持研究假设。研究人员根据先前的证据、理论、自身的临床经验和在研究中使用的方法来解释这些研究结果。解释还涉及对结果的临床意义得出结论，设想新证据如何用于护理实践，并阐明需要进一步研究的内容。

18. Communicating the Findings(传播研究结果)

This step of the research process is a very important one for nursing. A study cannot contribute evidence to nursing practice if the results are not shared. Even studies with nonsignificant findings should be published so that other researchers know the question was asked and studied. Research reports can take various forms：dissertations, journal articles, conference presentations, and so on. Journal articles usually are the most useful because they are available to a broad, international audience.

研究过程的这一步在护理中非常重要。如果不共享研究结果，则研究不能为护理实践提供证据。即使是没有重要发现的研究也应该发表，以便其他研究人员知道该问题已被提出和研究。研究报告可以采取多种形式：论文、期刊文章、会议报告等。期刊文章通常是最有用的，因为它们可被广泛的国际读者获得。

19. Utilizing the Findings in Practice(在实践中运用研究结果)

Ideally, the concluding step of a high-quality study is to plan for the use of the evidence in practice settings. Although nurse researchers may not be able to implement a plan for using research findings by themselves, he or she can make recommendations about how the findings could be integrated into nursing practice. Additionally, the researcher is actually helping promote utilization of study findings by disseminating these findings in as many ways as possible.

理想情况下，高质量研究的最后一步是计划在实践环境中使用证据。尽管护理研究人员自己可能无法实施运用研究结果的计划，但可以就如何将研究结果整合到护理实践中提出建议。此外，研究人员实际上正在通过尽可能多的方式传播这些研究结果，以帮助促进研究结果在实践中的运用。

Section Ⅳ　Major Steps in a Qualitative Study
第四节　质性研究的主要步骤

In qualitative studies, researchers have a much flexible approach, they do not know ahead of time exactly how the study will unfold themselves. During the research process, researchers continually examine and interpret data and make decisions about how to proceed based on what has already been discovered, so we cannot show the flow of activities precisely. However, we can help you understand how qualitative studies are conducted by describing some major activities and indicating when they might be performed.

在质性研究中，研究人员采用更为灵活的研究方法，且研究者自己也无法预知研究将如何展开。在研究过程中，研究人员不断地检查和解释数据，并根据已经发现的内容决定如何继续进行，因此我们无法准确显示质性研究活动的流程。但我们可以通过描述一些研究过程中的主要活动及其开展时间，以帮助更好地了解如何开展质性研究。

1. Identifying the Research Problem(确定研究问题)

Qualitative researchers usually begin with a broad topic area, focusing on an aspect of a topic that is poorly understood and about which little is known. Qualitative researchers often proceed with a fairly broad initial question, which may be further narrowed and clarified on the basis of self-reflection and discussion with others. The problem to be examined in a qualitative study may indicate the general nature of the phenomenon to be studied and the group or community that will be studied. And the reader might see a one-sentence statement of purpose.

质性研究人员通常从一个广泛的主题领域入手，专注于该主题知之甚少的方面。质性研究人员通常会提出一个较为广泛的初始问题，这些问题可能会在自我反省和与他人讨论的基础上进一步缩小范围和澄清。在质性研究中，要审查的问题可能会表明将要研究的现象的一般性质和将要研究的群体。同时，读者可能会看到一句话用以陈述研究目的。

2. Selecting the Research Design(选择研究设计)

The research design in a qualitative study depends on the phenomenon that will be studied. For example，in a statement of purpose，the researcher wants to understand the life experiences of children with asthma，this study would probably call for a phenomenological approach to data collection. If researchers want to understand the self-management process of people with schizophrenia and diabetes，they can use a grounded theory approach. Ethnographic studies may be an option if researchers are interested in the support and barriers to infant feeding in the NICU.

质性研究的研究设计取决于将要研究的现象。例如，在目的陈述中，研究人员想要了解哮喘儿童的生活体验，则这项研究可能需要一种现象学方法来收集数据。如果研究人员想要了解精神分裂症合并糖尿病患者的自我管理，则可以使用扎根理论方法。如果研究人员对新生儿重症监护病房婴儿喂养的支持及阻碍感兴趣，则可以选择民族志研究。

3. Reviewing the Literature(文献回顾)

Qualitative researchers debate about the timing of the review of literature. Not all of them agree about the value of doing an up-front literature review. Some researchers believe that a review of the literature prior to conducting research may help identify the gaps in knowledge and focus the study. Some believe that researchers should not consult the literature before collecting data because prior studies could influence conceptualization of the phenomenon. Those sharing this opinion often do a literature review at the end of the study.

质性研究人员对于文献回顾的时间有争论，研究者并不都认同前期文献综述的价值。一些质性研究人员认为，在开展研究之前进行文献回顾可能有助于确定研究空白并聚焦研究。而部分质性研究人员认为，研究人员在收集数据之前不应查阅文献，因为先前的研究可能会影响现象的概念化。持这种观点的人通常在研究结束时进行文献回顾。

4. Selecting the Sample(选择样本)

One of the main differences between qualitative and quantitative research is that the sample size in qualitative study is usually small. There are no fixed requirements for the necessary sample size for qualitative research. Some qualitative researcher claim that the quality of information obtained from each respondent is more important than the amount of data obtained. The guiding principles for considering sample size in qualitative research are the quality of the data and whether the information obtained is saturated and nothing new emerges.

质性研究与量性研究的主要区别之一是样本量通常较小。对于质性研究的必要样本量没有固定的要求。有些质性研究人员认为，从每个受访者那里获得的信息质量比获得的数据量更重要。在质性研究中考虑样本量的指导原则数据的质量和所获取的信息是否饱和，没有新的内容出现。

5. Selecting and Gain Entry to Research Site(选择并进入研究地点)

Before conducting the research, qualitative researchers must identify an appropriate research site. For example, if the research topic is the health beliefs of the urban poor, an inner-city neighborhood with low-income residents must be identified. Researchers may need to engage in anticipatory fieldwork to identify suitable environment for the study. However, before approaching potential research participants, the researcher must obtain permission from the IRB where she or he is employed, as well as the location from where the data are being collected.

在开展研究之前，质性研究人员必须确定一个合适的研究地点。例如，如果研究主题是城市贫民的健康信念，则必须确定市区内的低收入居民社区。研究人员可能需要提前进行实地考察，以确定适合开展研究的环境。然而，在接触潜在的研究参与者之前，研究人员必须获得其受雇单位的伦理委员会的许可，以及收集数据地的准许。

6. Conducting a Qualitative Study(开展质性研究)

In qualitative studies, the tasks of sampling, data collection, data analysis, and interpretation typically take place alternately. Interview is probably the most common type of data-collection method used in qualitative studies. Qualitative researchers begin by talking with or observing a few people who have first-hand experience with the phenomenon under study. The interviews used in qualitative research are generally semi-structured rather than structured.

在质性研究中，抽样、数据收集、数据分析和解释的任务通常会交替进行。访谈可能是质性研究中最常用的数据收集方法。质性研究人员首先会与一些对研究现象有第一手经验的人交谈或观察。质性研究中使用的访谈通常是半结构化的，而非结构化的。

Analysis and interpretation are ongoing, concurrent activities that guide choices about the kind of sample to select next and the types of questions to ask or observations to make. During interpretation, researchers pore over their data again and again, trying to find the meaning in the data. As analysis and interpretation progress, researchers begin to identify themes and categories, which are used to build a rich description or theory of the phenomenon.

分析和解释是持续的、同时进行的活动，以指导选择后续抽样对象的类型，以及要访谈的问题类型或要进行的观察。在解释的过程中，研究人员一次又一次地仔细研究他们的数据，试图找到数据中的含义。随着分析和解释的进展，研究人员开始确定主题和类别，这些主题和类别用于构建对现象的丰富描述或理论。

7. Disseminating and Utilizing Qualitative Findings(传播及运用质性研究结果)

Similar to quantitative research, qualitative researchers can also share their findings with others at conferences and in journal articles. Most nursing research journals contain qualitative research reports. Implications for nursing practice are usually included at the end of a qualitative research report. As with quantitative research, efforts should be made to apply the results of qualitative research to nursing practice.

与量性研究类似，质性研究人员也可以在会议和期刊文章中与他人分享研究结果。大多数护理研究期刊包含质性研究报告。对护理实践的影响通常包含在质性研究报告的末尾。同量性研究一样，也应该努力尝试将质性研究的结果运用于护理实践。

Studies Cited in Chapter 3(第三章参考文献)

[1] Fitzpatrick, J. J. Encyclopedia of Nursing Research [M]. 4th ed. Berlin：Springer Publishing Company, LCC, 2018.
[2] Fritz, H. A. Learning to do better：The transactional model of diabetes self-management integration[J]. Qualitative Health Research, 2015, 25(7)：875-886.

[3] Mabbott, I. The practice of nursing research: Appraisal, synthesis, and generation of evidence[J]. Nursing Standard Official Newspaper of the Royal College of Nursing, 2013, 27(31): 30.

[4] Peterson, S. J., Bredow, T. S. Middle range theories: Applications to nursing research [M]. 3rd ed. Philadelphia: Lippincott Williams & Wilkins, 2012.

[5] Polit, D. F., Beck, C. T. Nursing Research: Generating and Assessing Evidence for Nursing Practice[M]. 10th ed. Amsterdam: Wolters Kluwer, 2017.

[6] Patton, M. Qualitative research & evaluation methods[M]. 4th ed. New York: Sage Publications, 2015.

[7] Riegel, B., Dickson, V., Faulkner, K. The situation-specific theory of heart failure self-care: Revised and updated[J]. Journal of Cardiovascular Nursing, 2016, 31(3): 226-235.

[8] Saleem, J. J., Plew, W. R., Speir, R. C., et al. Understanding barriers and facilitators to the use of clinical information systems for intensive care units and anesthesia record keeping: A rapid ethnography[J]. International Journal of Medical Informatics, 2015, 84(7): 500-511.

[9] Willis, D. G., Grace, P. J., Roy, C. A. central unifying focus for the discipline: Facilitating humanization, meaning, choice, quality of life, and healing in living and dying[J]. Advances in Nursing Science, 2008, 31(1): E28-E40.

[10] Willis, D. G., Sullivan-Bolyai, S., Knafl, K. et al. Distinguishing features and similarities between descriptive phenomenological and qualitative description research[J]. Western Journal of Nursing Research, 2016, 38(9): 1185-1204.

PART 2：Conceptualizing and Planning a Study to Generate Evidence for Nursing

第二部分　概念化及制订研究计划，为护理实践提供证据

Chapter 4: Research Questions and Hypotheses
第四章 确定研究问题、提出研究假设

Identifying the research problem is the first and most important step to start the research. Think big and start small. The research direction should be long-term and the research problem should be specific. The process of selecting and refining a research question is usually a long one, which takes time and effort from the generation of initial ideas, to the reading of research literature and continuous thinking. It is better for researchers to start from the direction of interest and keep their passion for research.

确定研究问题是研究开始的第一步，也是最重要的一步。从大处着眼，从小处着手。研究方向要定得长远，研究问题要定得具体。选择和完善一个研究问题的过程通常较长，从产生初步的想法，到文献的阅读和不断的思考，都需要花费时间和精力。研究人员最好能从感兴趣的方向出发，保持对研究的热情。

Section Ⅰ Research Problems/Questions
第一节 研究问题

1. Overview of Research Problems(研究问题概述)

What is a research problem?

研究问题是什么？

Research field: the subject area of the research topic, or the subject range of the subject.

研究领域：一般指研究课题所在的学术领域，或课题所在的对象范围。

Research topic: The research topic is further condensed on the basis of the research field. The determination of research topics can lay a foundation for further determination of research problems.

研究主题：研究主题是在研究领域的基础上进一步凝练。确定研究主题可以为进一步确定研究问题奠定基础。

Research questions/problem：questions specifically answered or solved by researchers within the scope of the research topic.

研究问题：是研究主题范围内研究者具体回答或研究解决的问题。

Research questions are an area of concern where gaps exist in the knowledge base required for nursing practice, including meaning, context and problem statement. Researchers typically identify a broad topic, narrow down the questions, and identify questions that are consistent with the selection paradigm.

研究问题是护理实践所需的知识基础上存在缺口的一个关注领域，包括意义、背景和问题陈述。研究人员通常确定一个广泛的主题，缩小问题范围，并确定与选择范式相一致的问题。

Logic：Research field-Research topic-Research question（specific）

逻辑：研究领域—研究主题—研究问题（具体）。

Researchers may also identify several research goals or objectives. Goals include answering research questions or testing research hypotheses, but may also include broader goals（for example, developing effective interventions）.

研究人员也可能确定几个研究目的或目标。目标包括回答研究问题或测试研究假设，但也可能包含更广泛的目标（例如，开发有效的干预措施）。

【Example 1】Both alcohol consumption and diet seem to have significant effects on the composition of the human gut microbiota. However, whether alcohol consumption and diet habits during pregnancy were associated with the gut microbiota in mothers and newborns needs to be further investigated. Therefore, a population-based birth cohort study was performed to assess the influence of maternal alcohol consumption and diet during pregnancy on the gut microbiota of mothers and newborns. The results will confirm the relationship between maternal alcohol consumption, diet habits, and gut microbiota in both mothers and its offspring, which will provide a new angle to improve infants' health. The purpose of this study was to explore the effect of alcohol consumption and maternal diet during pregnancy on maternal and infant's gut microbiota（research purpose）（Wang, Y. et al., 2021）.

【例1】饮酒和饮食似乎对人类肠道微生物群的组成有显著影响。然而，怀孕期间的饮酒和饮食习惯是否与母亲和新生儿的肠道微生物群有关，还有待进一步研究。因此，我们进行了一项基于人群的出生队列研究，以评估母亲在怀孕期间饮酒和饮食对母亲和新生儿肠道微生物群的影响。研究结果将证实母亲的饮酒、饮食习惯和母亲及其后代的肠道微生物群之间的关系，这将为改善婴儿的健康提供一个新的角度。本研究旨在探讨妊娠期间母亲饮酒和饮食对母婴肠道菌群的影响（研究目的）（Wang，Y.等，2021）。

Quantitative methods are usually used for concepts that have been developed, for which there is existing evidence, and for which reliable measurements have been or will be developed. Qualitative research is more suitable for some unknown phenomena or behavior characteristics. To in-depth study the specific characteristics or behavior of the object, further explore its causes.

定量研究方法通常用于已经有所发展的概念上，这些概念已经有了现存证据，并且已经或将要发展出可靠的测量方法。而对于一些不甚了解的现象或行为特征等，更适合于使用定性研究方法。为深入研究对象的具体特征或行为，进一步探讨其产生的原因。

If quantitative research solves the question of "what", then qualitative research solves the question of "why".

如果量性研究解决"是什么"的问题，那么质性研究解决的就是"为什么"的问题。

2. Sources of Research Problems(研究问题的来源)

Nursing research problems often arise from researchers' own interests. Interest can inspire researchers in daily study, work and practice. Inspiration sources are as follows:

护理研究问题通常来源于研究者自身的兴趣。兴趣可以使研究者在日常学习、工作、实践中产生灵感。灵感来源大体为：

2.1　Clinical Experience(临床经验)

Researchers can find nursing research problems from personal experience formed by daily nursing practice and a large number of clinical case data. May be the recurring problems in the work whether there is a certain rule, can explore some adverse outcome factors, accustomed to the traditional operation is based on, is the basis credible?

从日常护理实践形成的个人经验和临床大量的病例数据中，研究者可以发现护理研究问题。可能是工作中反复出现的问题是否存在某种规律，能否探索一些不良结局的影响因素，习以为常的传统操作是否有依据，依据是否可信？

2.2 Quality Improvement Efforts(质量改进工作)

The quality improvement team will constantly summarize methods or procedures that need to be improved in their work, which will also provide a source of questions for research. Are improved methods or procedures effective? Is there any statistical difference compared with the traditional method?

质量改进小组会不断地总结工作中需要改进的方法或程序，这也会为研究提供问题来源。改进的方法或程序是否有效？与传统方式相比，是否有统计学差异？

2.3 Nursing Literature(护理文献)

Ideas for research often come from reading nursing literature. Researchers need to read high-quality core journals, such as academic journals and nursing professional journals. By reviewing research articles, researchers can identify areas of interest and determine what is known and unknown in that area. The research gap in this field provides the direction for future research. Researchers often make recommendations for further research when completing a research project. These recommendations provide opportunities for others to build on previous work and enhance knowledge in the field.

研究的想法通常来自阅读护理文献。研究者需要阅读高质量核心期刊，如学术期刊、护理专业期刊。通过查阅研究文章，研究者可以确定感兴趣的领域，并确定该领域中已知和未知的内容。该领域中的研究的空白为今后的研究提供了方向。研究人员在完成一个研究项目时，经常会提出进一步研究的建议。这些建议给其他人提供机会，可以以前人的工作为基础，加强该领域的知识。

2.4 Social Issues(社会问题)

The unexplained problems, phenomena, needs and so on in society are also sources of inspiration.

社会上尚未阐明的问题、现象、需求等也是灵感的来源。

2.5 Theories(理论)

Theories in nursing or other disciplines sometimes lead to research questions. Researchers can make predictions based on theories and test them with research.

护理学或其他学科的理论有时会引出研究问题。研究人员可以根据理论做出推测，而通过研究来验证推测。

2.6　Ideas from External Sources(来自外部资源的想法)

The idea of exogenous comes from formal academic exchanges and informal academic discussions. Through the guidance of the tutor, students can participate in academic exchange activities and high-level lectures from time to time, which can help students to have a deeper understanding of the frontier knowledge of the discipline, expand their thinking and inspire. It also allows researchers to detect errors in reasoning or information and break stereotypes.

外源的想法来源于正式的学术交流与非正式的学术探讨。通过导师对学生的指导，学生不定期参加学术交流活动、高水平讲座，有助于更深入地了解学科前沿知识，开拓思路，迸发灵感。同时也使研究人员能够发现推理或信息上的错误，打破思维定式。

3. Selecting Research Problems(选择研究问题)

A lot of ideas can come from these sources, so it's best to jot them down and categorize them as they come up. When you have a topic, you're interested in, find one to research by asking a few broad questions. For example: what phenomenon/event, etc. happened? Range of people/events, etc.? Is there an effect or cause? Is there a difference between it and it? Are the results likely to help/contribute?

通过以上来源，可能会迸发出很多灵感，当产生想法时，最好及时记录下来，并进行分类。当你有了感兴趣的话题，就可以通过提一些宽泛的问题，从中找到一个可研究的问题。比如：发生了什么现象/事件等？人群/事件等的范围？有影响或原因吗？两者相比有区别吗？结果可能产生帮助/贡献吗？

Researchers turn these questions into more specific ideas, where research questions may arise. For example, the phenomenon of decreased compliance of discharged patients taking antihypertensive drugs: Who are the discharged patients with decreased compliance? Is there a characteristic crowd? In what age group? Does it have anything to do with their profession? Why can't they take their blood pressure medication regularly? Is there any reason for this phenomenon? What do they think about taking their medication on time?

研究人员会将这些问题转为更具体的想法，研究问题可能会出现在其中。比如出院患者服用降压药依从性下降这一现象：依从性下降的出院患者都是哪些人群？人群有特征性吗？集中在哪一年龄段？与他们的职业有关系吗？他们为什么不能按时按量服用降压药物呢？有什么原因导致这个现象吗？对于按时服用药物他们有什么想法呢？

With these specific questions, researchers form research questions by consulting research literature and discussing with tutors or peers. Different research methods can be used for research problems. Some researchers will choose quantitative research, while others will choose qualitative research.

有了这些具体问题，研究者通过查阅研究文献，与导师或同行讨论，形成研究问题。而研究问题可以选用不同的研究方法，有的研究者会选择量性研究，而有的会选择质性研究。

3.1　Significance of the Problem(问题的重要性)

Nursing or social significance is a key factor in selecting research questions. In assessing the importance of an idea, ask yourself：Is the issue important to patients, nurses, healthcare systems, or society? Will these groups benefit? Do the findings support or challenge existing perceptions or practices? Can the results be put into practice? Meaningless questions should be abandoned in time.

对护理或社会有意义是选择研究问题的关键因素。在评估一个想法的重要性时，可以问问自己：这个问题对患者、护士、医疗保健系统或社会重要吗？这些人群会从中获得益处吗？研究结果是否会支持或挑战现有的认知或实践？研究结果可以用于实践吗？对于没有意义的问题，应该及时放弃。

3.2　Researchability of the Problem(问题的可研究性)

Questions of a moral or ethical nature are not suitable for study. For example, should euthanasia be legalized? These are just opinions. But some pertinent questions can be asked. For example, the attitude of patients with terminal cancer towards euthanasia? This question has nothing to do with euthanasia per se, but it does provide a better understanding of the psychology of patients with terminal cancer.

具有道德或伦理性质的问题，是不适合进行研究的。比如，安乐死应该合法化吗？这些只是一种观点。但是可以提出一些相关的问题。比如，癌症晚期患者对安乐死的态度。这一问题与安乐死本身没有关系，但是可以更好地理解癌症晚期患者的心理。

3.3　Feasibility of the Problem(问题的可行性)

Feasibility refers to the evaluation of whether a research project has the conditions for completion. The feasibility of the research question can be considered from the following aspects:

可行性是指评价研究项目是否具备完成的条件。研究问题的可行性可以从以下方面考虑:

(1) Technical feasibility: The technical capability required by the research team should be considered first. For example, relevant professional knowledge background, preliminary work basis, corresponding instruments and equipment and technical ability, appropriate measurement tools.

技术上的可行性:首先应考虑研究团队研究所需的技术能力。比如相关的专业知识背景、前期工作基础、相应仪器设备和技术能力、合适的测量工具。

(2) Financial feasibility: The cost of carrying out a research project varies greatly according to the size of the research and the items needed. When selecting research questions, financial considerations should be taken into account and the research budget should be carefully planned. It is better to be able to obtain funding support, such as applying for scientific research funding or various funds.

经费上的可行性:开展项目研究的花费根据研究的规模和所需物品等的不同而差异较大。选择研究问题时,应考虑经费问题,应谨慎规划研究预算。最好能够获得经费支持,比如申请科研经费或各种基金等。

Research funding should take into account personnel costs, participant costs, daily office supplies, printing and reproduction, equipment, laboratory costs for biochemical data analysis, etc.

研究经费应考虑人员费用、参与者费用、日常办公用品、打印和复制、设备、生物化学数据分析的实验室费用,等等。

(3) Operational feasibility: consideration should be given to the availability of the necessary conditions for each stage of implementation.

操作上的可行性:应考虑是否具备实施阶段中各环节所需的条件。

(4) Availability of research subjects: How to find suitable research subjects? How do you get access to your subjects? Was the subject interested and willing to participate in the study? Do you need incentives? Can a sufficient sample size be obtained in limited time?

研究对象的可获得性:如何寻找合适的研究对象?怎么接触到研究对象?研究对象有兴趣和意愿参与研究吗?是否需要奖励品激励?有限时间内能够获得足够的样本量吗?

(5) Feasibility of research team size and structure: Are researchers qualified? Are the

numbers sufficient?

研究团队人员数量和结构的可行性：研究者资质是否具备？人员数量是否充足？

（6）Time-based feasibility：Most studies must be completed within a certain timeframe. Estimates should be conservative, taking into account aspects such as the time point or seasonality of data collection to ensure adequate time for completion.

时间进程上的可行性：大多数研究必须在一定时间期限内完成。估计时间时应保守一些，考虑收集资料的时间点或季节性等方面，确保有足够的时间完成。

In addition to these aspects, ethical considerations should also be considered, and authorization and cooperation should be obtained if it is required in a community or institutional setting.

除了以上方面，还应考虑伦理问题，如需在社区或机构环境进行，还应获得授权，取得合作。

3.4　Researcher Interest(研究者的兴趣)

The researcher's interest in the problem is also an important prerequisite for research success. The interest of researchers will affect the input of research energy, the enthusiasm, initiative and creativity of researchers, thus affecting the quality of research results.

研究者对问题的兴趣也是研究成功的重要前提。研究者的兴趣会影响研究精力的投入，影响研究者的积极性、主动性和创造性，从而影响研究结果的质量。

4. Statement of Research Questions(研究问题的陈述)

4.1　Research Purpose(研究目的)

The purpose of the research is to write out the reasons and objectives for the research. "The purpose of this study is to..." English literature generally uses purpose, aim, goal, intent or objective to state, such as "The aim of this study was..." Objective statement words should be objective, should avoid certain, confirmed and other words.

研究目的是要写出进行此研究的理由和目标。中文一般陈述为"本研究的目的是……"英文文献一般使用purpose, aim, goal, intent 或 objective 来陈述，如 "the aim of this study was..." 目的的陈述用词应客观，应避免"确定""证实"等词汇。

In quantitative research, the statement of purpose identifies the key research variables and their possible interrelationships, as well as the population of interest. In qualitative research, a statement of purpose identifies key concepts or phenomena in the research as well as groups, communities, or backgrounds.

在量性研究中，目的陈述确定了关键的研究变量及其可能的相互关系，以及感兴趣的总体。在质性研究中，目的陈述表明了研究中的关键概念或现象，以及群体、社区或背景。

4.2　Research Objective(研究目标)

Research objectives are the specific contents determined to achieve the research objectives. The research objectives are determined according to the research objectives and research questions, and the research groups and variables should be clarified, and led out with action verbs.

研究目标是实现研究目的而确定的具体内容。研究目的根据研究目标和研究问题而确定，且要阐明研究群体和变量，并以行为动词引出。

4.3　Research Questions(研究问题)

Research questions are sometimes direct rewrites of statements of purpose, use questions rather than statements, and contain two or more variables.

研究问题有时是对目的陈述的直接改写，使用疑问句而不是陈述句，包含两个或多个变量。

A statement of the problem, usually clarifying the nature, background, and importance of the problem. State the quantitative research problem, usually including the problem itself, the background, the scope of the problem, the consequences of the problem, research gaps, and proposed solutions. State the qualitative research problem, usually including the nature, background, scope of the research problem, and information needed to solve the problem. Depending on the qualitative research method, terms and concepts may also be included.

问题的陈述，一般需阐明问题的性质、背景和重要性。陈述量性研究问题，通常包含问题本身、背景、问题的范围、问题的后果、研究空白、建议的解决方案。陈述质性研究问题，通常包含研究问题的性质、背景、范围和解决问题所需要的信息。根据质性研究方法的不同，还可能包含术语和概念。

Section Ⅱ　Research Hypotheses
第二节　研究假设

Research hypotheses is a formal statement of a possible（desired）relationship between two or more variables in a particular population. Predictions or inferences used to state the relationship between two or more variables can be transformed from research questions（to statements）. Research hypotheses are usually derived from theoretical or conceptual frameworks and help guide research design. But research hypotheses need to be tested against the results.

研究假设是对特定人群中两个或多个变量之间可能存在的(期望的)关系的一种正式的陈述。用于陈述两个或多个变量间关系的预测或推断，可以由研究问题转变而成(转为陈述句)。研究假设通常来自理论或概念框架，有助于指导研究设计。但研究假设需要接受研究结果的检验。

1. Function of Hypotheses in Quantitative Research(量性研究中研究假设的作用)

Research hypotheses are usually derived from theoretical or conceptual frameworks, and can also be derived from previous research and/or observations. Researchers start with theories, reason, form hypotheses, and test those hypotheses in the real world.

研究假设通常来自理论或概念框架，也可以来自前人的研究和/或观察。研究人员从理论出发，进行推理，形成假设，再从现实世界中检验这些假设。

If the hypothesis can be tested, the original theory is supported by real data and has credibility. The confirmation also allows the researchers to relate the results of earlier studies to existing research. If the hypothesis cannot be confirmed, the data do not support the conjecture. This allows researchers to critically think about analytical theories or previous studies, limitations of this study, or find alternative explanations.

如果假设可以得到检验，则说明原始的理论得到了真实数据的支持，获得了可信度。推测的证实也使研究人员将早期研究结果与现有研究联系起来。如果假设不能得到证实，则说明数据无法支持所做的推测，从而使研究人员批判地思考分析理论或之前的研究、本研究的局限性或发现其他的解释。

Assumptions also reduce the risk of misinterpreting false results. If there are no assumptions and only the research is conducted under the guidance of the research question, any results need to be accepted, and the subsequent explanation is not convincing.

假设还能降低误解虚假结果的风险。如果没有假设，只在研究问题的指导下进行研究，则需接受任何结果，事后的解释也是没有说服力的。

2. Research Hypotheses(研究假设)

To put forward a good research hypothesis, we should grasp the main characteristics of the hypothesis. The research hypothesis should be scientific, definite and testable. Hypotheses should not be put forward subjectively, but should conform to laws and logic, based on scientific theory or facts. State your assumptions clearly and concisely. The expected relationship of the research hypothesis can be confirmed by the research and subsequent practice.

要提出一个好的研究假设，应把握假设应具备的主要特点。研究假设应具有科学性、明确性和可检验性。假设的提出不应主观臆断，而是应符合规律和逻辑，建立在科学理论或事实的基础上。陈述假设时应清晰、简洁。研究假设的期望关系可以被研究及以后的实践所证实。

Testable hypotheses state the expected relationship between the independent variable (the reason for the prediction) and the dependent variable (the predicted result of the change in the independent variable). A relationship requires at least two variables.

可检验的假设陈述了自变量(预测的原因)和因变量(因自变量变化而发生变化的结果)之间的预期关系。一个关系至少需要两个变量。

Predictive relationships can be expressed in terms of words, such as greater than, less than, different, related, etc. Without such terms, without predictions of expected relationships, it may not be suitable for statistical testing.

预测的关系可以通过词语来体现，如大于、小于、不同、相关等。没有此类词语，没有对预期关系的预测，则可能不适合接受统计检验。

Hypotheses can be generated by induction and deduction. The induction hypothesis is derived from observation. Researchers make predictions based on certain associations or features between observed phenomena. Clinical experience and qualitative research are its important sources. The deductive hypothesis starts with an existing theory. If this theory is correct, then certain results can be expected over time (hypothesis). If this hypothesis is supported by research, the original theory will be confirmed and the conviction will be strengthened.

假设可以通过归纳和演绎方式产生。归纳假设是从观察中推导出的。研究人员通过观察到的现象间的某种关联或特征做出预测。临床经验和定性研究是其重要来源。而演绎假设是以已有的理论作为起点。如果这个理论是正确的，那么就可以预期某些结果（假设）。如果这一假设通过研究得到支持，那么此原始理论就会得到证实，信服力也会加强。

The development of nursing knowledge is inseparable from inductive hypothesis and deductive hypothesis. Theory comes from practice (induction), and practice is guided by theory (deduction). Nursing researchers should maintain critical thinking, constantly seek evidence, and push nursing theory and practice forward together.

护理知识的发展离不开归纳假设和演绎假设。理论来源于实践（归纳），实践又受理论（演绎）指导，相辅相成，交叉地发展和前进。护理研究人员应保持批判性思维，不断寻求证据，推动护理理论和实践共同前进。

The hypothesis can be expressed in many ways, but each statement should include the population, independent variables, dependent variables, and expected relationships between variables. The hypothesis can be directed or directionless.

假设可以用多种方式来表述，但不管哪种表述，都应包含人群、自变量、因变量和变量间的预期关系。假设可以是有方向性的，也可以是无方向性的。

The assumptions that come out of the theory are basically directional assumptions. Because existing theory and research provide the basis for the orientation hypothesis. Researchers prefer to use directional assumptions when the basis is sound. And when there is no relevant theory or research, or contradictory findings, the use of non-directional assumptions is recommended. The directionless assumption would be fairer.

从理论中得出的假设基本是方向性的假设。因为现有的理论和研究为方向性假设提供了基础。当基础合理的情况，研究人员更偏向使用方向性假设。而当没有相关理论或研究，或出现矛盾的发现时，更建议使用无方向性的假设。无方向性的假设会更公正。

There are two kinds of hypotheses to be written in statistical test：one is null hypothesis, H_0, also known as null hypothesis and null hypothesis；The other hypothesis is the alternative hypothesis, H_1, or the alternative hypothesis. The null hypothesis is opposed to the alternative hypothesis.

统计检验中建立假设，要写出两种假设：一种是原假设，H_0，也称无效假设、零假设；另一种是备择假设，H_1，也称对立假设。零假设与备择假设是相对立的。

The null hypothesis assumes that there is no relationship between the independent variable and the dependent variable, such as irrelevant or equally likely. Just like the assumption of innocence, if a person becomes the defendant, then the judge will first consider that the person is innocent, at this time the plaintiff needs to produce evidence to prove that the defendant is guilty. The null hypothesis is a step in statistical testing and should not be stated as a hypothesis in articles and reports.

零假设是假设自变量和因变量之间没有关系，比如无关或可能性一样大。就像无罪假设，如果一个人成为被告，那么法官就会首先认为这个人是无罪的，此时原告需要拿出证据来证明被告是有罪的。零假设是统计检验中的一步，而不应在文章和报告中作为假设陈述。

Hypothesis testing is to provide statistical evidence for research hypotheses and prove that research hypotheses are correct with a high probability.

假设检验是以统计学方法为研究假设提供依据，证明研究假设有很高的概率是正确的。

Hypothesis testing is to use the principle of "small probability events" to test through reductive proof with some probability properties. The idea of low probability is that a low probability event will almost never happen in an experiment. The idea of proof by contradiction is to put forward the test hypothesis first, and then determine whether the hypothesis is tenable by using appropriate statistical methods and the principle of small probability. That is, in order to test whether a hypothesis H_0 is correct, the hypothesis H_0 is first assumed to be correct, and then a decision is made to accept or reject the hypothesis H_0 based on the research sample. Hypothesis H_0 should be rejected if the sample observations lead to "low-probability events", otherwise hypothesis H_0 should not be rejected. If H_0 is rejected and H_1 is accepted, the hypothesis relationship is statistically significant. If H_0 is not rejected, it is proved that the hypothetical relationship is not statistically significant.

假设检验是利用"小概率事件"原理通过带有某种概率性质的反证法进行检验。小概率思想是指小概率事件在一次试验中基本上不会发生。反证法思想是先提出检验假设，再用适当的统计方法，利用小概率原理，确定假设是否成立。即为了检验一个假设 H_0 是否正确，首先假定该假设 H_0 正确，然后根据研究样本对假设 H_0 做出接受或拒绝的决策。如果样本观察值导致了"小概率事件"发生，就应拒绝假设 H_0，否则应不拒绝假设 H_0。拒绝 H_0，接受 H_1，则证明假设的关系有统计学意义；不拒绝 H_0，则证明假设的关系无统计学意义。

In most quantitative studies, whenever statistical tests are used, it means that there is an underlying hypothesis, because statistical tests exist to test hypotheses.

大多数量性研究中，只要使用了统计检验，就意味着存在潜在的假设，因为统计检验是为了检验假设而存在的。

3. Critiquing Research Problems/ Questions and Hypotheses
（评价研究问题和研究假设）

Research problems should be evaluated in multiple dimensions. Consideration should be given to whether the research question is of nursing importance and whether the findings can contribute to evidence-based nursing practice. Through continuous in-depth development of research problems, a systematic research plan will be formed to make a breakthrough in a certain aspect. Methodological aspects should also be considered, such as whether the research question is appropriate with the selected research paradigm and corresponding methods, and whether the research purpose and the statement of the research question are correct, etc.

研究问题应该从多个维度进行评价。需要考虑研究问题是否对护理有重要意义，其研究结果是否能够促进循证护理实践。通过不断深入地开发研究问题，会形成一个系统的研究计划，而做出某一方面的突破。还需考虑方法学方面，如研究问题与所选择研究范式及相应方法是否合适，研究目的和研究问题的陈述是否正确，等等。

Taking quantitative research as an example, if there is no clear hypothesis in the paper, it is necessary to consider whether its absence is reasonable. If there is a hypothesis, it is necessary to evaluate whether it is logical with the research question and whether the existing evidence and theory can support the research hypothesis. The appropriateness of the statement of research assumptions should also be evaluated. The guidelines for evaluating research questions and hypotheses are as follows.

以量性研究为例，如果文章中没有明确的假设，则需要考虑其缺失是否合理；如果存在假设，则需要评价其与研究问题是否符合逻辑，现有证据和理论是否能够支持研究假设。还应评价研究假设的陈述是否合适。评价研究问题和假设可以参考以下指南。

4. Guidelines for Evaluating Research Questions and Hypotheses
（评价研究问题和假设指南）

（1）What are the research questions? Is the research problem clearly and persuasively stated?

研究问题是什么？研究问题的陈述是否清楚、有说服力？

（2）Are the research questions of nursing significance? What is your contribution to nursing practice, management, education or policy?

研究问题对护理有重要意义吗？对护理实践、管理、教育或政策等有何贡献？

(3)Is there a good match between the research problem and the research paradigm? Is there a good match between this problem and the qualitative research tradition (if applicable)?

研究问题和研究范式是否匹配？这个问题和定性研究的传统(如果适用的话)之间是否有很好的匹配？

(4)Does the paper formally state the research objectives, questions, and/or assumptions? Is the statement clear and concise? Is it logical?

文章是否正式陈述了研究目的、问题和/或假设？陈述是否清楚、简洁？是否符合逻辑？

(5)Are research objectives and problem statements appropriate? (For example, are key concepts/variables identified and populations of interest specified? Are verbs properly used to imply inquiry and/or study the nature of tradition?)

研究目的和问题陈述是否恰当？（例如，是否确定了关键概念/变量，以及是否指定了感兴趣的总体？动词是否恰当地用来暗示探究和/或研究传统的性质？）

(6)If there is no clear assumption in the article, is its absence justified? Assumptions are not stated, but were statistical tests used to analyze the data?

如果文章中没有明确的假设，其缺失是否合理？没有陈述假设，但是分析数据时是否使用了统计检验？

(7)If a hypothesis is stated, is it derived from theory or research? Are the assumptions based on sound evidence?

如果陈述了假设，其是否来源于理论或研究？假设的依据是否合理？

(8)If the hypothesis is stated, is the statement correct? (Do they state a predictive relationship between two or more variables? Are they directional or non-directional, and do they have a reason? Are they presented as a research hypothesis or as a null hypothesis?

如果陈述了假设，其陈述是否正确？（它们是否陈述了两个或多个变量之间的预测关系？它们是方向性还是无方向性，它们有理由吗？它们是作为研究假设提出的还是作为零假设提出的？）

📖 Studies Cited in Chapter 4(第四章参考文献)

[1]Wang, Y., Xie, T., Wu, Y., et al. Impacts of Maternal Diet and Alcohol Consumption during Pregnancy on Maternal and Infant Gut Microbiota[J]. Biomolecules, 2021, 11(3): 369.

Chapter 5: Literature Review
第五章 文献综述

In order to raise research questions or hypotheses, researchers must summarize and critically evaluate the literature on a subject in a concise way. Researchers usually conduct a comprehensive literature review in the early stages of research. This chapter will provide specific guidance and practical suggestions related to literature review, including literature retrieval, literature processing and literature review writing.

为了提出研究问题或假设，研究者必须以简洁的方式对某一主题的文献进行概述和批判性评价。研究人员通常在研究的早期阶段进行全面的文献综述。本章将提供与文献综述有关的具体指导和实际建议，包括文献检索、处理文献和文献综述写作。

Section Ⅰ Getting Started on a Literature Review
第一节 文献综述入门

1. Purposes and Scope of Research Literature Reviews(文献综述的目的和范围)

1.1 Purpose of the Literature Review(文献综述的目的)

Cooper (1988) defined the purpose of literature review in the classification of literature review, that is, to critically analyze the literature, integrate different viewpoints in the literature, and determine the central problems in the existing literature. In recent years, with the development of literature review, we have summarized the following purposes: master the current research status, integrating effective research, put forward reasonable comments and guide the writing of research proposals.

Cooper (1988) 在《文献综述分类法》中确定了文献综述的目的，即批判性分析文献，整合文献中不同的观点，并确定现有文献中的中心问题。近年来，随着文献综述的研究发展，我们归纳了以下几个目的：掌握研究现状、整合有效研究、提出合理的评述和指导研究计划书的撰写。

1.2　Scope of the Literature Review(文献综述的范围)

The scope of literature review includes the subject scope, time scope and content scope involved in the topic. The scope of literature review should not be too wide and miscellaneous. The more concentrated, clear and specific the content of the review, the better. In the review, the year from the beginning to the end of the cited literature shall be determined.

文献综述的范围包括专题涉及的学科范围、时间范围和内容范围。文献综述范围切忌过宽、过杂，综述的内容越集中、越明确、越具体越好。在综述中要确定引用文献起止的年份。

The content and form of the review are flexible and diverse, there are no strict regulations, and the length is different. As large as a discipline or field, it can be a monograph of hundreds of thousands or even millions of words; As small as a method or theory, it can only be more than a thousand. The review is not a simple literature list. The review should have the author's own synthesis and induction, and the scope of the review should be determined according to the author's research needs.

综述的内容和形式灵活多样，无严格的规定，篇幅大小不一。大到一个学科或领域，可以是数十万字甚至数百万字的专著；小到一个方法或理论，可仅有千余字。综述并不是简单的文献罗列，综述要有作者自己的综合和归纳，综述的范围应该根据作者的研究需要而定。

2. Classification and Information Types of Literature Review
（研究综述的类别和信息类型）

2.1　Classification of Literature Review（文献综述的分类）

Literature review can be divided into experimental review and theoretical review according to the content information, and can also be divided into literature review part in dissertation or research thesis and independent review according to the reporting object of literature review.

文献综述可以按照内容信息分为实验性综述和理论性综述，也可以按照文献综述论述对象分为学位论文或研究论文中的文献综述部分和独立性综述。

2.1.1　Experimental Review(实验性综述)

Experimental reviews generally investigate all available information related to the research topic and critically analyze what has not been covered in the research field. In this sense, such review is a description and evaluation of past and recent research, an in-depth discussion of the work of experts in relevant field, and presentation of theoretical and practical knowledge related to the proposed research problems. The more extensive the content of the review, the more accurate and systematic the research content will be. Therefore, this kind of literature review is one of the most key critical of the research.

实验性综述一般会调查与研究主题相关的所有可用信息，并对研究领域还未覆盖到的内容进行批判性分析。在这个意义上，这种综述是对过去和近期研究的描述和评价，深入讨论相关领域专家的工作，陈述与提出的研究问题有关的理论和实践知识。综述的内容越广泛，研究内容也会越精确，其系统性也越高，因此这类文献综述是研究中最关键的部分之一。

2.1.2　Theoretical Review(理论性综述)

Theoretical review is a kind of paper that introduces or comments on the basis of generalizing and summarizing the researchers' existing research results on an academic problem in a discipline, so as to express their own opinions. Theoretical literature review should systematically summarize the main purpose of the review and write it down.

理论性综述是在归纳、总结研究者对某学科中某一学术问题已有研究成果的基础上，加以介绍或评论，从而发表自己见解的一种论文。理论性文献综述应该有组织性地对综述主旨进行总结，并将其具体写下来。

2.1.3　The Literature Review Section of a Degree or Research Paper
　　　　　(学位或研究论文中的文献综述部分)

No matter the research report, dissertation or research paper, they are introduced by introducing the research topic. This part is the literature review of the article. Its main purpose is to make clear to the readers the necessity of the research. After all relevant literature has been collected, researchers should sort out the literature. The research topics related to this kind of literature are generally broad. Researchers should sort out the recent relevant research progress by topic or time sequence, so that readers can understand the background literature of the research in the field.

不管是研究报告、学位论文还是研究论文，它们都是通过介绍研究主题来引入的，这部分就是文章的文献综述，其主要目的是给读者讲清楚进行该项研究的必要性。在所有相关文献搜集完毕后，研究者应该对文献进行整理。这类文献所相关的研究主题一般比较宽泛，研究者应该分主题或按照时间先后整理近期相关研究进展，这样能让读者了解领域内研究的背景文献。

When writing the literature, the author should discuss each topic in chronological order, explain how the relevant research has developed over time, and emphasize the important progress in the field. The literature review should include the comparison and contrast of different studies. By discussing these controversial contents, we can better clarify the direction of further research, which is very necessary to make a statement of research problems and highlight the importance of research.

撰写文献时，作者应按时间顺序分别对各主题进行讨论，说明相关研究是如何随着时间推移而发展的，并强调领域内的重要进展。文献综述应包含不同研究的比较和对比。通过讨论这些具有争议性的内容，能更好地明确需要进一步研究的方向，这对做好研究问题陈述、凸显研究重要性来说非常必要。

2.1.4　**Independent Literature Review**（独立性文献综述）

Literature review can also be written separately. Independent literature review is usually divided into two categories：descriptive review and systematic review.

文献综述也可以是单独成文的形式。独立文献综述通常分为两大类：描述性综述和系统性综述。

（1）Descriptive review.（描述性综述）

The conclusion of descriptive literature review is slightly different from the literature review in the research paper. This part gives the main conclusions after analyzing all existing studies, and then puts forward the next research approach. The author needs a critical interpretation to increase the value of the existing literature. In addition, the author should also give ideas or assumptions that can explain the inconsistency of the research, and put forward solutions to the existing problems.

描述性文献综述的结论和研究论文内的文献综述部分略有不同，这部分是通过对所有现有研究进行分析后，给出主要结论，然后提出下一步研究途径。作者需要有批判性的诠释，从而增加现有文献的价值。此外，作者还应在此给出能够解释研究不一致性的想法或假设，并针对现有问题提出解决方案。

（2）Systematic review.（系统性综述）

Systematic review generally follows a well-designed methodology to make qualitative or quantitative analysis of limited set of research. Such reviews usually focus on a single problem, with clear research objectives and systematic methods. Unlike descriptive reviews, such studies are based on very clear strategies and are organized in slightly different ways.

系统性综述，一般遵循着精心设计的方法，对有限的研究进行定性或定量的分析。这类综述通常聚焦在单一问题上，研究目标非常明确，并用系统性方法进行研究。不像描述性综述，这类研究基于的策略非常明确，二者的组织方式也略有不同。

Systematic review is different from descriptive review. This kind of research needs to review the research methods, including comprehensive methodology, which will narrow the scope of the review literature at the beginning. After determining the selection criteria based on the research problem itself, the researchers retrieve the database based on these criteria, and then analyze it in detail.

系统性综述不同于描述性综述，这类研究需要对研究方法进行综述，包含综合性强的方法论，一开始会把综述文献的范围缩小。研究者基于研究问题本身确定好选择标准后，再基于这些标准对数据库进行检索，然后对其进行具体分析。

2.2　Information Types of Literature Review（文献综述的信息类型）

2.2.1　Primary Source（主要来源）

The primary source refers to the original literature created based on the author's research results, such as journal articles, research reports, patent specifications, conference papers, etc. These literatures are innovative, practical and academic, and are the main basis for comparative analysis of literatures. The knowledge and information recorded by the main sources are relatively novel, specific and detailed.

主要来源是指以作者本人的研究成果为依据而创作的原始文献，如期刊论文、研究报告、专利说明书、会议论文等。这些文献具有创新性、实用性和学术性等明显特征，是进行文献对比分析的主要依据。主要来源所记载的知识和信息比较新颖、具体、详尽。

2.2.2　Secondary Source（次要来源）

Secondary source refers to the literature that is processed and sorted from the main source and compiled through comprehensive analysis, such as review, thematic review, annual summary of discipline, progress report, data manual, etc. These literatures have high practical value to review the existing achievements and predict the development trend. Secondary sources are obviously collected, systematic and retrievable. They can be used to reflect the review literature of research trends in a certain field, and understand its research history, development trends and level in a short time.

次要来源是对主要来源进行加工整理后，经过综合分析而编写出来的文献，如综述、专题述评、学科年度总结、进展报告、数据手册等。这些对现有成果加以评述并预测其发展趋势的文献，具有较高的实用价值。次要来源具有明显的汇集性、系统性和可检索性，可以用来反映某一领域研究动态的综述类文献，在短时间内了解其研究历史、发展动态、水平等。

3. Major Steps and Strategies in Doing a Literature Review (文献综述的主要步骤和策略)

Literature review generally includes three steps：searching the literature, reading and sorting out the literature and writing literature review.

文献综述包括三个步骤，分别是检索文献、阅读整理文献和撰写文献综述。

3.1　Search the Literature(检索文献)

Literature search is an important prerequisite for literature reading and review writing. The quality of a review largely depends on the author's knowledge of the latest literature on the subject matter.

检索文献是阅读文献和撰写综述的重要前提工作。综述的质量在很大程度上取决于作者对该主题的最新文献的掌握程度。

3.1.1　Principles of Literature Search(检索文献的原则)

（1）Comprehensiveness.（全面性）

Grasping a comprehensive and large number of literatures is the premise of writing a good review. Collect extensive literature, especially the first data, to ensure the objective and comprehensive research.

掌握全面、大量的文献资料是写好综述的前提，广泛收集文献资料，尤其是第一资料，以确保研究的客观全面。

(2) Representativeness. (代表性)

When searching the literature, there may be articles with similar viewpoints and conclusions, so attention should be paid to collecting literatures representing various viewpoints and drawing different or even contradictory conclusions as far as possible.

在检索文献时可能会出现观点雷同、结论相同的文章，应注意尽可能收集代表各种各样观点、得出不同甚至相互矛盾结论的文献。

(3) Reliability. (可靠性)

Through the retrieval, we can grasp the accuracy of the representative research and views. The reliability of literature can be identified by the impact factor (IF) of published journals, the number of citations, the research field and span of literature, and the number of research institutions.

通过检索，把握有关代表研究和观点的准确性。文献的可靠性可以通过文献发表期刊的影响因子(IF)、文献的被引用次数、文献的研究领域和跨度，以及文献的研究机构数量来鉴别。

3.1.2 The Process of Literature Search(检索文献的过程)

(1) Select database. (选择数据库)

(2) Develop a search strategy. (制订检索策略)

(3) Use literature management software. (使用文献管理软件)

Literature management software can bring great convenience and advantages for authors when they read and write papers.

文献管理软件可以为作者阅读和撰写论文带来极大的便利与优势。

3.2 Reading and Sorting Literature(阅读与整理文献)

The purpose of reading the literature is to sort out the literature so as to obtain the research progress in related fields. Reading literature and sorting out literature are inseparable in essence. In the process of reading literature, we realize the sorting of literature. To write a good literature review, we need to read the literature effectively, and then organize the literature through the process of reading and reviewing. To read the literature effectively, we must do the following:

阅读文献的目的是整理文献从而获得相关领域的研究进展。阅读文献和整理文献从本质上是不可分的，在阅读文献过程中，就可以对文献进行整理。撰写一篇好的文献综述，需要我们有效地阅读文献，然后通过阅读综述这个过程整理文献。要有效地阅读文献，必须要做到几点：

3.2.1 Clarify the Purpose of Reading（明确阅读目的）

When the subject has not been determined, we need to determine our own subject by reading the literature. Therefore, the purpose of reading is to find the unsolved problems in a certain field. Through the integration and comparison of several articles, we can find out the areas that have not been thoroughly studied in this field but are worth studying. After determining the subject and writing the paper, on the one hand, the purpose of reading literature is to solve the difficulties encountered, such as the problem of research methods; On the other hand, we can sort out our own results by reading literatures.

在课题尚未确定时，我们需要通过阅读文献确定自己的课题。因此阅读目的就是寻找某个领域目前尚未解决的问题。通过多篇文章整合和比较，找到该领域尚未被研究透彻但又值得研究的地方进行研究。在课题确定后及撰写论文时，阅读文献的目的一方面是解决遇到的困难，比如研究方法的问题；另一方面是我们可以通过阅读文献对自己的结果进行梳理。

3.2.2 Combine Intensive Reading with Extensive Reading（精读和泛读相结合）

Literature reading includes skimming and intensive reading. On the basis of extensive reading, we should carry out intensive reading, close reading and repeated reading of innovative, authoritative or high-quality literature.

文献阅读包括略读和精读。阅读文献时应在广泛阅读的基础上，对有创新性、权威性，或高质量的文献进行精读、细读和反复阅读。

In the process of reading a lot of literature, it is impossible to read every article intensively, nor can we skim every article. We must choose the reading method according to our own reading purpose and needs. Not knowing what is correct information is considered a barrier to reading and engaging in the available literature (Phillips & Glasziou, 2004). Skim the main topics, summaries and charts. After reading these three parts, we have basically mastered the main content of the article. Then see if there is a need for intensive reading of any part of the article or the whole article. If you want to understand the research trends in the field, you can read the background or introduction carefully; If you are interested in a result, you can carefully read the description and analysis of the result and relevant charts; If you have ideas about the thinkings or conclusions of the article, you can read the discussion carefully. In addition, the discussion part of the article will also put forward some unsolved problems of the article, which can expand ore own ideas.

　　大量阅读文献的过程中不可能每篇文章都精读，也不能每篇文章都略读，必须根据自己的阅读目的和需求来进行选择。不知道什么是正确的信息，被认为是阅读和着手现有文献的障碍（Phillips 和 Glasziou, 2004）。略读主要题目、摘要和图表。看了这三部分后基本就掌握了文章的主要内容。然后再看看是否有需要对文章的某部分或是整篇文章进行精读。如果想要了解领域研究动态，可以精读背景或引言部分；如果对某个结果感兴趣，可以精读结果部分，以及相关图表的描述和分析；如果对文章的思路或结论有想法，可以精读讨论部分。此外，有些文章的讨论部分还会提出一些该文章尚未解决的问题，可以拓展自己的思路。

3.2.3　Take Notes While Reading Literature（阅读文献时做好笔记）

Taking notes while reading literature can help us understand the literature and clarify the main points. It can also facilitate us to quickly find the literature for literature review.

　　阅读文献时做好笔记可以帮助我们理解文献并且明确要点，还可以方便我们快速地查找文献来进行文献回顾。

3.2.4　Classify and Sort Out the Literature（对阅读的文献进行分类和整理）

To sort out your own literature review through reading literature, you need to go through two steps：reading notes and sorting. Reading notes is to digest the content of an article, and sorting out is to organize a system of read articles according to our own understanding, which is a leap from quantitative change to qualitative change.

　　通过阅读文献整理出自己的文献综述，需经过阅读笔记和分类整理两个步骤。阅读笔记是消化一篇文章的内容，分类整理则是把读过的文章按自己的理解梳理出一个体系，是量变到质变的飞跃。

3.3　Writing and Revising Literature Reviews（撰写与修改文献综述）

3.3.1　Write Background or Preface（撰写背景或前言）

The literature review begins with a preface. In the preface, we should focus on the research background, research purpose and research methods, and focus on the following questions：

What is the current research status in this field? What are the problems? What methods do we plan to use in this study and what questions do we focus on? And possible implications and significances on for research in this field.

文献综述首先以前言开篇。在前言部分，应该着重从研究背景、研究目的、研究方法出发，着重阐述如下几个问题：目前该领域的研究现状如何？存在哪些问题？在本研究中我们拟采用什么方法，着重回答了什么问题？以及可能对本领域的研究产生的影响和意义。

3.3.2　Response Options(构建提纲和框架)

The outline and framework constitute the core structure of the article. Generally speaking, researchers can basically know what research content is included in this review by reading the title, abstract and the content title of the article. Therefore, the framework structure with clear logic and unique perspective is the core support of literature review.

提纲和框架构成文章的核心结构。一般来说，研究者通过阅读题目、摘要部分和文章的内容标题，基本就知道这篇综述内主要包含了哪些研究内容。因此，逻辑条理清晰，角度独特的框架结构是文献综述的核心支撑。

3.3.3　Write About Each Topic(撰写各主题)

After the topic selection and article framework are determined, they can be described in detail respectively. According to the writing outline, expand the content step by step, and pay attention to the consistency between the point of view and the content. In the process of writing, the structure and supplementary content can be adjusted as needed. After the introduction and specific content are completed, we should pay attention to the appropriate summary and high summary of the full text. It can systematically and objectively summarize the current research status, the latest progress and the existing problems, and put forward reasonable thoughts on the next research.

确定好了选题及文章框架之后，就可分别进行详细阐述。根据写作提纲，将内容逐步展开，并注意观点与内容的一致。在写作过程中，可根据需要调整结构和补充内容。在引言及具体内容完成之后，要注意对全文适当总结并高度概括。可以系统地、客观地总结目前的研究状态、最新进展以及当前存在的问题，对下一步的研究提出合理的思考。

Section Ⅱ　Locating Relevant Literature
第二节　查阅相关文献

1. Formulating a Search Strategy(制定检索策略)

Literature retrieval refers to the process of obtaining literature according to the needs of research content. The literature obtained through literature retrieval can have important refe。rence significance for the detailing of our research objectives. When we have a definite research goal, we can extract all the topics and research directions involved in a research goal, and then retrieve the topics and directions.

文献检索是指根据研究内容需要获取文献的过程。通过文献检索获得的文献资料对我们研究目标的详细化具有重要的参考意义。当我们有一个确定的研究目标时，我们可以提炼出一个研究目标所涉及的所有主题和研究方向，然后对主题和方向进行检索。

Through the principles of PICOS, subject terms / free terms, truncation operator, Boolean logic retrieval and other methods to develop accurate retrieval strategy and improve the accuracy of literature retrieval.

通过 PICOS 原则、主题词/自由词、截词符、布尔逻辑检索等方法制定准确的检索策略，提高文献检索的准确性。

1.1　The principles of PICOS(PICOS 原则)

In order to decompose the problem more clearly and accurately, and to find suitable and available evidence, researchers have summarized many retrieval methods, of which the most representative is the PICOS principle(see Table 5. 2. 1).

为了将问题分解得更加清晰明确，也为了更精准地找到合适可用的证据，研究者们总结出了很多种检索方法，而其中最具代表性的就是 PICOS 原则(见表 5. 2. 1)。

Table 5. 2. 1

What is the PICOS?

什么是 PICOS?

P	Population 研究对象	The subject population to be studied or represents a problem relevant to the subject. 需要研究的对象人群或代表与研究对象相关的问题。

I	Intervention 干预措施	Therapeutic interventions or observation indicators used in the study population. 对研究人群采用的治疗干预措施或观察指标。
C	Comparison 比较	Represents the control group and the indicators to be treated or observed. 代表对照组和将给予治疗措施或观察的指标。
O	Outcome 结局	Represents outcome measures and related problems. 代表结局指标和相关的问题。
S	Study design 研究设计	That is, what is the type of study, such as cohort study, case-control study and cross-sectional study. 即研究类型是什么，比如队列研究、病例对照和横断面研究。

【**Example 1**】 Case：A 75-year-old man suffered a stroke（left muscle strength weakened）and had difficulties in walking, eating, bathing, and dressing. He has a history of hypertension, which is well under control with diuretics. At present, everything is in good condition and the condition is stable. Doctors suggested transferring to the stroke unit for further treatment. The patient's family members hoped to continue treatment in the general medical ward and wanted to understand the benefits of stroke unit treatment.

【**例 1**】案例：一名75岁男性卒中患者(左侧肌力减弱)，行走、进食、洗澡和穿衣均有困难。有高血压史，服用利尿剂后控制很好。目前一切情况较好，病情稳定。医生建议转到卒中单元进一步治疗。患者家属希望继续在普通内科病房治疗，想了解卒中单元治疗有何益处。

Translated into clinical questions：For elderly stroke patients, does transferring to stroke unit treatment improve their quality of life and reduce the risk of death compared with ordinary ward treatment?

转换成临床问题为：对于老年卒中患者，转入卒中单元治疗与普通病房治疗相比能否改善其生活质量及降低死亡的风险？

The PICO format that guided their search for clinical questions was as follows：

指导他们搜索的临床问题的 PICO 格式如下：

P：Elderly stroke patients

P：老年卒中患者

I：Stroke unit therapy

I：卒中单元治疗

C：Treatment in general medical ward

C:普通内科病房治疗

O:Quality of life, death

O:生活质量、死亡

1.2 Subject Terms and Free Terms(主题词和自由词)

Literature retrieval language mainly includes natural language and artificial language. Natural language refers to the language originally used by literature authors, including literature title, abstract, key words, text, etc. Artificial language includes subject terms retrieval. Subject terms retrieval is a word or phrase selected and standardized from the main vocabulary of natural language for literature indexing or retrieval. Commonly used include MESH retrieval of PubMed and EMTREE of EMBASE.

文献检索语言主要包括自然语言和人工语言,自然语言是指文献作者原来使用的语言,包括文献题名、摘要、关键词、正文等。人工语言中则包括主题词检索。主题词检索是专门为文献的标引或检索而从自然语言的主要词汇中挑选出来并加以规范了的词或词组,常用的包括 PubMed 的 MESH 检索和 EMBASE 的 EMTREE。

Free words are not standardized words or phrases that have not been included in the subject vocabulary. Keywords are extracted directly from the title, abstract, hierarchical title or other content of the article, can reflect the concept of the topic of the paper word or phrase. The keywords are free words. Subject terms can be used as keywords, but keywords are not necessarily subject words.

自由词是未规范化的,即还未收入主题词表中的词或词组。关键词是直接从文章的题目、摘要、层次标题或文章其他内容中抽出来的,能反映论文主题概念的词或词组,关键词为自由词。主题词可以作为关键词使用,而关键词并不一定都是主题词。

1.3 Truncation Operator(截词符)

Word truncation is a symbol used to replace one or more characters in a search term. The word truncation retrieval is called word truncation retrieval. Its main function is to retrieve multiple same words with the same root or suffix and different spelling at the same time, so as to expand the scope of retrieval. Different retrieval systems have different symbols, such as " * " and " ? ", " ? " represents any character; " * " indicates multiple characters.

截词符是检索中用以代替检索词中一个或多个字符的符号。利用截词符检索称为截词检索,主要功能是同时对多个具有同一词根或词尾,以及对拼法不同的同一单词进行检索，从而扩大检索范围。不同的检索系统拥有不同的符号，如"＊"和"？"，"？"代表任意一个字符；"＊"代表多个字符。

1.4　Boolean operators(布尔运算符)

Boolean logic characters or Boolean logic retrieval are widely used and frequently used in literature retrieval. In a strict sense, Boolean retrieval refers to the method that uses Boolean operators to connect each search word, and then carries out the corresponding logical operation by the computer to find out the required information. Boolean logical operators are used to join search terms to form a logical search form. Common Boolean logic symbols include "AND" "OR" and "NOT".

布尔逻辑符或者布尔逻辑检索在文献检索中使用面广、使用频率高，严格意义上的布尔检索是指利用布尔运算符连接各个检索词，然后由计算机进行相应逻辑运算，以找出所需信息的方法。布尔逻辑运算符的作用是把检索词连接起来，构成一个逻辑检索式。常用的布尔逻辑符包括"AND""OR"和"NOT"。

2. Searching Bibliographic Databases(检索数据库)

When we want to explore a research field, we can search relevant research results through various databases, so as to understand who has studied the direction or topic, what the current development status is, and what the key problems are.

当我们想探索某个研究领域时，可以通过各种数据库搜索相关的研究成果，从而可以了解该方向或者课题都有哪些人研究过，当前的发展状况如何，以及目前存在的关键问题是什么。

3. Key Electronic Databases for Nurse Researchers
(护理研究人员常用电子数据库)

3.1　Common Electronic Databases(常用电子数据库)

When you want to know the details of a subject, you can select the subject qualification in the search qualification option on the home page of the electronic database, and enter the subject words to get the corresponding search results. At the same time, you can create a citation report on the search results, and then analyze the publication and citation of articles in recent years, understand the changes in the number of articles published over time, and understand whether the topic is a hot spot, whether it has attracted everyone's attention and whether it is a controversial point of view in recent years.

当想要了解一个主题的详细情况时，可以在电子数据库主页上的检索限定选项里选择主题限定，并输入主题词即可得到相应的搜索结果。同时，可以对搜索结果创建引文报告，进而分析近几年的文章发表和引用情况，了解随着时间的变化文章发表数量的变化，了解近几年该主题是否是热点，是否受到广泛的关注，是否有争议的观点。

The commonly used foreign language search databases in the medical field are: MEDLINE, PubMed, EMBASE, CINAHL, PsycINFO, Web of Science, Cochrane Library, Google Scholar.

医学领域常用的外文搜索数据库是：MEDLINE，PubMed，EMBASE，CINAHL，PsycINFO，Web of Science，Cochrane Library，Google Scholar。

3.2 Examples of Electronic Databases Commonly Used in Nursing

（护理常用电子数据库举例）

For nurse researchers, two particularly commonly used electronic databases are CINAHL (Cumulative Index to Nursing and Allied Health Literature) and MEDLINE (Medical Literature on-line).

对护理研究人员来说，两个特别常用的电子数据库是 CINAHL (Cumulative Index to Nursing and Allied Health Literature) 和 MEDLINE ((Medical Literature On-Line)。

3.2.1 Cumulative Index to Nursing and Allied Health Literature (CINAHL)

CINAHL collects nursing and auxiliary medical literature. It also includes books, papers and selected conference proceedings in nursing and related health fields. At present, the main collection of 1300 related academic journals. There are several versions of the CINAHL database, such as CINAHL, CINAHL Plus, and CINAHL Complete. CINAHL Complete has a literature collection of more than 4000 academic journals. CINAHL is mainly retrieved through the EBSCOhost platform.

CINAHL 主要收集护理及辅助医疗有关的文献，还包括护理和相关健康领域的书籍、论文和精选会议记录。目前主要收集 1300 份有关的学术期刊的文献。CINAHL 数据库有几个版本，如 CINAHL、CINAHL Plus、CINAHL Complete。CINAHL Complete 收集超过

4000 份学术期刊的文献。CINAHL 主要通过 EBSCOhost 平台进行检索。

On the main page of CINAHL database, you can change the language to simplified Chinese, and you can select restrictions in the accurate search results column to ensure that the scope of search results is reduced. Click the title of an article to enter the page. There is a PDF full text on the left and a series of tools on the right, focusing on the reference and export tools. There are 9 reference formats in the citation tool, which can be directly copied and pasted into the reference list at the back of the article to facilitate researchers to manage references when writing papers. If the 9 formats cannot meet the needs, you can select the export tool, confirm which reference management tools the library has purchased, and then select the corresponding column for export.

在 CINAHL 数据库主页面可以更改语言至简体中文，在精确搜索结果栏可以选择限制条件来缩小检索结果范围。点击一篇文章的标题进入页面，左侧有 PDF 全文，右侧有一系列工具，重点介绍引用和导出工具。引用工具中有 9 种参考文献的格式，可以直接复制粘贴到文章后面的参考文献清单中，方便研究者写论文时候管理参考文献。若 9 种格式无法满足需要，可选择导出工具，确认图书馆已购买的参考文献管理工具有哪些，然后选择相对应的栏目导出。

Click on my EBSCOhost to create a personal account and keep a record forever. After creating a new account, you can log in directly, and you can retrieve many types of resources on the EBSCO platform and save them in this folder. If you think the article is important, you can choose to add it to the folder and save it, and then log in to the folder above to see the results.

点击登录我的 EBSCOhost 可以创建个人账户，永久保存记录。创建一个新账号之后就可以直接登录，可以在 EBSCO 平台上检索多种类型的资源，保存在此文件夹中。如果认为该文章重要，可以选择添加至文件夹并保存，然后登录到上方的文件夹中查看结果。

3.2.2　The MEDLINE Database and the PubMed Database
（**MEDLINE** 数据库和 **PubMed** 数据库）

Founded in 1966 (dated back to 1946), MEDLINE is a journal documentation database developed by the National Library of Medicine (NLM). To date, MEDLNE has collected more than 5, 600 academic journals related to biomedical and life sciences, with more than 20 million literature records. In 1983, MEDLINE launched an electronic version, with online data updated every day and CD-ROM version updated every month. MEDLINE has a strict Literature

Selection Technical Review Committee (LSTRC) to select journals based on MEDLINE's Literature Selection guidelines, including originality, scientificity and the importance of a global audience. At present, the literature of MEDLINE is included in PubMed.

MEDLINE 始建于 1966 年(追溯收录至 1946 年)，是美国国家医学图书馆(National Library of Medicine，NLM)开发的期刊文献记录数据库。目前为止，MEDLNE 已经收录超过 5600 种生物医学及生命科学相关学术期刊，文献记录数量逾两千万条。1983 年，MEDLINE 推出电子版，网上数据每日更新，光盘版每月更新。MEDLINE 有严格的文献选择委员会(the Literature Selection Technical Review Committee，LSTRC)进行选刊，选刊标准基于 MEDLINE 选刊指南，包括原创性、科学性和全球读者重要性等方面。目前 MEDLINE 的文献都收录在 PubMed 中。

PubMed was born in 1996. As the most commonly used abstract database, PubMed has collected more than 25 million literature records so far. The collection scope includes not only MEDLINE, but also the processing data that will be included in MEDLINE, literatures that have been included in MEDLINE journals but have been prioritized for publication, literatures of authors funded by NIH Foundation and NCBI books, etc. PubMed also provides full-text links to the websites where the full text of the literature is located.

PubMed 诞生于 1996 年。作为目前最常用的文摘型数据库，PubMed 迄今为止已经收录了超过 2500 万条文献记录。其收录范围不仅包括 MEDLINE，还有即将收录至 MEDLINE 的处理中数据、期刊被 MEDLINE 收录但是文章已经优先出版的文献、NIH 基金资助作者的文献和 NCBI 书籍等。PubMed 还提供跳转到文献全文所在网站的全文链接。

MEDLINE supports subject word retrieval, restricted field retrieval, truncated word retrieval and free word retrieval. Searchers need to manually select appropriate retrieval methods for retrieval according to needs. PubMed not only has the retrieval method of MEDLINE, but also can perform automatic term mapping (ATM).

MEDLINE 支持主题词检索、限定字段检索、截词检索和自由词检索，需要检索人员根据需要人工选定合适的检索方式进行检索。PubMed 不仅具有 MEDLINE 的检索方式，还可以执行自动匹配(Automatic Term Mapping，ATM)。

Due to the large number of citations and fast update frequency of MEDLINE, researchers have developed a comprehensive set of semantic tags called MeSH (Medical Subject Headings) on all literature citation indexes. MeSH provides a consistent way to retrieve information that may use different terms for the same concept. Using MeSH, people can know the relationship between documents when reading documents. You can learn about relevant MeSH terms by clicking the "MeSH database" link on the home page.

由于 MEDLINE 引用量非常大而且更新频率快，研究人员在所有文献引用索引上开发了一套全面的语义标签，称为 MeSH(医学主题词)。MeSH 提供了一种一致的方式来检索可能对相同概念使用不同术语的信息，使用 MeSH，人们就可以在阅读文献时知道文献之间的关系。通过点击主页上的"MeSH 数据库"链接可以了解相关的 MeSH 术语。

When searching for free terms in PubMed, the entire collection range of PubMed will be retrieved, which is larger than that of MEDLINE. In particular, there will be new literature records that have been included in nearly half a year without being labeled with MeSH, which can only be retrieved with free words. When a MESH term or MEDLINE subset is defined in PubMed, only the MEDLINE data will be displayed in the search results. Entry Terms refer to the synonyms, thesaurus and polysemous words of medical subject headings. Click any medical headings of English translated words in the MeSH Database subject headings of the main page of Pubmed Database. In order to make the results more comprehensive and accurate, we can also use medical MeSH + free terms (Entry Terms)［Title/Abstract］and other qualified fields to search.

在 PubMed 中自由词检索时，会检索整个 PubMed 的收录范围，其范围大于 MEDLINE。尤其是会有新近半年被收录的文献记录并未被标注 MeSH，此时只能用自由词检索到。当在 PubMed 中限定 MeSH 词或 MEDLINE 子集时，其检索结果只会显示 MEDLINE 的数据。Entry Terms 指医学主题词的近义词、同义词和多义词，在 Pubmed 数据库主页中的 MeSH Database 主题词表中点击英文翻译词的任一医学主题词，即可出现 Entry Terms。为了使结果更加全面和精确，我们还可以采用医学主题词［MeSH］+自由词（Entry Terms）［Title/Abstract］等限定字段进行检索。

Section Ⅲ　Abstracting and Recording Information
第三节　文献信息提取及记录

1. Literature Management(文献管理)

After the researchers have consulted the relevant documents, they need to read and sort out the collected literature, and extract and record the information of the useful literature. Researchers often spend a lot of time and energy in sorting out a large number of references. At this time, it is necessary to use literature management software to achieve the purpose of saving time and effort. Literature management can simplify the process of literature sorting, so that researchers can directly insert references from various sources to facilitate sorting and reference, and modify them into various formats according to the needs of authors or journals, and can also insert the same references in articles with similar topics.

在研究者查阅出相关文件之后，需要将收集到的文献进行阅读整理，同时对有用的文献进行信息提取及记录。研究者往往会在整理大量参考文献时花费许多时间与精力，这时候就需要借助文献管理软件达到省时省力的目的。文献管理可以简化整理文献的流程，让研究者可以直接插入各种来源的参考资料，方便排序与参考，并按照作者或期刊需要修改为各种格式，也可以在类似主题的文章内插入相同的参考文献。

1.1　The Role of Document Management Software(文献管理软件的作用)

Literature management software can bring great convenience and advantages for authors when they read and write papers. Its main functions include：

文献管理软件可以为作者阅读和撰写论文带来极大的便利性与优势，其主要功能包括：

1.1.1　Sort Out Literature Information(整理文献信息)

Insert the cited papers, sort out the publication date, author, volume issue, abstract and other information of the literature.

插入引用论文，整理出该文献出版日期、作者、卷期、摘要等信息。

1.1.2　Adjust the Reference Format(调整引用格式)

It can be adjusted to the required citation format according to the journals.

可以依照各期刊调整为需要的引用格式。

1.1.3　Search for Research Information(搜索研究信息)

DOI, ISBN, PMID and other tag codes can be used to automatically search the latest information from the database.

可以利用 DOI、ISBN、PMID 等标签码从数据库中自动搜索最新信息。

1.1.4　Download the Full Text of the Literature(下载文献全文)

By connecting to the local library, the article of the cited literature can be downloaded directly.

通过连接当地图书馆，直接下载该引用文献的文本。

1.2　Literature Management Software（文献管理软件）

Common document management software includes EndNote，NoteExpress，Mendeley，
JabRef，Zotero and so on.

常用的文献管理软件有 EndNote、NoteExpress、Mendeley、JabRef、Zotero，等等。

1.2.1　EndNote

Endnote is the official software of SCI（Thomson Scientific Company）. It has powerful
functions. It is a software integrating literature retrieval，abstract and full-text management，
literature sharing and other functions. Endnote can directly connect thousands of databases，
improve the retrieval efficiency of scientific and technological literature，and manage hundreds
of thousands of references. Endnote can search relevant literature directly from the Internet and
import it into endnote's Literature Library. Endnote has the function of citation arrangement，
which can automatically help us edit the format of references. Endnote also has the function of
online search. Endnote can access most of the literature databases in the world，store the·
information connecting and searching these databases and directly provide them to users.

EndNote 是 SCI（Thomson Scientific 公司）的官方软件，自身具有强大的功能，是一款
集文献检索、文摘和全文管理、文献共享等功能于一身的软件。Endnote 能直接连接上千
个数据库，提高科技文献的检索效率，可以管理数十万条参考文献。EndNote 可以直接从
网络搜索相关文献并导入 Endnote 的文献库。EndNote 具有引文编排功能，可以自动帮助
我们编辑参考文献的格式。EndNote 还具有在线搜索功能，通过 Endnote 可以进入全世界
绝大多数的文献数据库，并将连接和搜索这些数据库的信息储存起来直接提供给使用者。

1.2.2　NoteExpress

NoteExpress is a domestic professional literature retrieval and management system. Its core
functions cover all links of knowledge management of "knowledge collection，management，
application and mining". It is a professional literature retrieval and management system in China.
It has a very powerful function of managing Chinese literature. It can realize the internal search
of the literature database of CNKI and batch download. It is especially convenient for scientific
research workers who have more Chinese literature and can improve work efficiency to a certain

extent.

NoteExpress 是一款国产专业级别的文献检索与管理系统，其核心功能涵盖"知识采集，管理，应用，挖掘"的知识管理的所有环节。是国内专业的文献检索与管理系统，具有很强大的管理中文文献功能，可以实现内部搜索知网的文献库，进行批量下载。对于中文文献较多的科研工作者来说尤为便利，可在一定程度上提高工作效率。

2. Record Literature Information(记录文献信息)

In a narrow sense, literature review may only be a simple summary of the source information, but it usually has an organizational pattern. Literature review combines abstract and synthesis. Abstract is an overview of the important information of the source, and synthesis is the reorganization of the information. Literature review can not only provide a new interpretation of source information, but also trace the knowledge progress, research advances and major events in this field. Because literature review is the summary of different literature, it is difficult to write it in an organized way, so a convenient way is needed to record literature information. Synthesis matrix is a method worth using. The synthesis matrix is particularly helpful for organizing literature reviews.

从狭义来看，文献综述可能只是对源信息进行的简单总结，但通常组织结构清晰。文献综述将摘要和综合结合起来，摘要是对重要信息的概述，而综合是对该信息的重新组织。文献综述可以对源信息进行一轮新的解释，也可以用来追溯该领域的知识进步、研究进展、重大事件。由于文献综述是对不同文献的总结，因此很难编写得有条理，那就需要一种便捷的方式来记录文献信息。综合矩阵便是很值得使用的一个方法。综合矩阵对组织文献综述特别有帮助。

Use the matrix to organize the literature review. Before the review, it is necessary to review different literature in many fields, so as to determine the overlap and deficiency of the current information in this field, and then synthesize them to better understand the overall situation of a field to a greater extent.

使用矩阵来组织文献综述。在综述前，必须查阅很多领域内不同的文献资料，从而确定该领域目前信息重叠的地方和不足的地方，然后对其综合起来，以便在更大程度上更好地了解某领域整体的情况。

A synthesis matrix is a table that allows researchers to rank and classify the different arguments that have been put forward on an issue. Table 5.3.1 is a common format for matrix tables. When you are reading a literature，simply record as much useful information as you can gather in a table，and summarize the main ideas. When writing a review，each piece of information collected needs to be processed horizontally. When you combine the information displayed in each line of the record，the entire literature review has formed in your mind.

　　综合矩阵就是一个表格，使研究人员可以对一个问题上提出的不同论点进行排序和分类。表5.3.1是矩阵表格的常用格式。当你在读一篇论文时，只需要在表格中记录收集到的尽可能多有用的信息，并对主要思想进行概括总结。在撰写综述时，需要将收集到的每条信息进行水平处理。当你把记录的每一行中显示的信息结合起来的时候，整篇文献综述已经在你脑海中成形了。

Table 5.3.1 **Matrix**（矩阵表格）

Citation	Problem/ Purpose	Design/ Sample	Instruments/ Measures	Results	Strengths/ Weaknesses
Authors	Purpose of study	Type of design	Instruments used； List them and what they measure and their reliability	Analysis	Strengths of study
Title	Theoretical framework	Sample； Number； Who； Characteristics	Demographics	Results	Weaknesses
Journal	Independent variable	Inclusion criteria			
Issue & Page	Dependent variables	Exclusion criteria			

Section Ⅳ　Analyzing and Synthesizing Information
第四节　文献分析综合

　　After comprehensively collecting and reading a large number of research literature，we need to summarize，analyze and identify these data and information，and systematically and comprehensively describe and comment on the research results，existing problems and new development trends of the research issues in a certain period of time. Literature review can be divided into the following categories:

在全面收集、阅读大量的研究文献后，我们需要对这些资料信息进行归纳整理、分析鉴别，对所研究的问题在一定时期内取得的研究成果、存在的问题，以及新的发展趋势等进行系统、全面的叙述和评论。文献综述的种类大概分为以下几种：

1. Theoretical Review(理论式综述)

Theoretical review is a review of different theories that explain the same phenomenon, introduce different theories respectively, compare the advantages and disadvantages of each theory, and evaluate their explanatory power to the phenomenon. When researchers need to integrate two theories or expand a theory, they often make a theoretical review.

理论式综述是对解释同一现象的不同理论进行综述，分别介绍不同理论，比较各理论的优势和劣势，并评价它们对该现象的解释力。当研究者需要整合两种理论或拓展某一理论时，往往会做理论式综述。

2. Background Review(背景式综述)

Background review is the most common type of literature review and usually appears at the beginning of the article. Background literature review introduces the significance and background of a research question, and places the research question in a larger relevant research context, so that the reader can understand the proportion and position of the research in the whole relevant research field. From the background review, readers can see the correlation between the research problem and the previous research, and understand the problems and deficiencies in the previous research.

背景式综述是文献综述中最常见的一种，通常在文章的开头部分出现。背景式文献综述介绍某一研究问题的意义、背景情况，将该研究问题置于一个大的相关的研究背景下，让读者了解到该研究在整个相关的研究领域中所占的比重和位置。读者可以从背景式综述中看到该研究问题与前期研究的相关性，并了解到前期研究中存在的问题和不足。

3. Historical Review(历史式综述)

Historical review is a kind of introductory review, mainly used to trace the formation and development of a certain idea or theory. Researchers often make a historical review of the most important issues in a field, which plays an important role in introducing a discipline. By reading the historical overview, the reader will have a basic comprehending and understanding of the whole picture of a certain subject.

历史式综述是一种介绍性的综述，主要用于追溯某一思想或理论形成和发展的来龙去脉。研究者们往往对某一领域中最重要的问题作历史性综述，历史性综述对介绍某一学科领域具有重要的作用。读者通过阅读历史性综述，会对某一学科的全貌有一个基本的了解和认识。

4. Methodological Review(方法式综述)

Methodological review is a review of the methodology of research results by researchers, to evaluate whether the research methods used in relevant studies are correct and appropriate, and to point out that different research designs, different samples and different measurement methods may lead to different research results.

方法式综述是研究者对研究成果的方法部分进行综述，评价相关研究中研究方法使用是否正确、得当，指出不同的研究设计、不同的样本、不同的测量方法可能会导致不同的研究结果等。

5. Integrated Review(整合式综述)

Integrated review is the integration of papers and research reports related to a research problem by researchers to show the research the current status of the research problem for readers.

整合式综述是研究者整合某一研究问题相关的论文和研究报告，为读者展现出该研究问题的研究现状。

Section V Preparing a Written Literature Review
第五节 文献综述的撰写

1. The Research Structure and Writing Process of Literature Review (文献综述的研究结构和撰写流程)

1.1 The Research Structure of Literature Review(文献综述的研究结构)

The research of literature review has two structural dimensions. One is the time structure dimension; the other is the spatial structure dimension.

文献综述的研究有两个结构维度。一个是时间结构维度，另一个则是空间结构维度。

1.1.1 The Time Structure Dimension(时间结构维度)

On the same research topic, researchers keep innovate with the development of time, so as to achieve the progress of research. For example, some papers organize literatures in chronological order. Generally speaking, there is a logical relationship between the literatures that appear successively in time, but this is not absolute and needs specific analysis.

在同一研究主题上，研究者伴随时间的发展不断创新，从而达到研究的进步。比如，有的论文按照时间顺序组织文献。一般来说，时间上先后出现的文献之间存在研究逻辑的先后关系，但这不是绝对的，需要进行具体分析。

1.1.2 The Spatial Structure Dimension(空间结构维度)

Researchers put multiple research topics together to form a research space. In this space, researchers continue to explore and innovate, thus enriching the research field. For example, some papers list the literature using different research methods, and compare the methods used with other methods to highlight the advantages and disadvantages of the methods used in this paper.

研究者将多个研究主题放在一起，共同构成一个研究空间。在这个空间里，研究者不断开拓创新，从而丰富了研究领域。比如，有的论文将采用了不同研究方法的文献罗列在一起，并在论文中将所用方法与其他方法进行比较，突出本文所用方法的优劣。

1.2　The Writing Process of Literature Review(文献综述的撰写流程)

After understanding that the research structure of literature review is the dimension of time and space structure, researchers can start to construct the writing process of literature review.

在理解文献综述的研究结构为时间和空间结构维度之后，研究者可以开始构建文献综述的撰写流程。

1.2.1　Identify Topics or Perspectives(确定主题或观点)

When writing a paper, the research status of the paper is not composed of the literature, but of the topic or perspective, and the literature is used as material to support the topic. Therefore, researchers need to first determine the topic or perspective, and then search for literature through the topic or perspective. Researchers should cite literature according to the needs of the thesis topic or perspective, so there will be a situation in which multiple literature supports a certain topic, and one part of the literature supports one subtopic while the other part supports another subtopic. In addition, it is not necessary to list all relevant literatures one by one, only cite representative literature.

撰写论文时，论文的研究现状不是由文献组成的，而是由主题或观点组成的，文献是作为材料来支持主题的。因此，研究者首先需要确定主题或观点，再通过主题或观点来查找文献。研究者应该根据论文主题或观点的需要来引用文献，所以论文会出现多个文献共同支持某个主题，以及文献的一部分支持某个子主题而另一部分支持另一个子主题的情况。此外，不需要将所有相关文献都一一列出，只需要引用具有代表性的文献即可。

1.2.2　Discovery Research Features(发现研究特征)

The characteristics of the research topic include sample size, research period, research area, reliability and validity, etc. Based on these characteristics, the researchers cited the literature and summarized and evaluated the literature. This characteristic evaluation comes from the author's professional accomplishment and experience accumulation. By refining topics and discovering the characteristic relationships between them, we can set up a research framework.

研究主题的特点包括样本量、研究周期、研究区域、信效度等方面。研究者基于这些特点引用文献并对文献进行总结归纳。这种特点的评价来自于作者的专业素养与经验积累。通过提炼主题、发现主题之间的特征关系，我们就可以搭建起研究框架。

1.2.3　Conduct Literature Evaluation(进行文献评价)

Finally, on the basis of existing research, we should reflect and evaluate the literature and point out their shortcomings. For example, the research consideration is not comprehensive, the inconsistencies and even contradictions between the literature, the gaps in the research field that have not been covered by the existing literature, and so on. The purpose is to connect different topics or perspectives. In addition, the last part of the research status must also clarify the research breakthrough point—point out the shortcomings of existing research on the basis of comprehensive evaluation, and then lead to the theme and value of this paper, which is also the most important purpose of writing literature review.

最后，在既有研究基础上，要对文献进行反思和评价，指出它们的不足。比如，研究考虑不全面，文献之间的不一致甚至矛盾之处，研究领域内尚未被现有文献覆盖的空白之处，等等。其目的是要将不同主题或观点衔接起来。此外，研究现状最后一部分还必须要明确研究突破点——在综合评价基础上指出已有研究的不足，继而引出本文所要研究的主题及其价值，这也是撰写文献综述最重要的目的。

2. Criteria for Literature Review(文献综述的标准)

Literature review writing is neither a direct paraphrase of the original literature, nor a simple literature report. It is necessary to integrate the research results of different authors and make analysis and comments. Therefore, literature review should have the following three criteria: comprehensive, commentary and progressiveness.

撰写文献综述既不是原文献的直接转述，也不是简单的文献报道，要把不同作者的研究成果加以整合，并做分析评论。因此文献综述应具有以下三个标准：综合性、评述性和先进性。

2.1　Comprehensive(综合性)

A literature review is a comprehensive summary of all the important research results on the same subject in a certain period. Therefore, it is necessary to collect all important research literature as much as possible, and make careful processing, sorting and analysis, so that various research points of view are clear. Therefore, before writing a literature review, we should sort out the literature, find the common and different points among the literature, construct the relationship between them and form a system.

文献综述是对某一时期同一主题的所有重要研究成果的综合概括。因此，要尽可能搜集所有重要研究文献，并作认真地加工、整理和分析，使各种研究观点清楚明晰。因此，撰写文献综述之前要梳理文献，发现文献之间的共同点和不同点，构建彼此之间的关系，形成一个体系。

Literature review should integrate the research of time and space dimensions, not only from the development of a topic to a vertical line of time, reflecting the progress of the current topic; But from domestic to foreign horizontal research, spatial comparison. Only in this way can the article be highly comprehensive. Through comprehensive analysis and induction, readers can fully understand the development status of a discipline or a field and predict the development trend.

文献综述要综合时间、空间两个维度的研究，既要以某一专题的发展为时间纵线，反映当前课题的进展；又要从国内到国外横向研究，进行空间的比较。只有如此，文章才具有较强综合性，经过综合分析，归纳整理，可以使读者全面了解某一学科或某一领域的发展现状并预测发展趋势。

2.2　Commentary(评述性)

Literature review should not be limited to introducing research achievements and transmitting academic information, but also comprehensively, deeply and systematically discuss a certain aspect, comprehensively analyze the contents of the review, and make appropriate and pertinent evaluation of various achievements, so as to show the author's views and opinions, give readers more enlightenment, and form a whole with the contents of the review. Due to the tendency of evaluation, the literature review will lead to the explanation of the future development trend or trend of the research topic. Therefore, when writing literature review, we should first report the important views of researchers from an objective standpoint. At the same time, when summarizing various views, we should grasp the key points and express them concisely.

文献综述不能局限于介绍研究成果，传递学术信息，还要比较全面深入系统地论述某一方面的问题，对所综述的内容进行综合分析，对各种成果进行恰当而中肯的评价，表明作者的观点和见解，给读者以更多的启示，并与综述的内容构成整体。由于评价的倾向性，通过文献综述，就会引导出对研究课题今后发展动向或趋势的说明。因此，撰写文献综述，首先要站在客观的立场上转述各研究者的重要观点；同时，在归纳各种观点时要抓住要点，表述时应简明扼要。

2.3　Progressiveness(先进性)

Literature review is not to write the history of research development, but to collect the latest information, obtain the latest content, and deliver the latest medical information and scientific research trends to the readers in a timely manner, which is the embodiment of the advanced nature of the review. In writing literature review, it is necessary to ensure that the results of literature review can give readers or researchers some inspiration and guide researchers to carry out the next research, so as to fill in the deficiencies of previous studies.

文献综述不是撰写研究发展的历史，而是要搜集最新资料，获取最新内容，将最新的医学信息和科研动向及时传递给读者，这就是综述先进性的体现。撰写文献综述要确保文献综述的结果能够给予读者或者研究者一定的启发，能够指引研究者开展下一步研究，从而填补前人研究的不足。

3. Components of a Literature Review(文献综述的组成部分)

Literature review is generally composed of title, author, abstract, key words, text and references. The text part includes the preface, the main body and the summary. Among them, the writing of the text and references is the most important.

文献综述一般由题名、作者、摘要、关键词、正文、参考文献几部分组成。其中，正文部分又包括前言、主体和总结。其中，正文和参考文献部分的撰写是最为重要的。

3.1　Writing of the Text(正文的撰写)

The text is the core part of literature review. When writing the text, we should introduce the useful information we have collected systematically on the basis of classification and arrangement. When writing this part, we should also pay attention to the following two points:

正文是文献综述的核心部分。撰写正文时，应在归类整理的基础上，对自己搜集到的有用资料进行系统介绍。撰写此部分时还应注意以下两点：

Firstly, the existing achievements should be classified and introduced with subheadings. The following are common classification clues: classified according to time and space, such as the research history and research status of this subject, foreign research status and domestic research status; classification according to different sub-topics involved in this subject; categorize different points of view according to existing results, etc.

首先，对已有成果要分类介绍，各类之间用小标题区分。以下是常见的分类线索：按时空分类，例如：本课题的研究历史与研究现状、国外研究现状与国内研究现状；按本课题所涉及的不同子课题分类；按已有成果中的不同观点进行分类，等等。

Secondly, there should be both to have a general introduction, and to focus on the introduction. According to their own classification, make a general introduction to all kinds of research, and then focus on the representative achievements in such research. It is required to point out the author's name, literature name and its specific views. Both the general introduction and the focus of the literature are required to reflect the sources of the literature in the references, but do not require one-to-one correspondence.

其次，既要有概括的介绍，又要有重点介绍。根据自己的分类，对各类研究先做概括介绍，然后对此类研究中具有代表性的成果进行重点介绍。重点介绍时点明作者名、文献名及其具体观点。无论是概括介绍还是重点介绍的文献资料均要求将文献来源在参考文献中反映出来，但不要求一一对应。

3.1.1 Writing of the Preface(前言的撰写)

This section generally does not have a special title, but directly serves as the opening part of the entire literature review. A concise introduction is an important part of a good paper. A good introduction can "sell" the research to editors, critics, readers, and sometimes even the media (Kotz & Cals, 2013). With 200 ~ 300 words, put forward the question, the content is to briefly introduce the writing purpose, significance and function of this research; major problems to be solved; summarize the history, current situation and development trend of the problem, and select the purpose and motivation, application value and practical significance of this topic. If the topic involves more cutting-edge theory, it should also be briefly introduced. If it is a controversial topic, indicate the point of contention.

此部分一般不用专设标题，而是直接作为整个文献综述的开篇部分。简明扼要的介绍是一篇好论文的重要组成部分。一个好的介绍可以向编辑、评论家、读者，有时甚至是媒体"推销"这项研究(Kotz 和 Cals, 2013)。用 200~300 字的篇幅，提出问题，内容是简要介绍本课题研究的写作目的、意义和作用；要解决的主要问题；综述问题的历史、现状和发展动态，选择这一专题的目的和动机、应用价值和实践意义。如果本课题涉及较前沿的理论，还应对该理论进行简要介绍；如果属于争论性课题，要指明争论的焦点所在。

In the preface, we should introduce the scope and sources of data collected by researchers, including what main works we have checked and read, which databases are queried in the network; and how to search, for example, by typing in "keyword" or "author name" or "article name"; the number of relevant papers searched in total; how many papers have direct reference value to themselves.

在前言中要介绍研究者搜集的资料范围及资料来源，其中要讲清查阅了哪些主要著作；在网络中查询了哪些数据库；并以怎样的方式进行搜索，比如通过输入关键词或作者名或文章名进行搜索；共搜索到的相关论文的篇目数量多少；对自己有直接参考价值的论文有多少等信息。

3.1.2　Writing of the Main Body（主体的撰写）

The main body of literature review mainly includes evidence and argumentation. By proposing, analyzing and solving problems, the author compares the similarities and differences of various views and their theoretical basis, so as to reflect the author's opinion. In order to explain the problem clearly and thoroughly, it can be divided into a number of sub-headings. This part should include historical development, current situation analysis and trend prediction. The main part has no fixed format, some according to the development history of the problem according to the chronological order of introduction, and some according to the status quo of the problem to be elaborated. No matter which method is adopted, the arguments and viewpoints of different studies should be compared, and the historical background, current situation and development direction of related issues should be clarified.

文献综述的主体部分主要包括论据和论证。通过提出问题、分析问题和解决问题，比较各种观点的异同点及其理论根据，从而反映作者的见解。为把问题说得明白透彻，可分为若干个小标题分述。这部分应包括历史演变、现状分析和趋势预测几个方面的内容。主体部分没有固定的格式，有的按问题发展历史依年代顺序介绍，也有的按问题的现状加以阐述。不论采用哪种方式，都应比较不同研究的论据与观点，阐明有关问题的历史背景、现状和发展方向。

（1）The general evolution of history.（历史演变）

The main body of literature review should be written in chronological order to briefly explain the proposal of this subject and the development of each historical stage, reflecting the research level of each stage.

文献综述主体的撰写要按时间顺序，简要说明这一课题的提出及各历史阶段的发展状况，体现各阶段的研究水平。

（2）The current situation analysis.（现状分析）

The main part will introduce the research status and views of this subject at home and abroad. Arrange and analyze the sorted and classified literatures and materials. The theories or hypotheses with creativity and development prospects should be introduced in detail and the arguments should be drawn out. For controversial issues, we should introduce various viewpoints or theories, make comparisons, show the focus of the problem and possible development trend, and put forward our own views. For questions familiar to ordinary readers, just mention them.

主体部分要介绍国内外对本课题的研究现状及观点。将整理、分类的文献和资料进行排列和必要的分析。对有创造性和发展前途的理论或假说要详细介绍，并引出论据；对有争论的问题要介绍各派观点或理论，进行比较，表明问题的焦点和可能的发展趋势，并提出自己的看法。对一般读者熟知的问题只要提及即可。

（3）The trend prediction.（趋势预测）

In the main body, we should also determine the research level, existing problems and different views of the reviewed topics, and put forward the outlook opinions. This part of the content should be written objectively and accurately. It should not only indicate the direction, but also to propose the trend forecast, to point out the direction for subsequent research.

在主体部分还要确定所综述课题的研究水平、存在问题和不同观点，提出展望性意见。这部分内容要写得客观、准确，不但要指明方向，而且要提出趋势预测，为后续研究指明方向。

3.1.3 Writing of the Summary(总结的撰写)

The summary mainly summarizes the main contents described in the theme part, focuses on comments, puts forward conclusions, and it is best to put forward your own opinions. The review mainly describes and evaluates the main characteristics, research trend and value of the above research results. This part should focus on the existing research foundation and remaining research space of this subject, such as what foundation or inspiration the existing achievements have laid for their own research, the gaps or weak links in the existing research of this subject, etc.

总结主要是对主题部分所阐述的主要内容进行概括，重点评述，提出结论，最好是提出自己的见解。评述主要是对上述研究成果的主要特点、研究趋势及价值进行描述与评价。此部分应着重点明本课题已有的研究基础与尚存的研究空间，比如已有成果为自己的研究奠定了怎样的基础或从中受到怎样的启发，本课题已有研究中存在的空白或薄弱环节，等等。

3.2 Writing of the Reference(参考文献的撰写)

Literature review should have enough references, which is the basis of writing literature review. In addition to showing respect for the research results of the cited and the basis of the cited materials, it is more important for the reader to provide clues to find relevant literature when exploring some problems in depth. The literature review explains the problem by comparing various points of view. If readers are interested in further research, they can consult the original text according to the references. Therefore, the author's name, literature name, literature source, time and other information should be fully marked according to the format of the references in the paper.

文献综述应有足够的参考文献，这是撰写文献综述的基础。它除了表示尊重被引证者的研究成果及表明文章引用资料的根据外，更重要的是使读者在深入探讨某些问题时，提供查找有关文献的线索。文献综述是通过对各种观点的比较说明问题的，读者如有兴趣深入研究，可按参考文献查阅原文。因此，应该按论文中的参考文献的格式将作者名、文献名、文献出处、时间等信息全面标示出来。

Section Ⅵ　Critiquing Research Literature Reviews
第六节　评判研究文献综述

1. Evaluation Index of Literature Review(文献综述评价指标)

Evaluation of research literature review can not only judge whether the literature review of a research field is comprehensive and representative, but also help researchers to review the maturity of their own review articles. By judging whether the research review cites a large number of empirical studies; whether these studies have resulted in fairly consistent and explanatory results; and whether these studies have reached a general consensus on understanding the nature of important relationships in this area. When evaluating the literature review, we need to focus on evaluating the literature as evidence to prove the innovation and rationality of the topic selection, research content and research conclusion. During the peer review, reviewers assess the quality of a paper based on two main criteria：contribution to the field and the adequacy of the research design (Bordage, 2001). Therefore, we can evaluate the research literature review by the three indexes of literature reliability, literature relevance and argumentation strength.

评判研究文献综述不仅可以判断一个研究领域的文献综述是否全面、有代表性，还可以帮助研究者回顾自己的综述文章是否成熟。通过判断该研究综述是否引用大量的实证研究；这些研究是否已经形成了相当一致且具解释力的结论；以及这些研究是否对于该领域重要关系性质的理解已经达成了普遍共识，可以评判该文献综述是否有缺陷。我们在评判文献综述的时候，需要重点评价文献作为证据证明选题、研究内容和研究结论的创新性、合理性。在同行评审期间，评审员根据两个主要标准评估论文质量：对该领域的贡献和研究设计的充分性（Bordage，2001）。因此我们可以通过文献可靠性、文献相关性及论证力度三个指标来评判研究文献综述。

1.1 Literature Reliability（文献可靠性）

As evidence of research, literature needs to be persuasive and reliable. The reliability of the literature can be reflected through the source of literature, that is, the journals that published the literature. It is generally believed that excellent journals in your professional field are the most reliable source. There are two main reasons.

文献作为研究的证据，需要有说服力和可靠性。通过文献的来源，也就是发表文献的期刊可以反映文献的可靠性。一般认为，你所在专业领域内的优秀期刊，是最可靠的来源。主要原因有两个。

First, each article in a published journal is reviewed by a peer review committee, and generally more than three reviewers. The peers who reviewed the papers were those who had previously published in the journal. They are reviewed by the journal's evaluation criteria to ensure the reliability of the literature.

首先，所发表期刊中的每一篇文献都会通过同行审议，并且一般有 3 位以上评审。而这些评审论文的同行，都是曾经在该期刊中发表过论文的。他们通过该期刊的评价标准来评审，可以保证文献的可靠性。

In addition, excellent journals in a professional field often have higher requirements for the research level of papers. The higher the research quality of the paper, the more reliable the general research results are.

此外，一个专业领域内优秀的期刊，往往对论文的研究水平要求更高。论文的研究质量越高，一般研究成果就越可靠。

1.2　Literature Relevance(文献相关性)

The cited literatures will be concentrated in three places of the paper: research questions and hypotheses related to the research background and purpose of the paper, research methods and implementation hypotheses related to the research content of the paper, and discussions and conclusions related to the research conclusions of the paper.

引用的文献会集中出现在论文的三个地方：与论文研究背景和目的相关的研究问题和研究假说、与论文研究内容相关的研究方法和实现假说、与论文研究结论相关的讨论和结论。

Literature relevance includes two aspects. First, the references cited are relevant to the contents of these three places. Second, the cited literatures are placed in the appropriate place.

文献相关性包括两个方面。所引用的文献是与这三个地方的内容相关的；所引用的文献被放在了对应的地方。

For example, as part of your research for a paper, you adopted a certain theory in your research, which is a methodological theory in psychology or education. Then, you should provide the concept and background of the theory, and cite the literature to provide evidence that the theory can be applied to your research. If you cite literature that doesn't say anything about the theory, you haven't provided evidence.

例如，作为论文的研究内容之一，你在研究中采用了某种理论，该理论属于心理学或教育学专业的方法学理论。那么，你就应该提供该理论的概念和背景，并引用文献来提供证据证明这种理论可以应用在你的研究中。如果你引用的文献中根本就没有关于这种理论的，那么你就没有提供证据。

In short, we use the literature as evidence. Even if the irrelevant literature is listed, it has no proof effect. If the relevant literature is placed in the wrong place, it cannot prove the effect.

总之，我们是用文献作为证据证明用的，不相关的文献就算是罗列出来也没有证明的效果，相关的文献被放在了错误的地方也起不到证明效果。

1.3　Argumentation Strength(论证力度)

As the evidence for writing papers, literature can be used to organize the internal logic of literature review and to prove the novelty and value of literature. The process of such a proof is an argumentation. Only by making strong arguments and providing reliable and relevant literature can researchers publish good papers.

文献作为撰写论文的证据，可以组织好文献综述的内部逻辑，为证明文献的新颖性和价值而使用。这种证明的过程就是论证。只有通过强有力的论证，同时提供可靠和相关的文献，研究者才能发表出好的论文。

To achieve strong argument, it must have the following characteristics:

要做到强论证就要具有以下几个特点：

(1) Comprehensive coverage. （覆盖全面）

(2) Generalize and classify in detail. （归纳和分类详细）

(3) Clear indexing of major issues. （重大问题的标引清楚）

(4) Propose the future direction. （提出未来的方向）

2. Features of an Excellent Literature Review(一篇优秀的文献综述的特点)

Literature review reflects the researchers' mastery of the literature in the research field and their ability of theoretical thinking. There are no hard and fast standards for literature review, but there are certain characteristics that make for a good literature review.

文献综述反映研究者对所研究领域文献的掌握程度和理论思维能力。评述研究文献综述并没有硬性标准，但是优秀的文献综述需要具备一些特点。

2.1 Leading Edge(前沿性)

The literature review should pay attention to the latest academic development, and the literature cited in the review should be the latest, on the one hand to pursue novelty, and on the other hand to prevent the omission of the latest achievements. But the latest means the number of citations is unlikely to be high. Then it can be judged from other aspects, such as whether the source journal is recognized as the top journal in the field.

文献综述应该关注学术的最新发展，综述引用的文献最好是最新的，一方面是追求新颖性，另一方面是防止遗漏最新成果。但是最新的意味着引用次数不可能高。那么可以从其他方面评判，比如来源期刊是否是领域内公认的顶级期刊。

2.2 Coverage(覆盖性)

A good literature review should cover all the important literature, explore all perspectives around the central problem of the research, including one's own opposing views. In particular, we should not ignore the literature or theories that are inconsistent with our own assumptions or findings. First of all, it's only when you're on the opposite side that you can really weigh your views carefully. Second, if you can refute a dominant idea or influential theory, your research will carry more weight. Third, the existence of the opposite at least suggests that your conclusion is not obvious.

一个好的文献综述应该涵盖所有重要文献，围绕研究的中心问题，探索方方面面的观点，包括与自己观点相反的观点。对与自己的假设或发现不一致的文献或理论，尤其不能忽略。首先，只有站在对立面上，才能真正深思熟虑地斟酌自己的观点。其次，如果你能驳倒某个主流的观点或有影响力的理论，那么你的研究将更有分量。再次，对立面的存在至少说明你的结论并非显而易见。

2.3　Relevance(相关性)

Literature review is a comprehensive discussion of the relevant literature on a subject in a certain period of time. It is not a pile of complex literature, nor is it a quotation of pure literature. On the basis of adhering to "comprehensiveness", we can not take all the documents indiscriminately. Excellent literature review only needs to review the literature directly related to this study, or at least indirectly related to it, and avoids discussing irrelevant literature.

文献综述是针对某个课题在某段时间的，内容相关的文献的综合论述。它并不是一堆复杂文献的堆砌，也不是一段纯文献的引用。在坚持"全面"的基础上，我们又不能对所有文献不加选择地包揽。优秀的文献综述只需要回顾与本研究直接相关的或至少间接相关的文献，避免讨论不相关文献。

2.4　Coherence(连贯性)

A good research review should focus on one main line from beginning to end, developing the research hypothesis step by step to serve the author's thinking. Coherence emphasizes the avoidance of literature stacking and disorganization in literature review. The most important way to avoid literature stacking is classification. Adding subheadings is of course the most important method of classification. At the same time, the writing of each subheading also needs to be classified. This classification may be based on different research contents, different influencing factors, different research methods, different research conclusions, and different schools of views. The most important thing is that the classification needs to use some transition statements to ensure coherence, the most commonly used transition relations are parallel and transition, with a logical relationship of transition statements, the article will be clearer.

　　好的研究综述应该是自始至终围绕一条主线，为作者的思路服务，一步一步推演出研究假设。强调文献综述要连贯，避免文献堆砌、杂乱无章。避免文献堆叠的最重要的方法就是分类，添加子标题是最重要的分类手段，同时，在每个子标题的行文里，也需要进行分类。这种分类可能是基于不同的研究内容，不同的影响因素，不同的研究方法，不同的研究结论，不同的观点流派。而最重要的是分类需要用一些过渡语句来保证连贯性，最常用的过渡关系是并列和转折，有了带有逻辑关系的过渡语句，文章就会更加清晰。

📖 Studies Cited in Chapter 5（第五章参考文献）

[1] Cooper, H. M. Organizing knowledge synthesis: A taxonomy of literature reviews[J]. Knowledge in Society, 1988, 1(1): 104-126.

[2] Phillips, R. S., Glasziou, P. What makes evidence-based journal clubs succeed? [J]. Acp Journal Club, 2004, 140(3): A11-12.

[3] Fernández-Castillo, R. J., Gil-García, E., Vázquez-Santiago, M. S. et al. Chronic non-cancer pain management by nurses in specialist pain clinics[J]. British journal of nursing (Mark Allen Publishing), 2020, 29(16): 954-959.

[4] Kotz, D., Cals, J. Effective writing and publishing scientific papers—part i: how to get started[J]. Journal of Clinical Epidemiology, 2013, 66(4): 397.

[5] Bordage, G. Reasons reviewers reject and accept manuscripts: the strengths and weaknesses in medical education reports [J]. Academic Medicine Journal of the Association of American Medical Colleges, 2001: 76.

Chapter 6: Theoretical Framework
第六章 理论框架

Section I The Nature of Theories and Conceptual Models
第一节 理论和概念模式的性质

Theories and conceptual models have much in common, such as origin, general properties, purpose, and function. In this section, we discuss some characteristics of theoretical and conceptual models.

理论和概念模式有很多共同之处，如起源、一般性质、目的、作用等。在本节，我们将讨论理论和概念模式的一些特征。

1. Theories, Models and Frameworks(理论、模式和框架)

Theory is a systematic understanding of natural and social phenomena, which is also a set of interrelated concepts that provides a systematic explanation of a phenomenon. Levels of theories include grand, middle-range, and micro theories. Model is a fewer formal means of organizing phenomena than theories. It is defined as a graphic or symbolic representation of a phenomenon. A framework is related to a specific event or question being studied and it refers to the overall conceptual underpinnings of a study.

理论是人们对自然界及人类社会现象的规律的系统认识，也是一组相关概念对一种现象的系统描述。理论分为广域理论、中域理论和局域理论。相比于理论，模式是一种不太正式的组织现象的方法。模式是一个现象的图解或符号表示。框架围绕某个具体被研究的事件或问题，是一个研究的整体概念基础。

2. Nature of Theories and Models(理论和模式的性质)

Theories and models are invented by humans, so they may change following with the change of human values. This means, some theories and models may fall into disfavor because of the development of the society, and may be modified with having new evidence.

理论和模式是人类发明的，因此，它们可能会随着人们价值观的改变而改变。这就意味着，有些理论和模式可能会随着社会的发展而被淘汰，也可能会因为新证据的出现而被修改。

3. The Role of Theories and Models(理论和模式的作用)

Theories and models play an important role in the progress of a science. Firstly, they are effective mechanisms to help aggregate data from isolated and separated investigations. Secondly, theories and models can not only guide researchers to understand what natural phenomena under study are, but also help them understand why the phenomena happen. Because of this predictability, theory is a vital resource for developing nursing intervention strategies. Finally, theories and models can provide directions for research.

理论和模式在科学发展中起着重要作用。首先，它们是帮助从孤立和分离的调查中收集数据的有效机制。其次，理论和模式不仅可以指导研究者理解所研究的自然现象是什么，还可以帮助其理解现象发生的原因。正因为有这样的预测性，理论是发展护理干预策略的重要资源。最后，理论和模式可为研究提供方向。

4. Relationship Between Theory and Research(理论与研究的关系)

Theory and research are reciprocal and mutually beneficial. On the one hand, theories and models are developed based on generalizations of observations in research. On the other hand, theories are evaluated by testing hypotheses in research. Therefore, research plays a reciprocal and continuous role in theory building and testing. Theory provides guidance for research, while, research evaluates the value of the theory and provides a basis for new theories.

理论和研究之间密不可分、互惠互利。一方面，理论和模型的形成是基于研究中观察的概括。另一方面，理论通过在研究中检验假设来评价。因此，研究在理论构建和检验中起到了密切和持续的作用。理论为研究提供指导和思路；而研究评估理论的价值，并为新理论的发展提供基础。

Section Ⅱ Conceptual Models and Theories Used in Nursing Research
第二节 护理研究中使用的概念模式和理论

Nurse researchers often use both nursing and non-nursing models to provide a conceptual context in their studies. In this section, we discuss several common models.

护理研究者常常在研究中使用护理或非护理的理论模式，提供所研究的概念背景。在本节中，我们将讨论几种常见的理论模式。

1. Conceptual Models and Theories of Nursing(护理概念模式和理论)

Four core concepts are emphasized in modern nursing: human beings, environment, health, and nursing. Different conceptual models and theories interpret the relationships among the four concepts differently, and identify different processes as being central to nursing. For example, in Roy's Adaptation Model, human being is regarded as an adaptive system, with biological, psychological, and social attributes. Environment is the stimulus that comes from within and around human being. Human being keeps interacting with the environment, through their internal and external changes, to maintain the integrity as a whole. Health is viewed as a process and state of being and becoming integrated and whole. While, nursing is to promote client adaptation by controlling the stimuli.

现代护理强调了四个基础概念：人、环境、健康及护理。不同的概念模式和理论对四个概念之间关系的诠释不同，并认为护理的核心不同。例如，在罗伊的适应模式中，人被认为是一个具有生物属性、心理属性和社会属性的适应系统。环境是来自人自身和周围的刺激。人通过内部和外部的变化与环境保持着互动以保持整体的完整性。健康是处于和成为一个完整的和全面的人的状态和动态的过程。而护理，则是通过控制刺激，促进个体的适应性。

2. Other Models and Middle-range Theories Developed by Nurses
(其他由护士发展的模式和中域理论)

Many nurse scholars developed middle-range theories used in the nursing field, such as Kolcaba's Comfort Theory, Peplau's Theory of Interpersonal Relations, Theory of Unpleasant

Symptoms, Theory of Transitions, Symptom Management Model, Pender's Health Promotion model, Beck's Theory of Postpartum Depression, Mishel's Uncertainty in Illness Theory, and Reed's Self-transcendence Theory. Here, we discuss Theory of Unpleasant Symptoms. The Theory of Unpleasant Symptoms was developed by Lenz et al. in 1995, which includes three core concepts of symptoms, influencing factors, and performance, addressing on interactions among concepts. It is often used to assess patients' physical and psychological performance related to uncomfortable or unpleasant symptoms. For example, in a study of understanding fatigue symptoms and influencing factors in patients with rheumatoid arthritis, authors identified the influencing factors based on the Theory of Unpleasant Symptoms, and further explored impacts of the influencing factors on fatigue.

很多护理学者发展了用于护理领域的中域理论, 如科尔卡巴的舒适理论、佩普劳的人际关系理论、不悦症状理论、转变理论、症状管理模式、潘德的健康促进模式、贝克的产后抑郁理论、米歇尔的疾病不确定感理论, 以及里德的自我超越理论等。在这里, 我们讨论不悦症状理论。不悦症状理论是 1995 年由 Lenz 等人提出, 包括症状、影响因素及结局表现三个核心概念, 强调了概念间相互影响。该理论常用于评估患者面对不舒适或不愉悦的症状时所出现的身体和心理表现。例如, 在一项类风湿关节炎患者疲乏症状及影响因素研究中, 作者基于不悦症状理论确定研究中的影响因子, 并进一步探讨这些影响因素对疲乏的影响。

3. Other Models and Theories Used by Nurse Researchers
（护理研究者使用的其他模式和理论）

There are a number of models and theories used by nurse researchers. Here, we discuss two non-nursing models or theories commonly used in nursing studies. The first is the Health Belief Model (HBM) developed in the early 1950s, which is one of the most widely used theoretical frameworks for understanding health behaviors. The main components of the HBM include perceived susceptibility, perceived severity, perceived benefits, perceived barriers, cue to action, and self-efficacy, which are important to change individuals' health behaviors. The second is Lazarus's Theory of Stress and Coping. The theory describes that how major life events affect people's emotions, with the main focus on individual cognitive evaluation and dealing with stress (coping). Cognitive evaluation consists of three types: primary appraisal, secondary assessment, and reassessment. Based on the assessment results, three different ways of dealing with stress are discussed, including the problem-oriented way, the emotion-oriented way, and the assessment-oriented way.

护理研究者经常使用一些非护理理论和模式。在这里，我们讨论两种常用于护理研究的非护理模式或理论。首先是 20 世纪 50 年代早期发展起来的健康信念模式（HBM），是用于理解健康行为的使用最广泛的理论框架之一。HBM 的主要组成部分包括感知易感性、感知严重性、感知益处、感知障碍、行动线索和自我效能，这些对改变个体的健康行为很重要。其次是拉扎勒斯的压力与应对理论。该理论阐述了生活中的重要事件如何影响人们的情绪，主要集中在个体的认知评价和压力处理（应对）。认知评价包括了三种方式：初级评价、次级评价，以及重新评价。根据评估结果，探讨了三种不同的压力处理方式，即以问题为导向的方式、以情绪为导向的方式，以及以评估为导向的方式。

4. Select a Theory or Model for Nursing Research（为护理研究选择理论或模式）

There are no rules for selecting appropriate theories or models to guide specific nursing research, however, there are two suggestions for researchers. Firstly, read relevant theoretical literature and be familiar with a variety of grand theory and middle-range theory, such as Orem's self-care theory, Roy's adaptation model, Watson's theory of care, Newman's system model, and Kolcaba's comfort theory, which are commonly used in nursing research. Secondly, we can find the theories used in similar research topics. After we learn as much as possible about the most promising theories, we choose the appropriate one for our own study. During deciding the theory, it is very important to determine whether the theory fits the research problem well, that is, whether the selected theory can explain, predict, or describe structures that are key to the research problem.

如何选择合适的理论或模式指导具体护理研究工作尚无规则可遵循，但有两个建议可供研究者们参考。第一，阅读相关理论文献，熟悉一些广域理论和中域理论，如常用于护理研究的奥瑞姆的自护理论、罗伊的适应模式、华生的照护理论、纽曼的系统模式、科尔卡巴的舒适理论等。第二，可以借鉴相似主题研究所使用的理论，尽可能多地了解几个最可能使用的理论后，选择适宜的理论用于自己的研究。在确定理论时，很重要的一点就是理论和研究问题能否很好地契合，即所选择的理论是否能够解释、预测或描述研究问题所揭示的结构。

Section Ⅲ Testing, Using and Developing a Theory or Framework in Nursing Research
第三节 护理研究中理论或理论框架的测试、应用和发展

There are three ways in which theories or frameworks are used in nursing research. Firstly, theory is generated as the outcome of a nursing study, appearing in qualitative research. Secondly, theory is used as a research framework, as the context for a study, being used in both qualitative and quantitative research. Thirdly, research is conducted to test a theory, being used in quantitative research. We discuss them separately in this section.

理论或理论框架在护理研究中的使用包括三个方面，第一，理论是护理研究的结果，出现在质性研究中；第二，理论被用作研究框架，作为研究的情境，可用于质性或量性研究；第三，理论被研究检验，用于量性研究。我们在这一节分别进行讨论。

1. Theories and Qualitative Research(质性研究与理论)

Theory almost always appears in qualitative studies, such as ethnography, phenomenology, grounded theory and so on. These qualitative research traditions provide an overarching framework, giving a theoretical grounding for specific qualitative studies. For example, most ethnographers adopt the following two cultural theories: (1)Ideational theories, which state that cultural conditions and adaptations originate from people's mental activities and ideas; (2) Materialistic theories, which suggest that material conditions, such as resources, money, and production, are the source of cultural developments. While, grounded theory is a method to study social interaction under the guidance of symbolic interaction. On the other hand, theory-generating research is a process of developing generalizations from specific observations. The research methods used for theory generation include conceptual analysis, phenomenology, grounded theory, case studies, ethnography, and historical inquiry. In particular, grounded theory researchers aim to develop their own substantive theories.

理论几乎总是出现在质性研究中，如民族志、现象学、扎根理论研究等。这些质性研究方法提供了一个总体框架，为具体质性研究提供了理论基础。例如，大多数民族志研究者采纳了以下两种文化理论：(1)观念理论，这一理论认为文化条件和适应源于人们的精神活动和想法；(2)唯物主义理论，认为资源、金钱和生产等物质条件是文化发展的源泉。

而扎根理论则是在象征互动理论指导下研究社会互动的一种方法。另一方面，理论生成研究是一个从特定的观察中形成一般化的过程。用于理论生成的研究方法包括概念分析、现象学、扎根理论、案例研究、民族志和历史探究等。特别是，扎根理论研究者的目的是形成自己的理论。

2. Theories and Models in Quantitative Research（量性研究中的理论和模式）

Quantitative researchers also often use theories or models in their studies. Here, we introduce two common approaches. Testing theories is a classic method in quantitative research. For example, Health Promotion Model proposed the factors influencing behaviors, such as perceived benefits of action, perceived barriers to action, perceived self-efficacy, and others. Based on this model, nursing researchers might hypothesize that patients who believe that dietary control is good for them will be more likely to change their eating habits than those who do not believe it is good for them. Such a conjecture can serve as a starting point for testing the model. On the other hand, scholars can use a theory or model as the organizational structure for research. Researchers assume that the theory or model is valid and then use its constructs to provide an interpretive context. For example, in O'Neill's study, researchers used the theory of planned behavior（TPB）as a framework to select attitudes, subjective norms, and perceived behavior control as factors, which can influence nursing staff intentions regarding early detection of the deteriorating health of a resident and providing subacute care in the nursing home. Then, they conducted A TPB survey, which consisted of 23 items related to early detection of deteriorating health and providing subacute care. Finally, multiple regression analysis was conducted with the attitude, subjective norm and perceived behavioral control as the predictors of behavioral intention.

量性研究者也常将理论或模式用于相关研究中。这里，我们介绍常见的两种方式。检验理论是量性研究中使用理论的经典方法。例如，HBM 中提出了感知到行为益处、感知到行为障碍、自觉自我效能等多个影响行为改变的因素。基于此，护理研究者可能会提出这样的假设：相比较那些不相信饮食控制对自身有好处的患者，相信该观点的患者会更愿意去改变其现有的饮食习惯。这样的假设可作为检验模式的起点。另一方面，学者们使用理论或模式作为研究的组织结构。研究者假设所运用的理论或模式是有效的，进而使用理论或模式的结构以提供一个解释研究结果的情境。例如，在 O'Neill 等人的研究中，研究者运用计划行为理论作为研究框架，确定态度、主观规范和感知行为控制是影响养老院护士早期发现患者身体状况恶化、并提供亚急性护理意图的因素。于是，他们制作了计划行为理论问卷调查，包括 23 项与早期发现身体状况恶化和提供亚急性护理有关的条目。最后，以态度、主观规范和感知行为控制作为行为意向的预测因子，进行多因素回归分析。

Section IV　Critiquing Frameworks in Research Reports
第四节　评判研究报告中的理论框架

When evaluating the theoretical framework in qualitative research reports, there are a number of issues that need to be addressed. For example, in a phenomenological study, it is necessary to assess whether or not the researcher emphasizes the philosophical underpinnings of the study. In a grounded theory study, it is necessary to evaluate whether the emerging theory is logical and whether the evidence supporting it is persuasive. Theoretical frameworks do not need be present for quantitative studies, such as studies to determine the optimal frequency of turning patients. However, if it is an intervention study, it is necessary to use a theoretical framework to guide the study. In quantitative research, if an explicit theoretical framework is used, it is necessary to evaluate whether the particular framework is appropriate, that is, the logic of using the framework, and the authenticity of the connection between the research questions and the theory. The questions can be asked, such as, do the research hypotheses arise from the theory? Do the results contribute to the validation of the theory? and so on.

评判质性研究报告中的理论框架时，我们需要关注一些问题。如在现象学研究中，要评价研究者是否强调了研究的哲学基础。而在扎根理论研究中，我们要评估所形成的理论是否合乎逻辑，以及支持其的证据是否具有说服力。对于量性研究而言，理论框架不一定出现，如检测卧床患者翻身的最佳频率的研究。但如果是干预性研究，有必要运用理论框架作指导。在量性研究，如果运用了明确的理论框架，要评估这个特定框架是否合适，即使用该框架的逻辑性，研究问题与理论之间联系的真实性。如提出问题："研究假设问题是来源于理论吗？研究结果是否有助于验证理论？"等。

📖 Studies Cited in Chapter 6（第六章参考文献）

[1] Champion, V. L., Skinner, C. S. The health belief model. In Glanz K., Rimer B. K., Viswanath K. (Eds.), Health behavior and health education: Theory, research, and practice[M]. San Francisco: Jossey-Bass, 2008.

［2］Lazarus, R. Stress and emotion: A new synthesis［M］. New York: Springer, 2006.

［3］Lenz, E. R., Suppe, F., Gift, A. G., et al. Collaboratiive development of middle-range nursing theories: Toward a theory of unpleasant symptoms［J］. Advances In Nursing Science, 1995, 17(3): 1-13.

［4］LoBiondo-Wood, G., Haber, J. Nursing research: Methods and critical appraisal for evidence-based practice［M］. 9th ed. St. Louis, Missouri: Elsevier, 2018.

［5］Morse, J. M. Strategies for sampling. In J. M. Morse (Ed.), Qualitative nursing research: A contemporary dialogue［M］. Newbury Park, CA: Sage Publications, 1991.

［6］Polit, D. F., Beck, C. T. Nursing research: Generating and assessing evidence for nursing practice［M］. 9th ed. Philadelphia: Lippincott Williams & Wilkins, 2012.

［7］O'Neill, B. J., Dwyer, T., Reid-Searl, K. et al. Nursing staff intentions towards managing deteriorating health in nursing homes: A convergent parallel mixed-methods study using the theory of planned behaviour［J］. Journal of Clinical Nursing, 2018, 27 (5-6): e992-e1003.

［8］李峥, 刘宇. 护理学研究方法: 第 2 版［M］. 北京: 人民卫生出版社, 2018.

［9］吴肃然, 李名荟. 扎根理论的历史与逻辑［J］. 社会学研究, 2020, 35(2): 75-98.

［10］郑素素. 基于不悦症状理论的类风湿关节炎患者疲乏症状及影响因素研究［D］. 沈阳: 中国医科大学, 2020.

Chapter 7: Ethics, Research Integrity and Academic Morality in Nursing Research
第七章 护理研究中的伦理原则、科研诚信及学术道德

With the development of nursing research, the legal, ethical and social issues in nursing research have been paid more attention. This chapter will discuss ethical principles and protective procedures for conducting nursing research, as well as research integrity and academic ethics in nursing.

随着护理科研的发展，护理科研中的法律、伦理和社会问题不断受到关注。本章将讨论进行护理研究的伦理原则、保护程序，以及护理中的科研诚信和学术道德。

Section I Ethics and Research
第一节 伦理与研究

The constraint function of ethics on human group in social activities cannot be ignored. Although ethical norms will change with social development and cultural evolution, on the whole, the binding force of ethics plays a positive role in regulating social behavior and maintaining social order. Ethical considerations in research are required not only to protect the rights of research participants, but also to ensure the effective exploitation and utilization of "knowledge" to enhance the knowledge base of humanity in all respects. If researchers conduct research in unethical ways, the research process can not only be called into question because of behavior toward study participants, but also affect the development of knowledge (Deventer, 2009).

伦理对于人类群体在社会活动中的约束作用不容忽视。虽然伦理规范会随着社会发展和文化演变而发生变化，但总体来说，伦理道德的约束力对规范社会行为、维护社会秩序

具有正面作用。研究过程中的伦理考虑不仅需要保护研究参与者的权利，还需要确保有效地开发利用"知识"，从而全面提高人类的知识基础。如果研究人员以不道德的方式进行研究，研究过程不仅会因为对研究参与者的行为而受到质疑，而且还会影响到知识的发展（Deventer，2009）。

1. Codes of Ethics(伦理准则)

1.1　Nuremberg Code(纽伦堡法典)

The *Nuremberg Code* was the first international convention on a code of conduct for human medical research, introduced after World War Ⅱ, to guide physicians, researchers and others in conducting experiments involving human subjects (Katz, 1996).

《纽伦堡法典》是在第二次世界大战后提出的关于人体医学研究行为准则的第一个国际性公约，以指导医师、研究人员等进行涉及人类受试者的实验(Katz，1996)。

During the World War Ⅱ, Nazi doctors carried out many cruel human experiments, involving low temperature, negative pressure, poison, and prolonged starvation without the consent of the subjects to observe the symptoms of the human body under these conditions. Such experiments not only did no good to the subjects but also resulted in pain, disability and death for a large number of them. Such actions are purely out of war and aggression, not science.

第二次世界大战期间，纳粹医生在未经受试者同意的情况下，进行了许多残酷的人体实验，包括低温、负压、下毒、长时间饥饿等，以观察人体在这些条件下的症状。这样的实验不仅对受试者没有任何益处而且导致了大量受试者的痛苦、伤残和死亡。这类行为仅仅是出于战争和侵略的需要，毫无科学而言。

The brutality, racism and brutality of these studies triggered a profound international rethink of modern medicine's use of living people in experiments, attracting unprecedented attention from the public, the medical and scientific community, and public authorities. To prevent such atrocities from happening again, the famous *Nuremberg Code* was enacted in 1946.

在这些研究中，野蛮残忍、种族歧视和暴虐行为引发了国际社会对现代医学使用活人来做实验的深刻反思，引起了公众、医学和科学界人士，以及公共权威的前所未有的关注。为了防止这类暴行的再次发生，在 1946 年颁布了著名的《纽伦堡法典》。

1.2　Declaration of Helsinki(赫尔辛基宣言)

In 1964, the *Declaration of Helsinki* was read and adopted at the 18th World Medical

Congress held in Helsinki, Finland (Goodyear et al., 2007). The *Declaration of Helsinki* sets out detailed ethical principles for human research. It stresses that researchers must be aware of the relevant ethics, laws and regulations before undertaking relevant research, and provides clear ethical guidance for researchers and medical practitioners. The publication of the declaration also establishes authoritative and binding agreements, without which the results of research cannot be announced at meetings of biological research institutions. In addition, the Declaration provides a basis for exposing biomedical research that violates ethical principles, so that inhumane research can be punished and curbed through media and other means.

1964 年，在芬兰首都赫尔辛基召开的第 18 届世界医学大会上宣读并通过了《赫尔辛基宣言》(Goodyear et al., 2007)。《赫尔辛基宣言》制定详尽的关于人体研究的伦理原则，它强调了研究者在从事有关的研究之前必须了解相应的伦理、法律和法规，并为研究者与医疗从业人员提供了明确的伦理指导。宣言的发表还建立了权威和有约束力的协议，如果没有这些协议，就不能在生物研究机构的会议上宣布其研究成果。此外，宣言还为揭露违背伦理原则的生物医学研究提供了基础，以便通过媒体和其他手段对不人道的研究予以鞭挞和遏制。

1.3　Belmont Report(贝尔蒙报告)

In 1978, the *Belmont Report* was presented by the American Biomedical and Behavioral Sciences Research Council. The report proposes three basic ethical principles for the protection of human subjects in medical research, namely, the principle of "respect for people", the principle of "benefit" and the principle of "justice", which have become the basic principles of biomedical research ethics.

1978 年由美国生物医学和行为科学研究委员会提出了《贝尔蒙报告》。该报告提出了医学研究中的保护人类受试者的三条基本的伦理学原则，即"尊重人"的原则、"受益"的原则和"公正"的原则，已成为生物医学研究伦理学的基本原则。

2. Ethical Dilemmas in Conducting Research(开展研究中的伦理困境)

Nursing research is an important impetus for the development of nursing discipline, as well as a guarantee for nurses to improve their own quality and provide better nursing services for patients. However, the rights of the research object are in direct conflict with the research in some cases, which will lead to the ethical dilemma of nurses.

护理研究是护理学科发展的重要推动力，也是护士提高自身素质，从而为患者提供更好护理服务的保障。然而在一些情形中，研究对象的权利和研究会发生直接的冲突，从而会导致护士陷入伦理困境。

Ethical dilemmas faced by nursing researchers include：as researchers, they would ask patients not to withdraw from the study to ensure the accuracy of the study results, but find that this conflicts with their responsibilities as nurses to respect patients' autonomy, so they fall into ethical dilemmas. In addition, sometimes patients' autonomy is at stake, for example, patients think they must attend and sign informed consent when they need immediate surgery in severe emergencies. In these cases, guaranteeing the interests of research or patients makes nursing researchers in a dilemma.

护理研究人员面临的伦理困境包括：作为研究者，他们会要求患者不要退出研究以保证研究结果的准确性，但发现这与其作为护士尊重患者自主权的责任是相违背的，因此陷入伦理困境。此外，有时患者自主权受到威胁处于危险境地，比如重症急诊需立即手术等情况时，患者认为自己必须参加而签署知情同意书。在这些情况下，保证研究的利益还是保证患者的利益让护理研究者陷入困境。

Section Ⅱ　Ethical Principles for Protecting Study Participants
第二节　保护研究参与者的伦理原则

1. Beneficence(有利原则)

"Beneficence" requires researchers to evaluate the benefits and risks of the study before carrying out the study, so as to minimize the harm and maximize the benefits for the subjects. Therefore, the principle of advantage has two complementary rules.

"有利原则"要求研究者在开展研究前评估研究的益处和风险，尽量减少伤害，而为受试者提供最大化的利益。因此，有利原则有两条互补的规则。

1.1　The Right to Be Free from Harm and Discomfort(免受伤害和不适的权利)

Before the implementation of the study, researchers should carefully evaluate the possible benefits and risks of the study to the study subjects, and maximize the benefits and reduce the risks. In human studies, risks include physical risks (e.g., injury, fatigue), emotional risks (e.g., stress, fear), social risks (e.g., lack of social support), and economic risks (e.g., loss of wages). If the risks outweigh the benefits, the content of the study should be modified to minimize harm. Research may not be carried out on subjects that may cause serious or permanent harm, no matter how beneficial the results may be.

在研究实施之前，研究者应谨慎评估该项研究可能给研究对象带来的受益和风险，并最大限度地增大受益和降低风险。在对人类的研究中，风险包括生理上的（如伤害、疲劳）、情感上的（如压力、恐惧）、社会上的（如社会支持的缺乏）和经济上的（如工资的损失）。如果风险大于受益，应修改研究的内容，将伤害降到最低。如果研究可能会给研究对象造成严重或永久性伤害，无论研究结果会带来多大的效益，也不可以对研究对象实施。

When evaluating the risk of research and benefit, you can consult relevant experts and assess the risk based on your own clinical experience and expert opinions. In the study design, researchers should customize corresponding countermeasures to deal with the occurrence of some injuries.

在评估研究风险与受益的风险时，可以咨询有关专家，根据自身的临床经验和专家的意见进行有关风险的评估。在研究设计方案中，研究者应制定相应的对策以应对某些伤害的发生。

1.2　The Right to Protection from Exploitation（不受剥削的权利）

The researcher and other members of the research team should strictly protect the personal information of the research object, and avoid the disclosure of information that may harm the social status, reputation and personality of the research object. Researchers should fully respect the rights and privacy of research subjects in the investigation, and the relationship established between research participants and researchers should not be arbitrarily used.

研究者和研究小组的其他成员应严格保守研究对象的个人信息，避免信息泄露导致研究对象的社会地位、名誉、人格等受到伤害。研究者在调查中应充分尊重研究对象自身权益及隐私，研究参与者与研究人员建立起的关系不应该被随意利用。

2. Respect for Human Dignity（尊重原则）

"Respect for human dignity" requires researchers to regard research objects as independent individuals, respect people's autonomy, let them have the right to make their own choices about whether to participate in research, and protect those vulnerable groups whose autonomy is limited.

"尊重原则"要求研究者把研究对象视为独立自主的个体，要尊重人的自主性，让他们有权自己做出是否参与研究的选择，对那些自主能力受限的弱势人群要给予保护。

2.1 The Right to Self-determination（自主决定权）

Self-determination means that subjects can voluntarily decide whether to participate in the study, and have the right to ask questions, refuse to provide information, and withdraw from the study. As an investigator, participants should also be informed that they can voluntarily decide whether to participate in the study or not.

自主决定权是指研究对象可以自愿决定是否参加研究，有权提出问题、拒绝提供信息，并退出研究。作为研究者，也应告知参与者可以自愿决定是否参加研究。

Self-determination includes freedom from compulsion, from punishment for not participating in research or from undue rewards for agreeing to participate. Subjects have the right to withdraw from the study at any time without penalty throughout the study.

自主决定权包括不受强迫，不会因为不参与研究而受到惩罚或因同意参与而获得过度奖励。在整个研究中，受试者有权在任何时候退出研究而不受到惩罚。

2.2 The Right to Full Cognitive（充分认知权）

The right to be fully cognitive means that researchers should fully inform participants of the specific content of the study, the right to make voluntary decisions, the possible benefits and risks, and let them decide whether to participate in the study or not.

充分认知权是指研究者要对参与研究的对象充分告知研究的具体内容、自主决定的权利、可能的获益和风险，并让研究对象自己决定是否参与研究。

However, full access to information can create problem with bias and sample collection problems. Research subjects may refuse to participate in the research or conceal the real situation after knowing the research content, which may be the content needed by our research. Such full cognition may affect the development of the research.

然而，充分的知情权可能会造成偏倚和样本收集的问题。研究对象可能在知晓研究内容后拒绝参与研究或隐瞒真实情况，而这些可能正是我们研究所需要的内容。那么这种充分知情会影响研究的开展。

In such cases, researchers sometimes use covert methods to collect data. When some social phenomena are rarely known to the public, the hidden participatory observation method is usually used for observation under the premise of knowledge, which can ensure obtaining relatively real information. However, this method may violate the privacy of the subjects and cannot be used when dealing with sensitive topics. Therefore, researchers need to ensure that participants face little risk and much benefit before using this method; the researcher is after using other methods cannot improve the validity of the premise; and when needed, researchers must inform participants about covert methods and reasons.

在这种情况下，研究者有时会采用隐蔽法收集资料。当有些社会现象很少被人所知时，在知情的前提下，通常采用隐蔽型的参与观察法进行观察，可以确保获得相对真实的信息。然而这种方法可能会侵犯研究对象的隐私权，在涉及敏感性话题时不能适用。因此，研究者在使用这种方法前需要保证参与者面临的风险很小而获益很多；研究者是在使用其他方法不能提高研究有效性的前提之下；以及一旦需要，研究者必须告知参与者隐蔽的手段和原因。

2.3　The Right to Anonymity and Confidentiality(匿名权和保密权)

Anonymity means that the subject's identity cannot be linked to his or her personal responses. The research kept the subjects anonymous, unable to contact them for additional information without specific approval.

匿名是指受试者的身份不能与他或她的个人回答联系起来。研究人员保持受试者匿名，未经特别批准无法联系受试者获得更多信息。

Confidentiality means that the investigator manages the subject's private information and does not share it with others without the subject's authorization. In most studies, researchers want to know the identities of their subjects and promise to keep their identities secret. Breaches of confidentiality can occur when researchers unintentionally or knowingly allow unauthorized access to the raw data of a study. Breaches of confidentiality can harm the psychological and social interests of the subjects and reduce their trust in the researchers.

保密是指研究人员对受试者的私人信息进行管理，未经受试者授权不得与他人共享。在大多数研究中，研究人员希望知道他们的研究对象的身份，并承诺将会对他们的身份进行保密。当研究人员无意或有意允许未经授权的人访问研究的原始数据时，就可能发生违反保密性的情况。违反保密性会损害受试者的心理和社会利益，并降低他们对研究人员的信任度。

3. Justice(公正原则)

The principle of justice means that every research subject should be treated fairly and should get what they deserve. The principle of justice includes distributive, egalitarian, egalitarian and other connotations (Raus, 2016). In a study, the selection and treatment of subjects during the study should be fair.

公正原则是指每位研究对象都应该得到公平对待，应该得到自己应得的东西，公正原则包括分配主义、平等主义、自由主义等内涵(Raus, 2016)。在研究过程中受试者的选择和治疗应该是公平的。

3.1　The Right to Fair Treatment(公平对待的权利)

The selection of population and specific study subjects should be fair, and the risks and benefits of a study should be fairly distributed according to the efforts and needs of subjects. When conducting the study, the investigator should treat the subjects fairly, make appointments with the subjects on time for each appointment if data collection is required, and terminate the data collection process at the appointed time. In addition, study participants should receive the same benefits regardless of their age, race and socioeconomic status.

对人群和具体研究对象的选择应该是公平的，一个研究的风险和利益应该根据受试者的付出和需求进行公平的分配。在进行研究时，研究者应该公平地对待受试者，如果数据收集需要与受试者进行预约，那么每次预约都要准时，并在约定的时间终止数据收集过程。此外，无论参加研究的受试者年龄、种族和社会经济地位有什么差异，都应该获得同等的利益。

3.2　The Right to Privacy(隐私权)

Privacy means that researchers need to carefully review data collection methods to protect the privacy of subjects, and data should not be collected without the knowledge of subjects, and subjects also have the right to protect their privacy.

隐私权是指研究者需要对数据收集方法进行仔细审核，以保护受试者的隐私，并且不能在受试者不知情的情况下收集数据，受试者也有权利保护自己的隐私。

Section Ⅲ Procedures for Protecting Study Participants
第三节 保护研究参与者的程序

1. Risk/Benefit Assessments(风险/获益评估)

In order to protect study participants, researchers and study reviewers must conduct a risk/benefit assessment, which is the ratio of possible harm to the benefits of study participation. The purpose of this assessment is to evaluate whether the risks of participating in the study are consistent with the benefits and whether the balance of risks and benefits in the study is maintained.

为了保护研究参与者，研究者和研究审查人员必须进行风险/获益评估，即参与研究的可能危害与获益的比率。该种评估旨在评价参与研究的风险是否与获益一致，是否保持研究中风险和获益的平衡。

The risk-benefit assessment consists of several components：

风险-获益评估包括几个部分：

（1）Determining whether the study design method is capable of generating scientific, reasonable and valuable conclusions and reducing unnecessary research interventions.

确定研究设计方法是否能够生成科学、合理且有价值的结论，并减少不必要的研究干预。

（2）Make an empirical judgment of possible risks and benefits based on existing research.

根据现有研究对可能的风险和获益做出经验判断。

（3）Normative assessment of possible risks in the study.

针对研究可能出现的风险进行规范性评估。

Researchers should not only assess and weigh possible risks and potential benefits, but also communicate the risks and benefits of the study to recruited participants so that they can assess whether participation is in their best interest. And as far as possible to reduce the risks that participants may bear, increase the relevant benefits.

研究人员不能仅仅对可能存在的风险和潜在获益进行评估和衡量，还应向被招募的参与者表明研究的风险和利益，以便他们能够评估参与是否符合他们的最佳利益。并且尽可能地减少参与者可能承担的风险，增加相关利益。

1.1 Assessment of Risks(风险评估)

Researchers need to assess the number, type, and severity of possible risks associated with study participants' participation. Research risk types depend on the purpose and process of research.

研究者需要评估研究对象参与研究可能产生风险的数量、类型和严重程度。研究风险类型取决于研究的目的和研究的过程。

All studies involve some risk, which can increase from small to large. Minimum risk refers to the risk which is not greater than the risk of daily life or during the performance of routine physical or psychological examinations or tests. When risks are increasing, researchers must begin to pay attention and take all possible measures to reduce risks and maximize benefits.

所有的研究都涉及一定的风险，风险可以从小到大不断增加。最小风险是指不影响日常生活或研究过程中经常发生的风险。当风险不断增加时，研究者必须开始注意，采取一切可能的方法来减少风险和最大化利益。

In the study, the potential risks of the subjects included:

在研究中，研究对象的潜在风险包括：

(1)Physical injury or discomfort, including side effects and fatigue.

生理上受到伤害或出现不适，包括副作用和疲劳等。

(2) Because of self-reflection, fear of the unknown, discomfort to strangers, fear of consequences, and fear of being.

因为自我的反思、对未知的恐惧、对陌生人的不适、害怕后果和对于被问的问题感到愤怒或尴尬而引起的心理情绪困扰。

(3)Social risks of loss of status, stigmatization and negative impact on relationships.

丧失地位、被污名化，以及对人际关系产生不利影响的社会风险。

(4)Loss of privacy affects your life.

失去隐私而影响自己的生活。

(5)Lost time and money.

损失时间和经济。

1.2 Assessment of Benefits(获益评估)

Research benefits include the benefits of individual, family and society. Both therapeutic and non-therapeutic studies affect the potential benefits of participants. In therapeutic care studies, treatments such as skin care, touch, and other nursing interventions are administered that benefit the participants themselves. Non-therapeutic research can indirectly benefit the discipline and plays an important role in generating and improving practical nursing knowledge.

研究获益包括研究对象个体、家庭和社会的获益。无论是治疗性的还是非治疗性的研究，都会影响参与者的潜在利益。在治疗性护理研究中，实施的治疗方法如皮肤护理、触摸和其他护理干预措施会使参与者自身受益。非治疗性研究可以间接为该学科带来利益，为产生和完善实践护理知识起着重要作用。

In the study, the potential benefits of the subjects included:

在研究中，研究对象的潜在获益包括:

(1) Potential benefits through participation in intervention research.

通过参与干预性研究，获得潜在的获益。

(2) You can share your situation or ideas with friendly and impartial people.

可以与友善、公正的人分享自己的情况或想法。

(3) Increase your knowledge of disease and health through participation in research, self-learning, or direct communication with researchers.

通过参与研究进行自我学习，或与研究人员的直接交流，来增加疾病和健康的相关知识。

(4) The information provided may help others in similar situations.

提供的信息可能会帮助其他有类似情况的人。

(5) Obtain material benefits such as money and spiritual benefits such as health education knowledge.

获得金钱等物质获益和健康宣教知识等精神获益。

2. Informed Consent and Participant Authorization(知情同意和参与者授权)

A particularly important procedure for protecting study participants is to obtain their informed consent. Subjects have the ability to voluntarily agree or refuse to participate in the study, and researchers should fully inform subjects of their right to voluntarily withdraw from the study. Informed consent has become an integral part of medical research to protect the interests of all stakeholders (Chatterjee 和 Das, 2021).

保护研究参与者的一个特别重要的程序就是获得他们的知情同意。研究对象有能力自愿同意或拒绝参与，研究者应充分告知研究对象有自愿中途退出的权利。知情同意已经成为医学研究的一个组成部分，以保护所有利益攸关方的利益（Chatterjee & Das，2021）。

2.1　The Content of Informed Consent（知情同意的内容）

（1）Subjects have the right to withdraw from the trial at any stage without discrimination or retaliation, and their equal medical treatment and rights will not be affected.

研究对象有权利在试验的任何阶段退出而不会遭到歧视或报复，其医疗平等的待遇和权益不会受到影响。

（2）The personal data of subjects participating in and participating in the study will be kept confidential. Personnel of the professional management department and members of the ethics committee can only access the data of the research object participating in the experiment when necessary, according to regulations.

研究对象参加试验及在试验中的个人资料均会被保密。专业管理部门人员和伦理委员会成员只能在必要时按规定查阅参加试验的研究对象的资料。

（3）The research object can know the research purpose, research process, research time and potential benefits and risks of the research object, and inform the research object that they may be assigned to different groups of the experiment.

研究对象可知晓研究目的、研究过程、研究时间，以及研究对象潜在的获益和风险，告知研究对象可能被分配到试验的不同组别。

（4）During the study, the subject can know the information related to it at any time.

研究期间，研究对象可随时了解与其有关的信息资料。

（5）In the event of trial-related injury, the subject will receive treatment and corresponding compensation.

如发生与试验相关的损害时，研究对象可以获得治疗和相应的补偿。

2.2　The Process of Participant Authorization（参与者授权的过程）

2.2.1　The Awareness of Participants（参与者的知晓）

Informed consent was not a simple matter of filling out a paper or electronic form. First, researchers are required by law to provide sufficient information to each patient. Second, pay attention to giving each subject the opportunity to ask questions and make suggestions.

参与者的知情同意并不是简单地填好一份纸质或者电子的知情同意表。首先，研究者必须向每一位患者提供充足的信息。其次，要注意给每位研究对象提问和建议的机会。

2.2.2　**Signing of Informed Consent**（知情同意书的签署）

After the study subject is fully informed about the study and agrees to participate，the study subject and the investigator conducting the informed consent discussion must sign the name and date on the informed consent before any activities related to the study can begin.

在研究对象对有关研究的情况做出充分了解并同意参加之后，研究对象和进行知情同意讨论的研究者必须在知情同意书上签署姓名和日期，然后才能开始任何与研究有关的活动。

2.3　The Requirements for Researchers（对研究者的要求）

Subjects should be given sufficient time to read the informed consent in a quiet environment and ample opportunity to learn the details of the study. The informed consent process should adopt language and writing that the research object can understand.

研究者应给予研究对象充足的时间在安静的环境下阅读知情同意书，并为受试者提供充足的机会了解研究的详细资料。知情同意过程应采用研究对象能理解的语言和文字。

The investigator must allow the subject sufficient time to consider whether or not he/she wishes to participate in the study，and should provide such introductions and instructions to his/her legal representative if the subject is unable to give consent.

研究者必须给研究对象充分的时间以便考虑是否愿意参加研究，对无能力表达同意的受试者，应向其法定代理人提供上述介绍与说明。

3. Confidentiality Procedures（保密程序）

Protecting the privacy and anonymity of research participants is an important protection method. Researchers should consider how to obtain relevant information of subjects needed for research and at the same time protect their privacy. How to store this information securely and ensure that it is not leaked；How to ensure that there is no relationship between participants and researchers other than the study.

保护研究参与者的隐私权和匿名权是重要的保护方法。研究者应思考如何既获取研究所需要的被试者的相关信息，同时又保护其隐私；如何安全地存储这些信息而确保不被泄露；如何保证参与者和研究者之间没有除研究外的其他关系。

Researchers should keep the condition，privacy and other information of the research object confidential, encode the general information of the research object, and do not involve the disclosure of important information of the research object before the presentation of statistical results. At the same time, study participants have the right to know that the data and answers they provide will be kept strictly confidential.

　　研究者应该对研究对象的病情、隐私等情况予以保密，对研究对象一般信息进行编码，统计结果呈现前不涉及研究对象重要信息的泄露。研究参与者有权知道他们提供的数据和回答将得到严格的保密。

4. Treatment of Vulnerable Group(如何对待弱势群体)

Researchers should protect the rights of participants in the study, and additional procedures may be required for special vulnerable groups. Researchers should be aware of informed consent and risk/benefit assessment and try to study vulnerable populations when the risk/benefit ratio is low or when there are no other options. Common vulnerable groups in nursing research include：

　　研究人员应在研究中保护参与者的权利，并且对于特殊脆弱群体可能需要额外的程序来保护。研究人员应该了解有关知情同意和风险/获益评估的内容，尽量在风险/受益比很低或没有其他选择时才对弱势群体进行研究。护理研究中常见的弱势群体中包括：

4.1　Children(儿童)

Legally and ethically, the child is not capable of giving informed consent. If the child is a participant, the informed consent must be obtained from his or her legal guardian. When the child is mature enough to understand basic informed consent information and make a decision to consent to participate in the study, consent must also be obtained to show respect for the child's self-determination.

　　在法律和伦理上，儿童没有能力进行知情同意，如果儿童作为参与者，必须征得其法定监护人的知情同意并签署知情同意书。当儿童足够成熟，能够了解基本的知情同意信息并做出同意参加研究的决定时，还必须征得其本人同意，以表示对该儿童自主决定权的尊重。

Therefore, researchers must protect these children during the study period, and researchers should design the study specifically to maximize the incentive for children to participate in the study, this includes providing young children with specific information about upcoming studies, working with parents to understand the involvement of children, and understanding the hesitation and rejection of participants (Brown et al., 2017).

因此，研究人员必须在研究期间保护这些儿童，应该针对性地设计研究，以最大限度地激励儿童参与研究，包括向幼儿提供关于即将进行的研究的具体信息、与父母合作了解孩子的参与情况，以及对参与者的迟疑和拒绝表示理解(Brown 等，2017)。

4.2　Pregnant Women(孕妇)

Researchers should protect pregnant women who may be at high physical and psychological risk. This and other studies should be examined carefully and need to take into account the full range of pregnancy exposures in the study, rather than broadly excluding all pregnant women (American College of Obstetricians and Gynecologists, 2015). Pregnant women are advised not to participate in studies that are not designed to meet their health needs and that pose the least risk to both the pregnant woman and the fetus.

研究人员应保护可能面临高度身体和心理风险的孕妇。对该类研究和其他研究应该进行仔细的检查，需要在研究中考虑怀孕暴露的各种情况，而不是广泛排除所有孕妇(American College of Obstetricians and Gynecologists, 2015)。如果研究目的不是满足孕妇的健康需求，并且对孕妇和胎儿的风险最小，孕妇最好不要参与研究。

4.3　Patients with Impaired Mobility(行动力受损的患者)

For patients with severe capacity, researchers should carefully assess their ability to participate in the study. Physical, communication, and social constraints can cause researchers to misunderstand their ability to engage in meaningful communication and engage in inclusive research, and therefore, when conducting research on this group of people, requires careful attention to the ethical and practical considerations of competence and informed consent (Hills, 2019). If the ethics committee agrees in principle and the investigator considers that it is in the interest of the subjects to participate in the study, these patients may also be admitted to the study and should sign and date the informed consent form with the consent of their legal guardian. For participants who are unable to read or write due to physical disorders, special methods such as video recording should be used to document the informed consent process.

对于病情严重、缺乏行为能力的患者，研究者应谨慎地评估他们参与研究的能力。身体、沟通和社会的限制可能会造成研究者对他们参与有意义的沟通和参与包容性研究的能力的误解，因此，在对这类人群进行研究时，需要仔细地关注其能力和知情同意方面的伦理和实际考虑(Hills, 2019)。如果伦理委员会原则上同意并且研究者认为受试者参加试验符合其本身利益时，这些患者也可以进入试验，同时应该通过其法定监护人同意，在知情同意书上签名并注明日期。对于因身体障碍而无法读写的参与者，应使用录像等特殊方式记录知情同意的过程。

4.4　People with Mental or Emotional Disorders(有精神或情感障碍的患者)

For patients with mental or emotional disorders, researchers should obtain written consent from the legal guardian. To the extent possible, the informed consent or consent of the participant himself should be sought as a supplement to the consent of the guardian. In addition, the method of acceptance of these subjects needs to be clearly stated in the trial protocol and relevant documentation, with prior agreement of the ethics committee.

对于患有精神或情感障碍的患者，研究人员应获得法定监护人的书面同意。在可能的范围内，应寻求参与者本人的知情同意或同意，作为监护人同意的补充。此外，需要在试验方案和有关文件中清楚说明接受这些受试者的方法，并事先取得伦理委员会同意。

4.5　The Terminally Ill(终末期患者)

Most end-stage patients participate for reasons other than their own benefit from the study, so researchers need to carefully evaluate the risk/benefit ratio. Measures must be taken to ensure that end-stage patients are healthy and comfortable to participate in the study and to reduce the impact of treatment.

终末期患者参与研究的原因大多数不是自己可以从研究中获益，因此研究者需要仔细评估风险/获益比。研究人员必须采取措施，确保终末期患者参与研究的健康舒适度，以及减少患者接受治疗的影响。

5. External Reviews(外部审查)

Researchers may not be objective in assessing the risks/benefits of their studies or in protecting participants' rights. Research is usually subject to external ethical review due to the possibility of biased self-evaluation. Informed consent is the most important part of any ethics committee review, because it is a document to guide subjects to participate in the study and to protect their rights and safety.

研究者在评估其研究的风险/收益或保护参与者权利时可能并不客观。由于可能存在有偏见的自我评价，研究通常需要接受外部伦理审查。知情同意书是所有伦理委员会审核的重中之重，因为它是引导受试者参加研究及保护受试者权益和安全性的证明文件。

The institutional review boards should be composed of more than 5 members with multidisciplinary professional background and one member who is not affiliated with the institution and has no close relationship with the project researcher. The ethics review committee may include experts and scholars in the medical field, research methodology, ethics, law and other fields. Such composition requirements can ensure the minimum representation of all groups of the study to protect the rights and interests of the subjects. Experts in specific areas may be retained as independent consultants if necessary.

在伦理委员会的组成中，应由 5 名以上多学科专业背景的委员组成，应该有一名不属于本机构且与项目研究人员并无密切关系的委员。伦理审查委员会可以包括医药领域和研究方法学、伦理学、法学等领域的专家学者。这样的组成要求可以最低限度保证研究的各个方面都有代表，保护受试者的权益。必要时可聘请特殊领域专家作为独立顾问。

Section Ⅳ　Other Ethical Issues
第四节　其他伦理问题

1. Ethics Issues in Scientific Research(科研伦理问题)

Misconduct in scientific research is also an ethical issue, belonging to a subjective thought and behavior of scientific researchers. The issue of scientific misconduct has come under increasing scrutiny in recent years as stories of researchers cheating and misrepresenting themselves have come to light. In view of this ethical problem, it is necessary to advocate the moral consciousness of scientific researchers and strengthen the guidance of public opinion, especially to pay attention to the moral education of young scientific researchers.

科研不端行为也是一个伦理问题，属于科研人员的一种主观思想和行为。近年来，随着研究人员欺骗和歪曲事件的曝光，科研不端行为的问题受到了越来越多的关注。针对该伦理问题，需要提倡科研人员的道德自觉意识并加强舆论的引导，特别是要重视对年轻科研人员的道德规范教育。

Scientific misconduct is defined by the *U. S. Public Health Service Regulations as* "fabrication, falsification, or plagiarism in presenting, conducting, reviewing, or reporting research findings." Scientific misconduct must be a marked departure from accepted practice and must occur knowingly and with the knowledge of the researcher. In the process of research planning and implementation, errors or deficiencies caused by reasons of research level and ability, as well as errors unrelated to scientific research activities, shall not be identified as scientific misconduct.

科研不端行为被《美国公共卫生服务条例》定义为"在提出、开展、审查研究或报告研究结果时捏造、伪造或剽窃的行为"。科研不端行为必须是与公认的实践有明显的背离，而且是在研究人员知情的状态下有意发生的。对于在研究计划和实施过程中，由于研究水平和能力方面的原因造成的错误或不足，以及与科研活动无关的过失等行为，不能认定为科学不端行为。

2. Animal Ethics in Research(研究中的动物伦理)

A growing number of nursing researchers are conducting studies that require the use of animals to explore physiological mechanisms and interventions that may pose risks to humans. Researchers use animals, not humans, as their study subjects, usually to focus on physiological phenomena.

越来越多的护理研究者正在进行需要使用动物的研究，来探索可能对人类构成风险的生理机制和干预措施。研究者以动物而不是人类作为他们的研究对象，通常是要关注生理学现象。

The use of animals in research is a controversial issue that requires researchers to carefully consider two important questions：First, should animals be used as research subjects? Second, if animals are used in research, what mechanisms are in place to ensure that they are treated humanely? Researchers should consider using animals in ethical, well-planned and well-funded research, not just for convenience or novelty.

在研究中使用动物作为研究对象是一个有争议的问题，需要研究人员仔细考虑两个重要的问题：第一，动物是否应该被用作研究对象？第二，如果动物被用于研究，有什么机制可以确保它们得到人道的对待？研究人员应考虑在符合伦理的、精心策划的和资金充足的研究中使用动物作为实验对象，而不仅仅是因为方便或者新颖而使用动物模型。

Ethical principles of animal research revolve around three core principles：the principle of non-maleficence, the principle of beneficence and the principle of voluntary participation (Patter & Blattner, 2020). The protection of the rights and interests of experimental animals is justified and necessary in three aspects: practical utility, social responsibility and ethics.

动物研究的伦理原则围绕三个核心原则：不伤害原则、有利原则和自愿原则（Patter & Blattner, 2020）。保护实验动物的权益在实际效用、社会责任和伦理道德三个层面上都具有正当性和必要性。

In actual utility level, protect the basic rights of animals, including the following animals living habits, maintain a clean and comfortable living environment, not cruelty to animals, and properly handle the dead animal bones and so on animal breeding and the standard process of operation, to ensure the animals used in experiments itself in its natural normal physiological state. Only on this basis can reliable research be carried out to truly discover the effects of study variables on laboratory animals.

在实际效用层面，保护好动物的基本权益，包括遵循动物的生活习性、维持清洁舒适的生活环境、不虐待动物，以及妥善处理死亡动物的尸骨等动物养殖和操作的标准流程，保证了用于实验的动物本身处在其自然正常的生理状态。在此基础上才能进行可靠的研究，真正发现研究变量对实验动物产生的效应。

At the level of social responsibility, ensuring the health of animals, the cleanliness of the breeding environment and proper handling of the aftermath can reduce the transmission of diseases. If an animal is infected with a disease, it may not be able to be used in experiments and spread easily among humans, putting researchers' health at immediate risk.

在社会责任层面，保证动物的健康、养殖环境的清洁，以及妥善的善后处理，可以减少疾病的传染。如果动物受到疾病的传染，可能无法用于实验，并且容易在人群中传播，研究人员的健康也会面临直接威胁。

At the ethical level, it is also a human requirement for researchers to protect the rights and interests of experimental animals, especially to properly dispose of animal carcasses or organs. Animals have suffered a lot of pain in the process of experiment, and should not be subjected to extra pain when it is not necessary. Treat animals well, that is, treat every life well.

在伦理道德层面，保护好实验动物的权益，尤其是妥善处理动物的尸体或器官，也是对研究人员人性的要求。动物在实验过程中已经承受了很多痛苦，不应该在非必要的情况下让动物承受额外的痛苦。善待动物，也就是善待每一个生命。

Section Ⅴ　Research Integrity
第五节　科研诚信

1. The Concept of Scientific Integrity(科研诚信的概念)

Integrity is an important part of the working method of scientific researchers and a virtue that they should possess (Shaw & Satalkar, 2018). Scientific integrity, also known as scientific integrity or academic integrity, means that researchers should carry forward the scientific spirit of pursuing truth, seeking truth from facts, advocating innovation, openness and collaboration as the core, and abide by scientific values, scientific spirit and norms of conduct in scientific activities.

诚信是科研工作者工作方法的一个重要组成部分，是科研人员所要具备的美德(Shaw 和 Satalkar, 2018)。科研诚信，也可称为科学诚信或学术诚信，是指科研人员在科研活动中要弘扬以追求真理、实事求是、崇尚创新、开放协作为核心的科学精神，恪守科学价值准则、科学精神和科学活动的行为规范。

2. Dishonesty in Scientific Research(科研失信行为)

In conducting research, scientific research workers should seek truth from facts, refrain from deception and fraud, and abide by the principles of scientific value, scientific spirit and norms of conduct in scientific activities.

科研工作者在研究时，应该实事求是、不欺骗、不弄虚作假，恪守科学价值准则、科学精神和科学活动的行为规范。

2.1　The Object of Dishonesty in Scientific Research(科研失信行为的对象)

The objects of scientific research trust-breaking behavior include applicants, undertaking personnel, consultation, evaluation experts and other individuals participating in scientific research projects, as well as reporting units, undertaking units and third-party service agencies.

科研失信行为的对象包括参与科学研究项目的申报人员、承担人员、咨询评审评估专家和其他参与科研项目的个人，以及申报单位、承担单位、第三方服务机构等机构。

2.2 Records of Dishonesty in Scientific Research(科研失信行为的记录)

In China's relevant regulations, the relevant responsible subjects of scientific research projects in the process of project declaration, project establishment, implementation, management, acceptance, performance evaluotion and consulting review evaluation will be objectively recorded according to procedures.

在我国相关规定中，对科学研究项目相关责任主体在项目申报、立项、实施、管理、验收、绩效评价和咨询评审评估等过程中存在的失信行为都会按程序进行客观记录。

The responsible subjects of general trust-breaking acts shall be listed in the records of general trust-breaking acts after being identified or investigated by the Science and Technology Bureau. The subject responsible for serious trust-breaking acts shall be listed in the record of serious trust-breaking acts if they are dealt with as follows:

对于一般失信行为的责任主体，经科技局认定或查处的，列入一般失信行为记录。对严重失信行为的责任主体，且受到以下处理的，列入严重失信行为记录：

(1)Due to serious scientific misconduct such as forgery, tampering, plagiarism and other serious scientific misconduct, academic publications published at home and abroad have been retracted.

因伪造、篡改、抄袭等严重科研不端行为被国内外公开发行的学术出版刊物撤稿。

(2)It shall be investigated and dealt with by relevant science and technology administrative departments in science and technology planning, project management or supervision and inspection and issued in official documents.

由相关科技管理部门在科技计划、项目管理或监督检查中查处并以正式文件发布。

(3)Investigated and punished by audit, discipline inspection and supervision departments and officially notified.

受审计、纪检监察等部门查处并正式通报。

(4)Receive criminal punishment or administrative punishment and make an official announcement.

受到刑事处罚或行政处罚并正式公告。

(5)Other serious violations of discipline after verification and implementation of notification procedures. Generally, the punishment period for dishonesty is two years. General acts of trust-breaking occurring during the punishment period shall be determined as serious acts of trust-breaking. The punishment period for serious trust-breaking acts shall be determined by the Science and Technology Bureau in accordance with the punishment decision made by relevant departments or in accordance with the *Measures for Handling Misconduct in Scientific Research During the Implementation of the National Science and Technology Plan* (*Trial implementation*) and other relevant provisions.

经核实并履行告知程序的其他严重违规违纪行为。一般失信行为的惩戒期为两年。惩戒期内发生的一般失信行为，认定为严重失信行为。严重失信行为的惩戒期由科技局根据相关部门作出的处罚决定或根据《国家科技计划实施中科研不端行为处理办法(试行)》等相关规定确定。

Section VI Academic Morality
第六节 学术道德

1. The Concept of Academic Ethics(学术道德的概念)

Academic ethic is the basic requirement of academic research and the academic conscience of scholars. Its implementation and maintenance mainly depend on the conscience of scholars and the moral public opinion in the academic community. It has the characteristics of self-discipline and demonstration. The lack of academic morality undoubtedly means the generation and spread of academic anomie.

学术道德是治学的起码要求，是学者的学术良知，其实施和维系主要依靠学者的良知及学术界的道德舆论。它具有自律性和示范性的特性，学术道德的缺失无疑意味着学术失范现象的产生和蔓延。

2. Academic Misconduct(学术不端行为)

2.1 The Concept of Academic Misconduct(学术不端的概念)

Academic misconduct refers to the behavior in scientific research that violates the universally recognized academic norms, academic ethics and code of conduct for scientific research.

学术不端行为是指在科学研究中违反公认的学术规范、学术伦理和科学研究行为准则的行为。

2.2 The Content of Academic Misconduct(学术不端行为的内容)

According to *Measures for Prevention and Treatment of Academic Misconduct in Colleges and Universities*, behaviors in scientific research and related activities, after investigation and confirmation, will be identified as constituting academic misconduct, including:

根据《高等学校预防与处理学术不端行为办法》，在科学研究及相关活动中，经过调查和确认，会被认定为构成学术不端的行为包括：

(1) Plagiarism, copying or misappropriation of others' academic achievements.

剽窃、抄袭或侵占他人学术成果。

(2) Tampering with others' research results.

篡改他人研究成果。

(3) Falsifying scientific research data, materials, literature and notes, or fabricating facts and research results.

伪造科研数据、资料、文献、注释，或者捏造事实、编造虚假研究成果。

(4) Signature on research results or academic papers without participating in research or creation, improper use of others' signature without permission, joint signature of fictitious collaborators, or joint completion of research by several people without indicating others' work or contribution in the research results.

未参加研究或创作而在研究成果、学术论文上署名，未经他人许可而不当使用他人署名，虚构合作者共同署名，或者多人共同完成研究而成果中未注明他人工作、贡献。

(5) Providing false academic information in the application of projects, achievements, awards and job evaluation, degree application and other activities.

在申报课题、成果、奖励和职务评审评定、申请学位等活动中提供虚假学术信息。

(6) Buying and selling papers, writing by others or writing papers for others.

买卖论文、由他人代写或者为他人代写论文。

(7) Other rules formulated by institutions of higher learning, relevant academic organizations and relevant administrative institutions of scientific research.

其他根据高等学校或者有关学术组织、相关科研管理机构制定的规则。

📖 Studies Cited in Chapter 7(第七章参考文献)

[1] Van Deventer, J. P. Ethical considerations during human centred overt and covert research

[J]. Quality & Quantity, 2009, 43(1): 45-57.

[2] Katz, J. The Nuremberg code and the Nuremberg trial: A reappraisal[J]. Jama, 1996, 276 (20): 1662-1666.

[3] Goodyear, M. D. E., Krleza-Jeric, K., Lemmens, T. The Declaration of Helsinki[J]. BMJ, 2007, 335(7621): 624-625.

[4] Raus Kasper. An analysis of common ethical justifications for compassionate use programs for experimental drugs[J]. BMC Med Ethics, 2016, 17(1): 60.

[5] Chatterjee, K., Das, N. K. Informed consent in biomedical research: Scopes and challenges [J]. Indian Dermatology Online Journal, 2021, 12(4): 529.

[6] Brown, H. R., Harvey, E. A., Griffith, S. F. et al. Assent and dissent: Ethical considerations in research with toddlers[J]. Ethics & Behavior, 2017, 27(8): 651-664.

[7] Committee on Ethics. ACOG Committee Opinion No. 646: Ethical Considerations for Including Women as Research Participants[J]. Obstet Gynecol, 2015, 126(5): e100-7.

[8] Hills, K., Clapton, J., Dorsett, P. Ethical considerations when conducting research with people with nonverbal autism: A commentary on current processes and practices[J]. Journal of Social Inclusion, 2019, 10(2).

[9] Van Patter, L. E., Blattner, C. Advancing ethical principles for non-invasive, respectful research with nonhuman animal participants[J]. Society & Animals, 2020, 28(2): 171-190.

[10] Shaw, D., Satalkar, P. Researchers' interpretations of research integrity: A qualitative study[J]. Accountability in research, 2018, 25(2): 79-93.

PART 3：Designing and Conducting Quantitative Studies
to Generate Evidence for Nursing

第三部分　设计及开展量性研究，为护理实践提供证据

Chapter 8：Quantitative Research Design
第八章 量性研究设计

Causality is a hotly debated philosophical issue, and yet we all understand the general concept of a cause. For example, we understand that lack of sleep causes fatigue and that high caloric intake causes weight gain.

因果关系是一个激烈争论的哲学问题，但我们都理解原因的一般概念。例如，我们知道缺乏睡眠会导致疲劳，高热量摄入会导致体重增加。

Several writers have proposed criteria for establishing a cause-and-effect relationship. Three criteria are attributed to John Stuart Mill (Lazarsfeld, 1955).

一些作家提出了建立因果关系的标准。约翰·斯图亚特·密尔提出了三个标准 (Lazarsfeld, 1955)。

(1) Temporal：A cause must precede an effect in time. If we test the hypothesis that smoking causes lung cancer, we need to show that cancer occurred after smoking commenced.

时间：在时间上，原因必须先于结果。如果我们检验吸烟导致肺癌的假设，我们需要证明癌症是在吸烟后发生的。

(2) Relationship：There must be an empirical relationship between the presumed cause and the presumed effect. In our example, we must show an association between smoking and cancer—that is, that a higher percentage of smokers than nonsmokers get lung cancer.

关系：假定的原因和假定的结果之间必须存在经验关系。在我们的例子中，我们必须表明吸烟和癌症之间的联系，即吸烟者比不吸烟者患肺癌的比例更高。

(3) No confounders：The relationship cannot be explained as being caused by a third variable. Suppose that smokers tended also to live in urban environments. There would then be a possibility that the relationship between smoking and lung cancer reflects an underlying causal connection between the environment and lung cancer.

不要混淆：这种关系不能被解释为是由第三个变量引起的。假设吸烟者也倾向于生活在城市环境中，那么，吸烟和肺癌之间的关系就有可能反映了环境和肺癌之间潜在的因果关系。

Researchers testing hypotheses about casual relationships must provide persuasive evidence about meeting these various criteria through their study designs. Some designs are better at revealing cause-and-effect relationships than others. In particular, experimental designs (randomized controlled trials or RCTs) are the best possible designs for illuminating causal relationships—but, it is not always possible to use such designs for various ethical or practical reasons. Much of this chapter focuses on designs for illuminating causal relationships.

研究人员在测试关于随意关系的假设时，必须通过他们的研究设计提供有说服力的证据来满足这些不同的标准。有些设计比其他设计更能揭示因果关系。特别是，实验设计(随机对照试验或 RCT)是阐明因果关系的最佳设计，但是，由于各种伦理或实际原因，并不总是可以使用这种设计。本章的大部分内容都集中在说明因果关系的设计上。

It is easy to get confused about terms used for research designs because there is inconsistency among writers. Also, design terms used by medical and epidemiologic researchers are often different from those used by social scientists. Early nurse researchers got their research training in social science fields such as psychology before doctoral training became available in nursing schools, and so social scientific design terms have prevailed in the nursing research literature.

人们很容易混淆用于研究设计的术语，因为不同作者之间存在不一致的看法。此外，医学和流行病学研究人员使用的设计术语通常与社会科学家使用的术语不同。早期的护理研究人员在护理学校提供学术培训之前，就已经接受了心理学等社会科学领域的研究培训，因此，社会科学设计术语在护理研究文献中占了上风。

Nurses interested in establishing an evidence-based practice must be able to understand studies from many disciplines. We use both medical and social science terms in this book. The first column of Table 8.1.1 shows several design terms used by social scientists and the second shows corresponding terms used by medical researchers.

对建立循证实践感兴趣的护士必须能够理解许多学科的研究。在这本书中，我们使用了医学和社会科学术语。表8.1.1 的第一列显示了社会科学家使用的几个设计术语，第二列显示了医学研究人员使用的相应术语。

Table 8.1.1 **Research Design Terminology in the Social Scientific and Medical Literature**
(社会科学和医学文献中的研究设计术语)

Social scientific term(社会科学术语)	Medical research term(医学研究术语)
Experiment, true experiment, experimental study (实验,真实验,实验研究)	Randomized controlled trial, RCT (随机对照试验,RCT)
Quasi-experiment, quasi-experimental study (准实验,准实验研究)	Controlled trial, controlled trial without randomization (对照试验,非随机对照试验)
Social scientific term(社会科学术语)	Medical research term(医学研究术语)
Nonexperimental study, correlational study (非实验研究,相关研究)	Observational study (观察性研究)
Retrospective study (回顾性研究)	Case-control study (病例-对照研究)
Prospective nonexperimental study (前瞻性非实验研究)	Cohort study (队列研究)
Group or condition (e.g., experimental or control group/condition) (组或条件(例如,实验组或对照组/条件))	Group or arm (e.g., intervention or control arm) (组或臂(例如,干预或控制臂))
Experimental group (实验组)	Treatment or intervention group (治疗或干预组)

Section Ⅰ General Design Issues
第一节 一般设计问题

1. The Basic Elements of Study Design(研究设计中的基本要素)

Quantitative studies can be divided into experimental studies, quasi-experimental studies and non-experimental studies according to whether the subjects are intervened, grouped or randomized. Medical research consists of three basic components, namely treatment (study factor), subject, and experimental effect.

量性研究按照对研究对象是否进行干预、是否分组或应用随机原则分为实验性研究、类实验性研究与非实验性研究三大类。医学研究由三个基本部分组成,即处理因素、研究对象和实验效应。

1.1　Treatment, Study Factor(处理因素)

Treatment, study factor refers to the factor that is intended to be applied or observed according to the research purpose and can act on the research object and cause direct or indirect effects, also known as experimental factor. The treatment factor can be some external intervention (or measure) imposed subjectively by the experimenter, such as using or not using a certain drug, etc. It can also be objective, such as observing the relationship between the pollution degree of culture medium in the air and season. "Different seasons" is the "treatment factor" of the experiment, and "season" is not artificially imposed but objectively existing.

处理因素指根据研究目的欲施加或观察的、能作用于研究对象并引起直接或间接效应的因素，又称实验因素。处理因素可以是实验者主观施加的某种外部干预(或措施)，如使用或不使用某种药物等；也可以是客观存在的，如观察培养基在空气中的污染程度与季节的关系，"不同季节"就是该实验的"处理因素"，而"季节"这个处理不是人为施加的而是客观存在的。

1.2　Subject(研究对象)

People, animals or other experimental materials treated and observed in experiments are the objects of treatment factors, also known as experimental objects. According to different research purposes, different research objects can be selected. The following three aspects should be paid attention to when selecting research objects: (1) Whether subjects are sensitive to treatment factors; (2) Whether the response of the research object to the treatment factors is stable; (3) Research objects shall have strict inclusion and exclusion criteria. Research, for example, some nursing measures for patients with high blood pressure, the intervention effect of all patients with high blood pressure should be the object of study in theory, but in fact, in order to ensure that the object of study of homogeneity, eliminate confounding factors on the results of interference, the choice of research object needs to have qualification, such as select only 30 ~ 65-year-old patients with stage Ⅱ primary hypertension. Secondary hypertension and cardiopulmonary insufficiency were excluded.

实验中接受处理并作为实验观察的人、动物或其他实验材料，是处理因素作用的对象，又称实验对象。根据不同的研究目的，可选用不同的研究对象，选择研究对象时应注意以下三方面：(1)研究对象是否对处理因素敏感；(2)研究对象是否对处理因素的反应稳定；（3）研究对象要有严格的纳入标准与排除标准。例如，研究某种护理措施对高血压患者的干预效果，理论上所有高血压患者都应是研究对象，但实际上为了保证研究对象的同质性，排除混杂因素对结果的干扰，研究对象的选择需要有限定条件，如只选择30~65岁的Ⅱ期原发性高血压患者，且排除继发性高血压、心肺功能不全者等。

1.3 Experimental effect(实验效应)

Experimental effect refers to the response or result of treatment factors on experimental subjects, which is generally expressed by experimental indicators. The research index should reflect the effect of the treatment factors. If the index is improperly selected or the method of measuring the index is improper, the research result is not scientific. Therefore, the selection of research indicators and measurement methods is critical to the success or failure of the research. Research indicators should be relevant, objective, valid and accurate.

实验效应指处理因素作用于实验对象的反应或结果，一般通过实验指标来表达。研究指标应能反映处理因素的效应，如果指标选择不当或测定指标的方法不当，未能准确地反映处理因素的作用，则获得的研究结果就缺乏科学性。因此研究指标和测定方法的选择事关研究的成败。研究指标应具有关联性、客观性、有效性和准确性。

1.3.1 Relevance(关联性)

The selected indicators must be closely related to the problems to be solved in the study, that is, the selected indicators are essentially related to the purpose of the study. For example, electrocardiogram as an indicator of the pumping function of the heart is obviously not correct, and the cardiac output should be more appropriate.

选用的指标必须与研究要解决的问题有密切的关系，即选用的指标与本次的研究目的有本质上的联系。例如心电图作为心脏泵血功能的指标显然是不正确的，而应该选择心排血量较为合适。

1.3.2 Objectivity(客观性)

Research indicators can be divided into subjective indicators and objective indicators. Objective indicators refer to measurements made with instruments to reflect the objective state or observation results of the research object, such as body temperature, pulse and blood pressure. Objective index should be the first choice in experimental research. Subjective indicators, such as pain, dizziness and improvement, were used to describe the observation results by the respondent's answers or the qualitative judgment of the observer. Subjective indicators are easily affected by the psychological factors of the observer and the observed, and contain subjective knowledge, often with randomness and contingency. Sometimes, it is difficult to ensure the authenticity and stability of indicators, so they should be used cautiously in the research design.

　　研究指标有主观指标与客观指标之分，客观指标是指借助仪器等进行测量来反映研究对象的客观状态或观察结果，如体温、脉搏、血压等均属客观指标。实验研究中应以客观指标为首选指标。主观指标是由被观察者回答或观察者定性判断来描述观察结果，如痛感、头晕、好转等均为主观指标。主观指标易受观察者和被观察者的心理因素影响，含有主观上的认识，往往带有随意性、偶然性，有时难以保证指标的真实与稳定，因此在研究设计中要谨慎使用。

1.3.3　Effectiveness(有效性)

Including sensitivity and specificity. Sensitivity refers to the degree to which the selected index can reflect a certain effect in the presence of a certain treatment factor. Specificity refers to the degree to which the selected index does not show the treatment effect in the absence of a treatment factor. The index with high sensitivity can truly reflect the change degree of micro-effect in the study object. The indexes with high specificity can reveal the essence of things and are not easily disturbed by non-processing factors, thus making the experimental effect more real and effective. For example, the detection rate of mycobacterium tuberculosis in sputum is a specific indicator of open tuberculosis, while the increase of white blood cell count is not a specific indicator of urinary tract infection. Therefore, the selected research indicators should have both high sensitivity and specificity.

　　包括灵敏度与特异度两方面。灵敏度指某处理因素存在时所选指标能反映出一定效应的程度；特异度指某处理因素不存在时所选指标不显示处理效应的程度。灵敏度高的指标能真实反映研究对象体内微量效应变化的程度；特异度高的指标能揭示事物的本质，且不易受非处理因素的干扰，从而使实验效应更加真实有效。如痰中结核杆菌的检出率是开放性肺结核的特异性指标，而白细胞计数升高则不是泌尿道感染的特异性指标。因此，所选择的研究指标应同时具有较高的灵敏度与特异度。

1.3.4　Accuracy(准确性)

Including accuracy and precision. Accuracy refers to the degree to which the observed value is close to the real value, which is mainly affected by systematic error. Accuracy refers to the degree of closeness between the observed value and its mean value when an index of the same object is repeatedly observed under the same conditions, which is mainly affected by random factors. In nursing research, if a certain result has multiple indicators or a certain indicator has multiple measurement methods, the one with higher validity and reliability should be selected as the observation indicator or measurement method in the design.

包括准确度和精确度两方面。准确度，指观测值与真实值的接近程度，主要受系统误差影响。精确度，指相同条件下对同一对象的某指标进行重复观察时，观测值与其均值的接近程度，主要受随机因素的影响。护理研究中，如果某一结果有多种指标，或某一指标有多种测定方法，则在设计时应尽量选择效度和信度均较高者作为观察指标或测定方法。

2. Internal Validity and External Validity of the Study (研究的内部效度与外部效度)

2.1 Internal Validity(内部效度)

Internal validity refers to the degree of clarity of causal relationship between independent variables and dependent variables in the study. Internal validity is often asked to answer the question, "Are the results authentic? Were the results caused by treatment factors?" Therefore, high internal validity of a study means that the change in the dependent variable is caused by a specific independent variable. Since any external variable except independent variable may have an impact on dependent variable, leading to confusion of research results, it is difficult to determine the certainty of the relationship between independent variable and dependent variable. Therefore, in order to have high internal validity, it is necessary to control various external variables. Common factors affecting internal validity include the following aspects.

内部效度指研究中的自变量与因变量之间因果关系的明确程度。内部效度通常需要回答的问题是："研究结果是否真实可信？研究结果是否由处理因素引起？"因此，一项研究的内部效度高，就意味着因变量的变化确系由特定的自变量引起的。由于除了自变量以外，任何外变量都可能对因变量产生影响，导致研究结果的混淆，这样就难以判定自变量与因变量之间关系的确定性。因此要使研究有较高的内部效度，就必须控制各种外变量。常见的内部效度影响因素有以下几方面。

2.1.1 Growth and Maturity(生长和成熟)

In addition to the independent variable may cause individual changes, the growth and maturity of the individual itself is also an important factor to make it change, especially in the case of children as subjects and the measurement before and after a single group of experiments, the influence of growth and maturity factors is greater.

除了自变量可能使个体发生变化外，个体本身的生长和成熟也是使其变化的重要因素，尤其是在以儿童为被试而又采用单组实验前后测量的情况下，生长和成熟因素的影响就更大。

2.1.2　Influence of Pre-test（前测的影响）

In general, there will be some differences between the results of the two measurements, and the score of the post-test will be higher than that of the pre-test. This includes practice factors, on-the-spot experience, and sensitivity to research objectives, thus improving post-test performance. Especially when the time of the last two measurements is relatively recent, the influence of this factor is more significant.

在一般情况下，前后两次测量的结果会有一定的差异，后测的分数将比前测的高。这中间包括练习因素、临场经验，以及对研究目的的敏感程度，从而提高了后测的成绩。特别是当前测和后测两次测量时间较近时，这一因素的影响就更显著。

2.1.3　Selection Bias of Research Objects（研究对象的选择偏倚）

In the grouping of research objects, if random sampling and random allocation are not used, they will not be homogenous in some aspects before experimental processing, resulting in confusion of research results and reduced internal validity.

在对研究对象进行分组时，如果没有用随机取样和随机分配的方法，在实验处理之前，他们在某些方面并不具备同质性，从而造成研究结果的混淆，降低了内部效度。

2.1.4　Loss of Subjects（研究对象的缺失）

Lost to follow up bias is commonly caused by subjects' migration, going out, refusal to continue to participate or death from non-endpoint diseases during a long follow-up observation period. Even though the samples of the subjects at the beginning of the study were randomly sampled and randomly assigned, the missing subjects could not represent the original samples due to the mid-course deletion of the subjects, thus reducing the internal validity. Generally speaking, a release rate of less than 5% has little effect on the results, while a release rate of 30% or more is considered to be extremely unreliable.

常见的是在一个较长的追踪观察期内，由于研究对象迁移、外出、拒绝继续参加或死于非终点疾病而造成的失访偏移。即使开始参加研究的被试者样本是经过随机取样和随机分配的，但由于被试者的中途缺失，缺失后的被试者样本难以代表原来的样本，降低了内部效度。一般来说，释放率小于5%对结果产生的影响不大，释放率达到30%或以上则认为研究结果极不可靠。

2.1.5　Inconsistency of Research Procedures（研究程序的不一致）

In the process of research, inconsistency of experimental instruments, control methods and changes of measurement methods and procedures will affect the stability of research tools, thus affecting the authenticity of results. For example, in an intervention study on weight control, the zero correction of the scale used in the measurement before and after the intervention was inconsistent, resulting in the weight measured after the intervention was larger than the actual value.

在研究过程中，实验仪器、控制方式的不一致，测量方法和程序的变化，均会影响到研究工具的稳定性，从而影响结果的真实性。如在一项体重控制的干预研究中，前后测量使用的体重计零点校正不一致，从而导致干预后测量的体重值比实际值偏大。

2.1.6　Diffusion of Treatment（处理扩散或污染）

Diffusion of treatment means that due to the communication between research objects in different groups, the treatment factors are not clear between the two groups, making it difficult to judge the influence of treatment factors on the dependent variable. Often meet with such problems in the research of clinical nursing interventions, such as in a ward postoperative patients with certain diseases of music therapy to alleviate postoperative anxiety research, intervention group was given music playback, the control will not be implemented, but because live in the same room, the control of the family may get the information and follow the implementation, leading to the result is not true.

处理扩散是指因不同组的研究对象互相交流，处理因素在两组间不分明，致使难以判断处理因素对因变量的影响。临床护理干预性研究中经常遇到此类问题，如对某病室某种疾病术后病人进行音乐疗法以减轻术后焦虑的研究，干预组给予音乐播放，对照组不予实施，但由于住在同一个病室，对照组的家属可能获取该信息而效仿实施，从而导致结果的不真实。

2.1.7 Experimenter Expectancy(实验者期望)

It refers to that the researcher strongly believes a certain hypothesis, but indirectly tells the experimental expectation to the subjects, not out of unethical behavior with ulterior motives, which leads to the distortion of research results. For example, if the researchers believe that by intravenous drug use HIV from family of drugs and AIDS double discrimination, is in the process of face to face questionnaire survey, may talk through eye contact, tone of voice, posture, biased response, and other forms of nonverbal communication, suggests that the object of study by the family of the double discrimination.

指研究者非常相信某个假设，并不是出于别有用心的不道德行为，而是间接地将实验期望告诉了受试者，从而导致研究结果的失真。比如，如果研究者深信经静脉注射吸毒的艾滋病病毒感染者受到了来自家庭对吸毒和艾滋病的双重歧视，则在面对面问卷调查的过程中，可能会通过目光接触、谈话语调、姿势、带有偏见性的回应方式，以及其他非语言的交流形式，暗示研究对象受到了家人的双重歧视。

2.1.8 Hawthorn Effect(霍桑效应)

This effect mainly refers to that the research object makes a certain reaction, which is similar to the processing effect because the research object feels that he is being paid attention to, rather than the real processing factor.

该效应主要指研究对象做出某种反应，并不是真正的处理因素的作用，而是因为研究对象感觉自己受到了关注而呈现的类似于处理效应的反应。

2.1.9 Placebo Effect(安慰剂效应)

It refers to what happens when subjects receive a placebo but receive the real treatment factor. For example, in a smoking cessation study, subjects were either given a drug to reduce their nicotine dependence or a placebo, and if the placebo subjects also stopped smoking, they thought they were getting the drug to reduce their nicotine dependence.

指当研究对象收到的是安慰剂，却出现接受真正处理因素时所发生的状况。例如，一个戒烟的实验中，研究对象不是接受药物处理以降低他们对尼古丁的依赖，就是收到安慰剂，如果接受安慰剂的研究对象也停止吸烟，说明研究对象认为他们接受的也是可以降低对尼古丁依赖的药物。

2.2　External Validity(外部效度)

External validity refers to the extent to which the research findings can be generalized to the whole population from which the samples come and other similar phenomena, that is, the general representativeness and applicability of the experimental results. External validity refers to the generalization of the relationship between independent variables and dependent variables, which involves the generality and external thrust of research conclusions. External validity generally involves three aspects, namely other populations, other environments and other times, i. e., to what extent conclusions drawn from one study can be generalized to different people, environments and times.

外部效度指研究发现能够普遍推广到样本来自的总体和其他同类现象中去的程度，即实验结果的普遍代表性和适用性。外部效度是自变量和因变量之间关系的推广程度，涉及研究结论的概括力和外推力。外部效度一般涉及三个方面，分别为其他总体、其他环境和其他时间，即在多大程度上，从一个研究所得出的结论能够同样推广到不同的人、环境和时间上。

2.2.1　**Other Populations**(其他总体)

For example, one study examined the relationship between weekly physical activity and the prevalence of diabetes. However, the study only looked at women. This raises the question of whether the women's findings can be generalized to men. To determine whether a conclusion is applicable to different populations, different populations must be considered as part of the study design. In factor design, different populations can be included as a factor. The study was redesigned to include gender as a variable and compare differences between four groups: physically active women, non-active women, physically active men, and non-active men. The interaction between gender and exercise in diabetes prevention suggests that exercise has different benefits for men and women.

例如，一项研究探讨了每周体育锻炼与糖尿病患病率之间的关系。然而，该研究只对女性研究对象做了调查。这就存在一个问题，即女性的研究结果是否可以推广到男性研究对象。判断一个结论是否适合于不同人群，必须把不同人群作为研究设计的一部分。在因素设计中，可以纳入不同人群作为一个因素。以上述研究为例予以重新设计，将性别作为一个变量，比较4组之间的差异：体育锻炼的女性、不锻炼的女性、体育锻炼的男性、不锻炼的男性。性别和锻炼之间对预防糖尿病的交互作用说明，锻炼对男性和女性具有不同的收益。

The possibilities for comparing a trait between different groups of people are almost infinite. From a policy and social perspective, important traits include gender, age, race, and socioeconomic status.

在不同人群之间比较某种特质，可能的选择几乎是无限的。从政策和社会的角度来看，重要的特质包括性别、年龄、种族和社会经济地位。

2.2.2 Other Environments(其他环境)

Some medical and nursing studies are carried out in laboratories with strictly controlled conditions or in specially controlled scenarios, so the research environment has certain particularity and artificiality, which is far from real life situations. One question for the research, then, is to what extent the results obtained can be generalized to real-life situations.

一些医学、护理学的研究，都是在严格控制条件的实验室或特定控制的场景中进行的，因此研究环境有一定的特殊性和人为性，和现实生活情景有很大的差距。这样，研究所面临的一个问题是，所获得的研究结果在多大程度上能够推广到现实生活情境中。

2.2.3 Other Time(其他时间)

Involved the study of social factors, such as, nursing psychology, nursing ethics, aesthetics, psychiatric nursing and other fields of study, there might be such a problem, that is in a particular social background in the history of research conclusion, is no longer applicable to the new social background have changed. In this case, it can be considered that the external validity of previous studies is low, so it is necessary for researchers to conduct new studies.

涉及社会因素的研究，如护理伦理学、护理美学、护理心理学、精神科护理学等领域的研究，可能会存在这样的问题，即在一个特定的社会时代历史背景中获得的研究结论，已经不再适用于已经发生变化的新的社会背景。这种情况下，可以认为先前的研究外部效度低，因此研究者有必要进行新的研究。

In conclusion, in most cases, improving the external validity of a study is not achieved by a single study, but by a series of extensional (extended to other populations, settings, and times) and even repeatable validation studies.

总之，多数情况下，提高研究的外部效度并不能单凭一项研究，而是需要凭借一系列拓展性(拓展到其他总体、环境、时间)甚至是重复验证性的研究工作才能做到。

2.3 Relationship Between Internal Validity and External Validity
（内部效度和外部效度的关系）

If internal validity ensures the authenticity of research results, what we explore is the depth of research, while external validity ensures the extensibility of research results, what we explore is the breadth of research. However, internal validity and external validity are not two independent subjects. The purpose of internal validity is to exclude alternative explanations, purify and highlight the relationship between research variables, and withstand repetition and verification, which is the prerequisite for external validity. There is no external validity without internal validity. Therefore, some factors that influence internal validity, such as subject effect and Hawthorne effect, are also influential factors of external validity. External validity opens up space for the promotion of internal validity. Without external validity, internal validity is relatively narrow. They are accompanied by each other, which is opposite to and unified with each other.

如果说内部效度确保了研究结果的真实性，探究的是研究的深度，那么外部效度确保了研究结果的可推广性，探究的是研究的广度。然而内部效度与外部效度不是两个独立的主体，内部效度的目的在于排除另类解释，使研究变量之间的关系纯化、凸显，能经得起重复、验证，是外部效度的先决条件，没有内部效度就无所谓外部效度。因此，影响内部效度的一些因素，如受试者效应、霍桑效应等也是外部效度的影响因素。外部效度为内部效度的推广开拓了空间，没有外部效度，内部效度就相对狭隘，它们相伴而生，既相互对立，又相互统一。

2.3.1 Relativity（相对性）

In order to obtain high internal validity, researchers must exclude, reduce or control external variables to prevent them from affecting research results. However, the control of external variables will make the research situation with strong artificiality, resulting in the research results may not be valid outside the research environment. Therefore, improving internal validity leads to decreasing external validity. Instead, to achieve high external validity, researchers often create research environments that closely resemble the real world. The risk of this kind of research is that there are too many chaotic and uncontrolled variables in the real world compared to the standardized laboratory environment, and efforts to improve external validity will allow external variables to creep into the research, leading to a decline in internal validity.

为了获得较高的内部效度，研究者必须排除、减少或控制外变量，以防止其影响研究结果。然而，对研究外变量的控制会使研究情境带有较强的人为性，致使研究结果在研究环境之外可能不成立。因此，提高内部效度会导致外部效度降低。相反，为了获得较高的外部效度，研究者通常会创设与现实世界非常相似的研究环境。这种研究的风险在于，与实验室标准化的实验环境相比，现实世界有太多混乱的、不受控制的变量，努力提高外部效度会使外变量潜入研究，从而导致内部效度的下降。

2.3.2　Unity(统一性)

Although they are opposite in the direction of ensuring research quality, they both aim to improve the accuracy and universal value of research and serve for research results. The pursuit of internal validity is "seeking truth" and the pursuit of external validity is "seeking goodness". Truth and goodness are fundamentally unified, so internal validity and external validity are also fundamentally unified. In this sense, the relationship between internal validity and external validity is not necessarily negative, and it does not necessarily show that the improvement of one party is at the expense of the reduction of the other party. They are both unified and mutually exclusive.

二者虽然在确保研究质量的方向上有对立的一面，但是都是为了提高研究的精度和普适价值，都是为研究结果而服务的。追求内部效度是"求真"，追求外部效度是"求善"，真与善从根本上讲是统一的，因此内部效度与外部效度从根本上讲也是统一的。从这种意义上讲，内部效度与外部效度之间并不必然是负相关，并不必然表现为一方的提高以另一方的降低为代价，它们之间是一种既相统一又相排斥的关系。

Section Ⅱ　Experimental Research
第二节　实验性研究

Experimental research, also known as interventional study, is a kind of interventional study in which researchers set intervention measures for research objects artificially according to the research purpose, control the influencing factors other than the intervention measures according to the principle of repetition, control and randomization, and summarize the effect of intervention measures. For example, in the study on whether health education can prevent primary school students from myopia, the primary school students are randomly divided into experimental group and control group, the experimental group of primary school students are given health education about the prevention of myopia, the control group is only once a day to do eye exercises, no health education. After observation for a period of time, the incidence of visual impairment of the two groups of pupils was compared.

实验性研究，又称干预性研究，是研究者根据研究目的人为地对研究对象设置干预措施，按重复、对照、随机化原则控制干预措施以外的影响因素，总结干预措施的效果。例如，在关于健康教育能否预防小学生近视的研究中，将小学生随机分为试验组和对照组，对试验组的小学生给予有关预防近视的健康教育，对照组则只是每天做一次眼保健操，不进行健康教育。观察一段时间后，比较两组小学生视力下降的发生情况。

Controlled experiments are considered the gold standard for yielding reliable evidence about causes and effects. Experimenters can be relatively confident in the authenticity of causal relationships because they are observed under controlled conditions and typically meet the criteria for establishing causality. Hypotheses are never proved by scientific methods, but RCTs offer the most convincing evidence about whether one variable has a casual effect on another.

对照实验被认为是获得关于因果关系的可靠证据的金标准。实验者可以对因果关系的真实性相对有信心，因为他们是在受控条件下观察的，通常符合建立因果关系的标准。假设从来没有被科学方法证明过，但是随机对照试验提供了最令人信服的证据来证明一个变量是否对另一个变量有偶然的影响。

A true experimental or RCT design is characterized by the following properties:

真正的实验或 RCT 设计具有以下特点：

(1) Manipulation: The researcher does something to at least some participants—that is, there is some type of intervention.

操纵：研究人员至少对一些参与者做了一些事情——也就是说，存在某种类型的干预。

(2) Control: The researcher introduces controls over the research situation, including devising a counterfactual approximation—usually, a control group that does not receive the intervention.

对照：研究者在研究情境中引入对照，包括设计一个反事实的近似——通常是一个不接受干预的控制组。

(3) Randomization: The researcher assigns participants to a control or experimental condition on a random basis.

随机化：研究者随机分配参与者到一个控制或实验条件。

1. Design Features of True Experiments(真实验研究的特点)

Researchers have many options in designing an experiment. We begin by discussing several features of experimental designs.

研究人员在设计一个实验时有很多选择。我们首先讨论了实验设计的几个特征。

1.1 The Experimental Intervention(实验干预)

Manipulation involves doing something to study participants. Experimenters manipulate the independent variable by administering a treatment (or intervention (I)) to some people and withholding it from others (C), or administering different treatments. Experimenters deliberately vary the independent variable (the presumed cause) and observe the effect on the outcome (O)—often referred to as an end point in the medical literature.

操纵指的是做一些事情来研究参与者。实验者通过对一些人进行治疗(或干预(I))，而对另一些人进行控制(C)，或使用不同的治疗来控制自变量。实验人员故意改变自变量(假定的原因)，观察结果(O)的影响——通常在医学文献中被称为终点。

For example, suppose we hypothesized that gentle massage is an effective pain relief strategy for nursing home residents (P). The independent variable, receipt of gentle massage, can be manipulated by giving some patients the massage intervention (I) and withholding it from others (C). We would then compare pain levels (the outcome [O] variable) in the two groups to see if receipt of the intervention resulted in group differences in average pain levels.

例如，我们假设轻柔的按摩对疗养院的居民来说是一种有效的镇痛策略(P)。可以通过对一些患者进行推拿干预(I)，对另一些患者进行推拿干预(C)来控制自变量，即接受轻柔按摩。然后，我们将比较两组的疼痛水平(结果(O)变量)，看看接受干预是否导致平均疼痛水平的组间差异。

In designing RCTs, researchers make many decisions about what the experimental condition entails, and these decisions can affect the conclusions. To get a fair test, the intervention should be appropriate to the problem, consistent with a theoretical rationale, and of sufficient intensity and duration that effects might reasonably be expected. The full nature of the intervention must be delineated in formal protocols that spell out exactly what the treatment is. Among the questions researchers need to address are the following:

在设计随机对照试验时，研究人员需要对实验条件做很多决定，这些决定会影响结论。为了得到一个公平的检验，干预应与问题相适应，与理论基础相一致，并有足够的强度和持续时间，使效果可以合理地预期。干预的全部性质必须在正式的协议中描述，明确说明治疗是什么。研究人员需要解决的问题包括：

（1）What is the intervention, and how does it differ from usual methods of care?

什么是干预，它与通常的护理方法有何不同？

（2）What specific procedures are to be used with those receiving the intervention?

接受干预的患者应采用什么具体程序？

（3）What is the dosage or intensity of the intervention?

干预的剂量或强度是多少？

（4）Over how long a period will the intervention be administered, how frequently will it be administered, and when will the treatment begin (e. g., 2 hours after surgery)?

干预将在多长时间内实施，实施频率如何，何时开始治疗（例如，手术后 2 小时）？

（5）Who will administer the intervention? What are their credentials, and what type of special training will they receive?

谁将进行干预？他们的证书是什么？他们将接受什么样的特殊培训？

（6）Under what conditions will the intervention be withdrawn or altered?

在什么情况下会撤回或改变干预？

The goal in most RCTs is to have an identical intervention for all people in the treatment group. For example, in most drug studies, those in the experimental group are given the exact same ingredient, in the same dose, administered in exactly the same manner—all according to well-articulated protocols.

大多数随机对照试验的目标是对治疗组中的所有人进行相同的干预。例如，在大多数药物研究中，实验组被给予完全相同的成分、相同的剂量、完全相同的方式——所有这些都是根据明确的方案进行的。

1.2 The Control Condition（对照）

The establishment of control is also called control. In intervention studies, in addition to the influence of intervention on research results, some non-intervention factors will also have an impact on the results. The establishment of control is to control the influence of non-intervention factors in the experiment. When setting up the control group, it is required that the non-intervention factors should be as same as possible except for the different intervention factors, so that the intervention effect can be correctly evaluated. For example, " The impact of individualized health education on the quality of life of patients after enterostomy" should be controlled for the age, gender, educational background, medical expenses payment, fistula time and other factors of the subjects.

设立对照又称控制，在干预性研究中，除了干预对研究结果产生影响外，还有一些非干预因素也会对结果产生影响，设立对照就是为了控制实验中非干预因素的影响。设立对照时要求所比较的各组间除干预因素不同外，其他非干预因素应尽可能相同，从而能够正确评价干预效果。例如"个体化健康教育对肠造瘘术后病人生活质量的影响"对研究对象的年龄、性别、教育背景、医疗费用支付情况、造瘘时间等因素都应尽量控制。

1.2.1 According to the Study Design Scheme Classification
（按照研究设计方案分类）

（1）Concurrent randomized control：Subjects were randomly assigned to the trial at the same time according to a strict randomization method group and control group. Due to the randomization grouping method, the equilibrium comparability between groups can be ensured, and the influence of potential unknown factors on experimental results can be effectively avoided. The simultaneous control can be used to observe each group at the same time, which effectively avoids the influence of the sequence of roles on the results and makes the results more convincing. Since most statistical methods are based on random samples, this design is more conducive to the statistical analysis of data. However, half of the subjects are required to act as controls for the randomization control, so the sample size is large. And in some cases there may be ethical issues involved.

同期随机对照：按严格规定的随机化方法将研究对象同期分配到实验组与对照组。同期随机对照由于采用了随机化分组方法，可以较好地保证各组之间的均衡可比，有效避免了潜在未知因素对试验结果的影响。设置同期对照，可以同时对各组进行观察，有效避免了因饰演先后顺序对结果的影响，使研究结果更有说服力。由于多数统计方法都是建立在随机样本的基础之上，采用本设计类型更有利于资料的统计分析。但是同期随机对照需要有一半对象充当对照，因此所需样本量较大；并且在有些情况下可能涉及伦理道德方面的问题。

（2）Non-randomized concurrent control：There were simultaneous controls, but the experimental group and the control group did not strictly follow the randomization criteria are grouped. For example, in a collaborative study, patients were grouped according to different wards, that is, one ward was used as the control group and the other ward as the experimental group. This method of setting comparison is simple and feasible, which can avoid some ethical problems related to inequity, and is easily accepted by researchers and research objects. However, due to non-random allocation, the baseline situation of the two groups may be inconsistent due to selection bias, resulting in poor comparability.

非随机同期对照：有同期对照，但试验组与对照组未严格按随机化原则进行分组。如在协作研究中按不同病房进行分组，即一所病房作为对照组，而另一所病房作为试验组。这种设置对照的方法简便易行，可避免一些与不公平相关的伦理问题，易被研究者及研究对象接受。但由于非随机分配，可能因选择偏倚导致两组基线情况不一致，可比性较差。

（3）Self-control: The research objects were divided into the former and the latter two stages, and compared after the intervention differences in variables between the two stages. Self-control is mainly used for the intervention study of chronic recurrent diseases with a long course of disease and little change in condition, but it is difficult to guarantee the condition consistency of the two stages, and there may be influence on the results of treatment sequence.

自身对照：将研究对象分为前、后两个阶段，施以干预措施后，比较两个阶段的变量差异。自身对照主要用于病程长且病情变化不大的慢性反复发作性疾病的干预性研究，但是难以保证两个阶段的病情完全一致，可能存在处理先后对结果的影响。

（4）Cross-over control: the two groups of subjects were divided into two stages for the experiment. The first group was in the first stage of the experiment Measure A: test measure B after an interval of elution period; In the second group, measure B was tested in the first stage, and measure A was tested after an interval of washout period, and then the effects of the two interventions were compared. In the cross-control, the same research object is both the experimental group member and the control group, which saves the sample number and makes the two groups better balanced and comparable. This method is also mainly used for the intervention of chronic recurrent diseases with long course and little change in condition.

交叉对照：将两组研究对象分为两个阶段进行试验，第一组第一阶段试验 A 措施，间隔一段洗脱期后再试验 B 措施；第二组第一阶段试验 B 措施，间隔一段洗脱期后再试验 A 措施，然后对比 A、B 两种干预措施的效果。交叉对照中同一个研究对象既作为试验组成员又作为对照，节省了样本数，又使两组均衡性、可比性更好。此种方法还主要用于病程长且病情变化不大的慢性反复发作性疾病的干预性研究。

（5）Historical control: It is a mistake to compare the results of new interventions with those of past studies A randomized, non-contemporaneous controlled study. Data for this type of comparison can be obtained from literature and hospital records. This method of setting contrast is easy to be accepted by patients and will not violate medical ethics; And save money and time, but a lot of literature lack the object of study about the characteristics of the records, some hospital medical record information is incomplete, it is difficult to determine whether compared two groups of comparable, and due to the progress of science, diagnostic tools, makes some light or atypical patients for early diagnosis, coupled with the progress of nursing techniques. The differences in outcomes between the two groups do not fully reflect the differences between the different interventions, making the conclusions incorrect.

历史性对照：将新的干预措施的结果与过去的研究做比较，这是一种非随机、非同期的对照研究。此类型对照的资料可来自文献和医院病历资料。这种设置对照的方法易被患者接受，也不会违背医德；而且节省经费和时间，但是不少文献资料缺乏研究对象有关特征的记载，有的医院病历资料残缺不全，难以判断对比两组是否可比，而且由于科学的进展，诊断手段的改进，使得一些轻型或不典型患者得到早期诊断，再加上护理技术的进步，对比两组结果上的差别并不完全反映不同干预措施的差异，从而使研究结论不正确。

1.2.2 According to the Treatment Measures of the Control Group
（按照对照组处理措施分类）

（1）Standard control: currently recognized effective treatment methods (such as a disease of routine nursing), effective the effect of the intervention (the new nursing approach) was compared with that of the experimental group. Such studies usually adopt a randomized double-blind design, in which the subjects are randomly assigned to the experimental group and the control group, which is a commonly used control method in clinical studies. The treatment applied to the control group by the standard control group was stable and caused few ethical problems.

标准对照：以目前公认的有效的处理方法（如某病的护理常规、有效的护理方法）施加给对照组，然后与试验组的干预措施（新护理方法）的效果比较。这类研究通常采用随机双盲设计，研究对象随机分配至试验组与对照组，是临床研究中常用的对照方法。标准对照施加给对照组的处理措施效果稳定，较少引起伦理方面的问题。

（2）Blank control: the control group was not given any treatment during the test, and they were only observed. The results were recorded and compared with those of the experimental group. The blank control is only applicable to patients with mild and stable disease, and there are no ethical issues even if no treatment is given. The placebo control is also a blank control in nature, but it can produce a placebo effect and the influence of subjective factors should be eliminated as much as possible in the trial.

空白对照：对照组在试验期间不给予任何处理，仅对他们进行观察、记录结果，并将其与试验组的结果进行比较。空白对照仅适用于病情轻且稳定的病人，即使不给予任何处理也不会产生伦理方面的问题。安慰剂对照（placebo control）本质上也是一种空白对照，但其可产生安慰剂效应，在试验中应尽量消除主观因素的影响。

1.3　Randomization（随机化）

Randomization is to avoid the interference of subjective factors from researchers and research objects and make the results deviate from the true value when selecting samples and grouping research objects. A special method is adopted to make the probability of occurrence of an event equal for each individual in the population or sample. Randomization includes two forms：（1）Random sampling：In the process of sampling, randomization method is adopted to ensure that all subjects in the population have an equal chance to be selected into the research sample and ensure that the sample has good representativeness.（2）Random allocation：In order to improve the balance between groups and reduce the interference of non-research factors, after the research sample is determined, further random allocation method is adopted to ensure that the research objects are equally allocated to the experimental group or the control group. Common randomization methods are as follows：

随机化是为了在选取样本和将研究对象分组时，避免来自研究者与研究对象两方面的主观因素的干扰而使结果偏离真实值，采用特殊方法使总体或样本中每个个体发生某事件的概率均等。随机化包括两种形式：（1）随机抽样：在抽样过程中采用随机化方法，使总体中所有对象都有同等的机会被抽取进入研究样本，保证了样本有较好的代表性。（2）随机分组：为提高组间的均衡性，减少非研究因素的干扰，在研究样本确定后，进一步采用随机的方法，使研究对象以同等的机会被分配进入试验组或对照组中。常用的随机化方法如下：

1.3.1　Simple Randomization（简单随机法）

There are many specific methods of this kind of randomization. The simplest is to draw lots or flip a coin or roll dice, but if the sample size is large, it is more troublesome. So, the most common allocation is by random table numbers. Currently available computer, especially often used large sample study, according to the software by the random number generator produces a random number of simple random method is suitable for the sample size of more than 100 research, when each group distribution of the sample is not equal, need to adjust, based on the principles of randomization, still need to make balance test in statistical analysis. Some researchers for convenience and sufferings choose order, hospital number, date, such as the patient's birthday, even grouping, called a random method, is not a randomized method, because when the researchers know in advance the next research object will be assigned to which group, some information of the research object of the certain choice, selection bias may be produced, should be careful.

此类随机化的具体方法有很多种。最简单为抽签或抛硬币或掷骰子，但若样本量大则比较麻烦。所以最常用的是按随机数字表数字进行分配。目前可用计算机进行，尤其大样本研究时常用，可按有关软件经随机数发生器产生随机数简单随机法适用于样本量超过100的研究，当各组间分配的样本数不相等时，需再按随机化原则进行调整，在统计学分析时仍然需要做均衡性检验。有些研究者为了方便，选择就诊顺序、住院号、就诊日期、病人生日等的奇偶数进行分组，称为半随机法，实际上不是随机化方法，因为当研究者预先知道下一位研究对象将被分配到哪一组时，主观上对研究对象的某些资料进行一定的取舍，可能产生选择偏倚，应慎用。

1.3.2　Stratified Randomization(分层随机法)

Firstly, the research objects are divided into groups (layers) according to a certain feature, and then the simple random method is adopted to extract the research objects from each layer to form samples, so as to achieve stratified random sampling. Or according to the method of simple random allocation in each layer, separate the test objects and control objects, and finally combine the test objects and control objects in each layer respectively as the experimental group and control group, realizing stratified and random grouping. Stratified random sampling can ensure that each "layer" has a certain number of research objects into the sample, improve the sample representativeness. Stratified random grouping can ensure that all "layers" have objects into the experimental group or the control group, and improve the balance between experimental groups.

先将研究对象按某一特征进行分组(层)，然后在各层中采用简单随机法抽取研究对象组成样本，实现分层随机抽样(stratified sampling)；或在各层中按简单随机分配的方法，分出试验对象与对照对象，最后将各层试验对象与对照对象分别合在一起作为试验组与对照组，实现分层随机分组(stratified allocating)。分层随机抽样可以保证各"层"都有一定研究对象进入样本，提高了样本的代表性；分层随机分组可以保证各"层"都有对象进入试验组或对照组，提高了试验组间的均衡性。

In stratifying random sampling, the factors that have a greater influence on the variation of observed values are often regarded as stratifying factors. In stratified random grouping, some characteristics that may cause confounding effects are mainly used as stratified factors, such as important clinical features or prognostic factors (including age, gender, disease condition and whether there are complications, etc.). In nursing research, stratification factors can be considered according to the following principles:

在分层随机抽样中，往往是以对观察值变异影响较大的因素作为分层因素；在分层随机分组中，主要以研究对象中某些可能产生混杂作用的特征作为分层因素，如研究对象的重要临床特征或预后因素(包括年龄、性别、病情、有无并发症等)。在护理学研究中，可根据以下原则考虑分层因素：

(1)the selection of risk factors for the disease or its complications under study;

选择所研究疾病或其并发症的危险因素；

(2)select the factors that have obvious influence on the dependent variables studied;

选择对所研究的因变量有明显影响的因素；

(3)following the principle of minimization, stratification factors should be controlled to the minimum. Excessive stratification will cause excessive dispersion of research objects within the group. Generally, 2 to 3 main layers are appropriate.

遵循最小化原则，将分层因素控制到最低限度，分层过多会造成组内研究对象过度分散，一般2~3个主层比较合适。

1.3.3　Blocked Randomization(区组随机分组法)

The subjects were divided into different groups, and then the subjects in each group were assigned by simple random method. The number of research objects in each area group is generally determined by multiples of the number of groups. If the study is divided into experimental group and control group, the number of block groups can be 2, 4, 6, 8, etc., but the larger the number of block groups, the more complex the arrangement and combination of research objects in allocation. For example, a study was divided into experimental group and control group, and the number of study groups was determined to be 4. Firstly, four research objects were divided into groups according to the sequence of entering the experiment, and then the four research objects in each group were randomly grouped according to the random number table. One of the characteristics of block randomization is the equal number of subjects in each group after grouping. However, when four objects in a block group are randomly allocated according to the random number table, it is likely that the number of cases in two groups is not equal, so it must be adjusted appropriately.

先将研究对象分为不同区组，然后再对每一区组内的研究对象用简单随机法进行分配。每一区组的研究对象数一般按分组数的倍数来确定。如研究分为试验组和对照组，则区组例数可选 2、4、6、8 等，但区组例数越大，研究对象在分配时的排列组合越复杂。例如某研究分为试验组和对照组，确定区组例数为 4。首先，研究对象按进入试验的先后顺序，每 4 个研究对象一组，然后再对每一区组的 4 个研究对象分别根据随机数字表进行随机分组。区组随机分组的特点之一就是分组后各组研究对象数相等。而对一个区组的 4 个对象按随机数字表进行随机分配时很可能出现两组例数不等的情况，必须进行适当调整。

To ensure the equal number of subjects in each group and facilitate the gradual accumulation of clinical cases, the subjects in each group can be grouped and the trial can be started. It is not necessary to group and start the trial after all samples are collected.

区组随机分组保证各组研究对象数量相等，并便于逐渐累积临床病例，即可每积累一个区组数的研究对象即进行分组及开始试验，不需要把所有样本全部收集齐后再来分组、展开试验。

1.3.4　Systematic Randomization（系统随机法）

Firstly, the observation units were numbered in order of some characteristics unrelated to the observation indicators (such as the order of admission, the number of admissions, and the number of house), and then divided into several parts according to the sampling proportion. The first observation unit was randomly selected from the first part, and then the second and third observation units were selected at a fixed interval… And other parts of the observation unit composition sample. For example, to select 100 constituent samples from 2000 observation units, that is, the sampling proportion is 5%(the sampling interval is 1/20), one observation unit can be randomly selected from the first to 20(the first part), such as No.12, and then one observation unit is selected every 20, that is: 32, 52, 72… Sample No.1992. If they all met the inclusion and exclusion criteria, they could be randomly divided into two groups equally.

先将总体的观察单位按某种与观察指标无关的特征(如按入院先后顺序、住院号、门牌号)顺序编号，再根据抽样比例将其分为若干部分，先从第一部分随机抽取第一个观察单位，然后按一固定间隔在第二、第三等各部分抽取观察单位组成样本。例如，欲从 2000 个观察单位中抽取 100 个组成样本，即抽样比例为 5%(抽样间隔为 1/20)，可先从第 1~

20(第一部分)随机抽出一个观察单位，如为 12 号，此后按每隔 20 抽取一个单位，即：32，52，72，…，1992 号组成样本。若其均符合纳入与排除标准，则可随机等分成两组。

1.3.5 Cluster Randomization(整群随机法)

Sampling or grouping is done in ready-made groups（communities，streets，townships，villages，hospitals，wards，etc.）rather than individual units. In cluster random sampling，all observation units from the selected population will be used as the study sample. For example，2 schools are randomly selected from 20 elementary schools in a district. All the students in these two primary schools were examined to understand the myopia rate of primary school students in this area. Similarly，in the whole group randomization，each observation unit in the group assigned to the experimental group was used as a test object，and each observation unit in the group assigned to the control group was used as a control object.

以现成的群体(社区、街道、乡、村、医院、病房等)而不是个体为单位，进行抽样或分组。在整群随机抽样中，所抽到群体中的所有观察单位都将作为研究样本。例如，从某地区的 20 所小学中随机抽取 2 所学校，并对这 2 所小学的全部阅读笔记学生进行视力检查，以了解该地区小学生近视率。同样，在整群随机分组中，被分到试验组的群体中的每个观察单位都作为试验对象，被分到对照组的群体中的每个观察单位都作为对照对象。

1.3.6 Multistage Random Sampling(多级抽样法)

A sampling method with multiple levels of sampling from large to small. First，a larger range of units are randomly selected from the overall population，known as first-level sampling units（such as provinces and cities），and then a smaller range of second-level units（such as districts and streets）are randomly selected from the first-level units. If the sampling stops here，it is called second-level sampling；if the sampling continues to a smaller range，it is called multi-level sampling.

一种从大到小多个级别进行的抽样方法。首先从总体中随机抽取范围较大的单元，称为一级抽样单元(例如省、市)，再从抽中的一级单元随机抽取范围较小的二级单元(如区、街道)，若抽样到此为止称为二级抽样，若再继续往小范围抽样，则称为多级抽样。

In some large-scale studies（national hypertension sampling Survey，national diabetes Prevalence Survey，etc.），multistage sampling has become the only practical sampling method. In practice，multistage sampling is often used in combination with the above basic sampling methods.

在一些大规模研究(全国高血压抽样调查、全国糖尿病患病率调查等)项目中，多级抽样成为唯一实用的抽样方法。在具体实施时，多级抽样常常与上述各种基本抽样方法结合使用。

2. Specific Experimental Designs(具体的实验设计)

2.1 Randomization Controlled Trail(随机对照试验)

Randomized controlled trail: subjects who met the inclusion and exclusion criteria were randomly assigned to the experimental group or the control group, two groups after baseline survey to accept different interventions, under the condition of same or environment, can be synchronously many times to study and observe the end of the two groups, the experimental results are scientific measurement, comparison and evaluation (Figure 8.2.1).

随机对照试验：采用随机分配的方法，将符合纳入与排除标准的研究对象分配到试验组或对照组，基线调查后两组分别接受不同的干预措施，在一致的条件下或环境中，可多次同步地进行研究和观察两组的结局，对实验结果进行科学的测量、比较和评价(图8.2.1)。

$$
\begin{array}{llllll}
R & E & O_1 & X_A & O_2 \\
R & C & O_1 & X_B & O_2 \\
or \\
R & E & O_1 & X_A & O_2 & O_3 & O_4 \\
R & C & O_1 & X_B & O_2 & O_3 & O_4
\end{array}
$$

Figure 8.2.1 Design principles of randomized controlled trial(随机对照试验的设计原理)

R=random group; E = experimental group; C = the control group; X = impose intervention or treatment factors; O_n =n time observation or measurement

R=随机分组；E=实验组；C=对照组；X=施加干预或处理因素；O_n=第 n 次观察或测量

Randomized controlled trials should be according to the type, data type (counting or measuring data), the research of the distribution of the number of clusters, data (normal or non-normal distribution), and influenced the results of related factors, such as selecting the corresponding statistical analysis methods, such as chi-square test, rank test, t test, analysis of variance and two more than two comparisons, factor analysis, time analysis, etc.

随机对照试验应根据研究类型、资料种类(计数或计量资料)、研究的分组数、资料的分布(正态或非正态分布)、影响研究结果的相关因素等,选择相应的统计分析方法,如卡方检验、秩和检验、t检验、方差分析及其两两比较、多因素分析、时效分析等。

2.2　Pretest-posttest Design(实验前后对照设计)

Pretest-posttest design: with the method of random distribution, will be met inclusion and exclusion criteria subjects assigned to the experimental group or control group, the first observation index of the baseline survey research variables, then experimental group accepted intervention measures, control group not given interventions, under the condition of same or environment, simultaneously study and observation of the end of the two groups. Scientific measurement, comparison and evaluation of experimental results (Figure 8.2.2) are also randomized controlled trials.

实验前后对照设计:采用随机分配的方法,将符合纳入与排除标准的研究对象分配到试验组或对照组,首先做研究变量观察指标的基线调查,然后试验组接受干预措施,对照组不给予干预措施,在一致的条件下或环境中,同步地进行研究和观察两组的结局,对实验结果进行科学的测量、比较和评价(图8.2.2),其实也是随机对照试验。

```
R  E  O₁  X  O₂
R  C  O₁     O₂
or
R  E  O₁  X  O₂  O₃  O₄
R  C  O₁     O₂  O₃  O₄
```

Figure 8.2.2　Design principles of pretest-posttest design(实验前后对照设计原理)

R = random group; E = experimental group; C = the control group; X = impose intervention or treatment factors; O_n = n time observation or measurement

R=随机分组;E=实验组;C=对照组;X=施加干预或处理因素;O_n=第 n 次观察或测量

2.3　Posttest-only Design(单纯实验后对照设计)

Posttest-only design adopts the method of random distribution, will be met inclusion and exclusion criteria subjects assigned to the experimental group or control group, and group accepted intervention, control group not given intervention or only given conventional measures, under the condition of same or environment, the experimental results are scientific measurement, comparison and evaluation (Figure 8.2.3), not to intervene in front of the baseline survey.

采用随机分配的方法，将符合纳入与排除标准的研究对象分配到试验组或对照组，然后试验组接受干预措施，对照组不给予干预措施或仅给予常规措施，在一致的条件下或环境中，对实验结果进行科学的测量、比较和评价（图 8.2.3），不进行干预前的基线调查。

$$
\begin{array}{lll}
RE & X & O_1 \\
RC & & O_1 \\
or & & \\
RE & X_A & O_1 \\
RC & X_B & O_1 \\
\end{array}
$$

Figure 8.2.3 Design principles of posttest-only design(单纯实验后对照设计原理)

R = random grouping; E = experimental group; C = control group; X = impose intervention or treatment factors; O_1 = observation or measurement

R = 随机分组；E = 实验组；C = 对照组；X = 施加干预或处理因素；O_1 = 观察或测量

2.4 Other types of randomized controlled trials(其他类型的随机对照试验)

2.4.1 Quasi-randomized Controlled Trial(半随机对照试验)

A randomized controlled trial is the difference between the distribution of the object of study in a different way, is as a random distribution, such as hospital as the research object's birthday, or of such confinement, etc. At the end of the number of odd or even number, number will be assigned to the experimental group or control group subjects, accept the corresponding intervention measures and control measures. Due to the distribution method, semi-randomized controlled trials are prone to be affected by selective bias, resulting in baseline imbalance, and their results are less authentic and reliable than randomized controlled trials.

与随机对照试验的区别是研究对象的分配方式不同，是按半随机分配方式，如按研究对象的生日、住院日或住院号等的末尾数字的奇数或偶数，将研究对象分配到试验组或对照组，接受相应的干预措施与对照措施。半随机对照试验由于分配方式的关系，容易受选择性偏倚的影响，造成基线情况的不平衡，其结果的真实性与可靠性不及随机对照试验。

2.4.2 Unequal Randomized Controlled Trial(不对等随机对照试验)

Due to limited sample sources and research funds, researchers hope to obtain results as soon as possible and randomly assign subjects to the experimental group or control group in a certain proportion (usually 2 : 1 or 3 : 2). The effectiveness of this method will be reduced.

由于样本来源和研究经费有限，研究者希望尽快获得结果，将研究对象按一定比例(通常为 2 : 1 或 3 : 2)随机分配入试验组或对照组。此种方法检验效能会降低。

2.4.3 Cluster Randomized Controlled Trial(整群随机对照试验)

A family, a couple, a group or even a town were randomly assigned to the experimental group or the control group to receive corresponding measures respectively for research. The design of the cluster randomized controlled trial is the same as that of the general randomized controlled trial, but the difference lies in that the calculation of sample content and analysis methods of results are different due to the different randomly assigned units, and the required sample content is large.

以一个家庭、一对夫妇、一个小组甚至一个乡镇等作为随机分配单位，将其随机分配到试验组或对照组，分别接受相应的措施，进行研究。整群随机对照试验在设计上与一般随机对照试验一样，不同之处在于因随机分配的单位不同，导致样本含量的计算和结果的分析方法有所差异，所需样本含量较大。

Experimental research can accurately explain the causal relationship between independent variables and dependent variables, reflecting the scientific nature and objectivity of the research. However, as most nursing problems are studied by people, the interfering variables in many studies, such as climate, environment, design ethics or privacy issues, cannot be completely controlled, leading to the poor universality of experimental research in nursing problems.

实验性研究能准确地解释自变量和因变量之间的因果关系，反映研究的科学性和客观性较强。但由于大多护理问题的研究对象是人，很多研究中的干扰变量如气候、环境、设计伦理或隐私等问题无法得到完全控制，导致实验性研究在护理问题的研究中应用的普遍性较差。

3. Strengths and Limitations of Experiments(实验的优点和局限性)

In this section, we explore the reasons why experimental designs are held in high esteem and examine some limitations. An experimental design is the gold standard for testing interventions because it yields strong evidence about intervention effectiveness. Experiments offer greater corroboration than any other approach that, if the independent variable (e. g., diet, drug, teaching approach) is varied, then certain consequences in the outcomes (e. g., weight loss, recovery, learning) are likely to ensue. The great strength of RCTs, then, lies in the confidence with which causal relationships can be inferred. Through the controls imposed by manipulation, comparison, and randomization, alternative explanations can be discredited. It is because of these strengths that meta-analyses of RCTs, which integrate evidence from multiple experimental studies, are at the pinnacle of evidence hierarchies for questions about treatment effects.

在本节中，我们将探讨实验设计受到高度尊重的原因，并探讨一些局限性。实验性设计是测试干预措施的黄金标准，因为它能提供干预措施有效性的有力证据。实验比任何其他方法都更能证明，如果自变量(如饮食、药物、教学方法)是不同的，那么结果中的某些结果(如减肥、恢复、学习)很可能随之产生。因此，随机对照试验的强大之处在于通过操纵、对照和随机化的控制，拥有能够推断出因果关系的信心。正是因为这些优势，整合了多个实验研究的证据的 RCT 荟萃分析，在治疗效果的问题上处于证据层次的顶峰。

Despite the benefits of experiments, this type of design also has limitations. First, there are often constraints that make an experimental approach impractical or impossible. A problem with RCTs conducted in clinical settings is that it is often clinical staff, rather than researchers, who administer an intervention, and therefore, it can sometimes be difficult to ascertain whether those in the intervention group actually received the treatment as specified and if those in the control group did not. Clinical studies are conducted in environments over which researchers may have little control—and control is a critical factor in RCTs.

尽管实验有好处，但这种设计也有局限性。首先，通常有一些限制因素使实验方法不切实际或不可能。在临床环境中进行的随机对照试验的一个问题是，它往往是临床工作人员管理干预，而不是研究人员，因此，有时很难确定干预组的人是否真的接受了特定的治疗，而对照组的人是否没有接受。临床研究是在研究人员几乎无法控制的环境中进行的，而控制是随机对照试验的一个关键因素。

Sometimes problems emerge when participants can "opt out" of the intervention. Suppose, for example, that we randomly assigned patients with HIV infection to a special support group intervention or to a control group. Intervention subjects who elect not to participate in the support groups, or who participate infrequently, actually are in a "condition" that looks more like the control condition than the experimental one. The treatment is diluted through nonparticipation, and it may become difficult to detect any treatment effects, no matter how effective it might otherwise have been.

有时候，当参与者可以"选择退出"干预时，问题就出现了。例如，假设我们随机将HIV感染患者分配到一个特殊的支持组或一个对照组。那些选择不参加支持小组的干预对象，或者那些很少参加的干预对象，实际上处于一个看起来更像控制小组而不是实验小组的"条件"中。由于不参与，治疗效果降低了，而且可能很难检测到任何治疗效果，无论它原本有多么有效。

Another potential problem is the Hawthorne effect, a placebo-type effect caused by people's expectations. The term is derived from a series of experiments conducted at the Hawthorne plant of the Western Electric Corporation in which various environmental conditions, such as light and working hours, were varied to test their effects on worker productivity. Regardless of what change was introduced, that is, whether the light was made better or worse, productivity increased. Knowledge of being included in the study (not just knowledge of being in a particular group) appears to have affected people's behavior, obscuring the effect of the treatments.

另一个潜在的问题是霍桑效应，这是一种由人们的期望引起的安慰剂效应。这个词来源于西方电力公司霍桑工厂进行的一系列实验，在这些实验中，不同的环境条件，如光线和工作时间，以测试它们对工人生产率的影响。不管引入了什么变化，无论光线是变好了还是变差了，生产力都提高了。研究对象对自己被纳入研究的认知(不仅仅是对身处某个特定群体的认知)似乎影响了人们的行为，掩盖了治疗的效果。

Section Ⅲ　Quasi-Experiments
第三节　类实验性研究

1. Quasi-Experimental Designs(类实验性研究)

Quasi-experiments, often called controlled trials without randomization in the medical literature, involve an intervention but they lack randomization, the signature of a true experiment. Some quasi-experiments even lack a control group. The signature of a quasi-experimental design, then, is an intervention in the absence of randomization. In quasi-experiments, researchers cannot completely control the grouping of research objects, that is, the design content must contain nursing intervention content for research objects, but may not be grouped according to the principle of randomness or no control group, or both conditions are not met.

类实验，在医学文献中通常被称为没有随机化的对照试验，涉及干预，但它们缺乏随机化，这是真正实验的标志，一些准实验甚至没有对照组。那么，准实验设计的特征就是在没有随机化的情况下进行干预。类实验是研究者不能完全控制研究对象的分组，即设计内容一定有对研究对象的护理干预内容，但可能没有按随机原则分组或没有设对照组，或两个条件都不具备。

1.1　Nonequivalent Control Group Design(不对等对照组设计)

Nonequivalent control group designs, also known as nonequivalent control group design in epidemiology. The experimental group and the control group are not randomly grouped, but artificially included in the experimental group or the control group by the researcher according to the relevant factors, and carried out a controlled trial at the same time. For example, suppose we wished to study the effect of a new chair yoga intervention for older people. The intervention is being offered to everyone at a community senior center, and randomization is not possible. For comparative purposes, we collect outcome data in a different community senior center that is not instituting the intervention. Data on quality of life are collected from both groups at baseline and again 10 weeks after its implementation in one of the centers. Researchers artificially met inclusion and exclusion criteria subjects assigned to the experimental group or control group, and group accepted intervention measures, the control group does not accept interventions or accept compared to conventional measures, under the condition of same or environment, simultaneously study and observation of the end of the two groups, the experimental results are scientific measurement, comparison and evaluation (Figure 8.3.1, Figure 8.3.2), and the results were basically the same as those of RCT.

不对等对照组设计，又称为流行病学的非随机同期对照试验，指试验组与对照组的研究对象不是采用随机的方法分组，而是由研究者根据有关因素人为地纳入试验组或对照组，进行同期的对照试验。例如，假设我们想研究一种新的椅子瑜伽对老年人的影响。社区老年人中心为每个人提供干预，不可能随机进行。为了进行比较，我们在没有实施干预

的不同社区老年人中心收集结果数据。两组的生活质量数据均在基线和其中一个中心实施
10 周后收集。研究者人为地将符合纳入与排除标准的研究对象分配到试验组或对照组，然
后试验组接受干预措施，对照组不接受干预措施或接受对照的常规措施，在一致的条件下
或环境中，同步地进行研究和观察两组的结局，对实验结果进行科学的测量、比较和评价
（见图 8.3.1、图 8.3.2），其结果分析基本同 RCT。

$$
\begin{array}{llll}
E & O_1 & X & O_2 \\
C & O_1 & & O_2
\end{array}
$$

Figure 8.3.1 Design principles of nonequivalent control group pretest-posttest design（不对等对照组前-后对
照设计原理）

E= experimental group；C = control group；X = impose intervention or treatment factors；$O_n = n$ time
observation or measurement

E=实验组；C=对照组；X=施加干预或处理因素；$O_n =$第 n 次观察或测量

$$
\begin{array}{lll}
E & X & O_1 \\
C & & O_1
\end{array}
$$

Figure 8.3.2 Design principles of nonequivalent control group posttest-only design

E= experimental group；C = control group；X = impose intervention or treatment factors；$O_n = n$ time
observation or measurement

E=实验组；C=对照组；X=施加干预或处理因素；$O_n =$第 n 次观察或测量

1.2 One-group Pretest-posttest Design（自身前-后对照设计）

There was no control group in the study. The subjects who met the inclusion and exclusion
criteria were randomly or artificially included into the study for baseline investigation, and then
received intervention measures to measure the results after intervention. Finally, the
measurement results before and after the intervention were compared（Figure 8.3.3）, and the
result analysis was basically the same as that of RCT. Suppose that a hospital implemented rapid
response teams（RRTs）in its acute care units. Administrators want to examine the effects on
patient outcomes（e.g., unplanned admissions to the ICU, mortality rate）and nurse outcomes

(e. g. , stress). For the purposes of this example, assume no other hospital could serve as a good comparison. The only kind of comparison that can be made is a before-after contrast. If RRTs were implemented in January, one could compare the mortality rate (for example) during the 3 months before RRTs with the mortality rate during the subsequent 3-month period.

研究没有设对照组，将符合纳入与排除标准的个体随机或人为纳入研究对象后做基线调查，然后接受干预措施，测量干预后的结果，最后将前后两次的测量结果进行比较(见图 8.3.3)，其结果分析基本同 RCT。假设一家医院在其急症监护室中实施了快速反应小组(RRTs)。管理者想要检查对病人结果(例如，意外入住 ICU，死亡率)和护士结局(例如，压力)的影响。为了本例的目的，假设没有其他医院可以作为一个很好的比较。唯一能做的比较是前后对比。如果在 1 月实施快速反应疗法，人们可以比较在快速反应疗法实施前 3 个月的死亡率与随后 3 个月期间的死亡率。

$$O_1 \quad X \quad O_2$$

Figure 8.3.3　Design principles of one-group pretest-posttest design(不对等对照组前-后对照设计原理)

X=impose intervention or treatment factors; O_n =n time observation or measurement

X=施加干预或处理因素; O_n =第 n 次观察或测量

1.3　Time Series Design(时间序列设计)

Time series design is an improvement of the one-group pretest-posttest design. This design can be used when the stability of its own variables is uncertain (Figure 8.3.4).

时间序列设计是自身实验前后对照设计的一种改进。当自身变量的稳定性无法确定时，可以采用此种设计(见图 8.3.4)。

$$O_1 \ O_2 \ O_3 \ O_4 \ X \ O_5 \ O_6 \ O_7 \ O_8$$

Figure 8.3.4　Design principles of time series design(时间连续性设计原理)

X=impose intervention or treatment factors; O_n =n time observation or measurement

X=施加干预或处理因素; O_n =第 n 次观察或测量

2. Strengths and Limitations of Quasi-Experiments
（类实验性研究的优点和局限性）

A major strength of quasi-experiments is that they are practical. In clinical settings, it may be impossible to conduct true experimental tests of nursing interventions. Strong quasi-experimental designs introduce some research control when full experimental rigor is not possible.

类实验的一个主要优点是它们很实用。在临床环境中，对护理干预进行真正的实验测试的可能性很小。当完全严格的实验不可能进行时，强大的类实验设计引入了一些研究控制。

Another advantage of quasi-experiments is that patients are not always willing to relinquish control over their treatment condition. Indeed, it appears that people are increasingly unwilling to volunteer to be randomized in clinical trials. Quasi-experimental designs, because they do not involve random assignment, are likely to be acceptable to a broader group of people. This, in turn, has positive implications for the generalizability of the results—but the problem is that the results may be less conclusive.

准实验的另一个好处是，病人并不总是愿意放弃对自己治疗状况的控制。事实上，人们似乎越来越不愿意自愿参与随机临床试验。类实验设计，因为它们不涉及随机分配，可能会被更广泛的人群所接受。这反过来又对研究结果的普遍性产生了积极的影响。但问题是，研究结果可能不那么具有决定性。

Researchers using quasi-experimental designs should be cognizant of their weaknesses and should take steps to counteract the weaknesses or take them into account in interpreting results. When a quasi-experimental design is used, there usually are rival hypotheses competing with the intervention as explanations for the results. Take as an example the case in which we administer a special diet to frail nursing home residents to assess its effects on weight gain. If we use no comparison group or a nonequivalent control group and then observe a weight gain, we must ask: Is it plausible that some other factor caused the gain? Is it plausible that pretreatment differences between the intervention and comparison groups resulted in differential gain? Is it plausible that the elders on average gained weight simply because the most frail patients died or were hospitalized? If the answer is "yes" to any of these questions, then inferences about the causal effect of the intervention are weakened. The plausibility of any particular rival explanation typically cannot be answered unequivocally. Because the conclusions from quasi-experiments ultimately depend in part on human judgment, rather than on more objective criteria, cause-and-effect inferences are less compelling.

使用类实验设计的研究人员应认识到他们的弱点，并应采取措施来抵消这些弱点，或在解释结果时考虑到它们。当使用类实验设计时，通常会有与干预相竞争的假设作为对结果的解释。举个例子，我们给虚弱的疗养院居民提供一种特殊的饮食来评估其对体重增加的影响。如果我们没有使用对照组或非等效对照组，然后观察到体重增加，我们必须问：是否有其他因素导致了体重增加？干预组和对照组之间的预处理差异是否可能导致差异收益？老年人的平均体重增加仅仅是因为最虚弱的病人死亡或住院吗？如果上述任何一个问题的答案是"是"，那么关于干预的因果效应的推论就被削弱了。任何与之相对的解释的合理性通常都不能得到明确的回答。由于类实验的结论最终部分地取决于人类的判断，而不是更客观的标准，因果推论就不那么有说服力了。

Section Ⅳ　Nonexperimental/ Observational Research
第四节　非实验性/观察性研究

Non-experimental study refers to a research method in which the study design does not impose any nursing intervention on the subjects. Many research questions—including ones seeking to establish causal relationships—cannot be addressed with an experimental or quasi-experimental design. For example, at the beginning of this chapter we posed this prognosis question: Do birth weights less than 1, 500 grams cause developmental delays in children? Clearly, we cannot manipulate birth weight, the independent variable. Babies are born with weights that are neither random nor subject to research control. One way to answer this question is to compare two groups of infants—babies with birth weights above and below 1, 500 grams at birth—in terms of their subsequent development. When researchers do not intervene by manipulating the independent variable, the study is nonexperimental, or, in the medical literature, observational.

非实验性研究指研究设计内容对研究对象不施加任何护理干预措施处理的研究方法。许多研究问题——包括那些寻求建立因果关系的问题——不能用实验或准实验设计来解决。例如，在本章开头，我们提出了一个预后问题：出生体重低于 1500 克会导致儿童发育迟缓吗？显然，我们无法控制出生体重这个自变量。婴儿出生时的体重既不是随机的，也不受研究控制。回答这个问题的一种方法是比较两组婴儿——出生时体重在 1500 克以上和 1500 克以下的婴儿——他们随后的发育情况。当研究人员不通过操纵自变量进行干预时，该研究是非实验性的，或者在医学文献中是观察性的。

Most nursing studies are nonexperimental, mainly because most human characteristics (e. g., birth weight, lactose intolerance) cannot be experimentally manipulated. Also, many variables that could technically be manipulated cannot be manipulated ethically. For example, if we were studying the effect of prenatal care on infant mortality, it would be unethical to provide such care to one group of pregnant women while deliberately depriving a randomly assigned control group. We would need to locate a naturally occurring group of pregnant women who had not received prenatal care. Their birth outcomes could then be compared with those of women who had received appropriate care. The problem, however, is that the two groups of women are likely to differ in terms of many other characteristics, such as age, education, and income, any of which individually or in combination could affect infant mortality, independent of prenatal care. This is precisely why experimental designs are so strong in demonstrating cause-and-effect relationships. Many nonexperimental studies explore causal relationships when experimental work is not possible—although, some observational studies have primarily a descriptive intent.

大多数护理研究是非实验性的，主要是因为大多数人类特征(如出生体重，乳糖不耐受)不能通过实验来控制。此外，许多在技术上可以被操纵的变量在道德上无法被操纵。例如，如果我们在研究产前护理对婴儿死亡率的影响，在为一组孕妇提供这种护理的同时，故意剥夺一组随机分配的对照组，这是不道德的。我们需要找到一组没有接受产前护理的自然怀孕妇女。然后可以将她们的分娩结果与那些接受了适当护理的妇女的分娩结果进行比较。然而，问题是，这两个群体的妇女在许多其他特征方面可能有所不同，例如年龄、教育和收入，其中任何一个单独或结合起来都可能影响婴儿死亡率，而不受产前护理的影响。这正是实验设计在证明因果关系方面如此强大的原因。许多非实验研究在实验工作不可能进行的情况下探索因果关系——尽管，一些观察性研究主要具有描述性的意图。

1. Descriptive Research(描述性研究)

The purpose of descriptive studies is to observe, describe, and document aspects of a situation as it naturally occurs and sometimes to serve as a starting point for hypothesis generation or theory development. Using the existing data or special investigation data, according to different areas, different time and different group characteristics, the distribution of disease or health status and exposure factors are truly described, through comparative analysis of the causes of the distribution difference of disease or health status, put forward further research direction or prevention and control strategies.

描述性研究的目的是观察、描述和记录自然发生的情况，有时作为假设生成或理论发展的起点。利用已有的资料或特殊调查的资料，按不同区、不同时间及不同分群特征分组，把疾病或健康状态和暴露因素的分布情况真实地描述出来，通过比较分析导致疾病或健康状态分布差异的原因，提出进一步的研究方向或防治策略。

1.1 Cross Sectional Study(横断面研究)

Investigation and analysis of the occurrence of a certain population event and its influencing factors in a specific time and space. Types of cross-sectional study:

指特定时间与特定空间内对某一人群事件的发生状况及其影响因素进行的调查分析。横断面研究的种类：

1.1.1 Census(普查)

To investigate or examine all subjects within a specified area at a specified time for a specified purpose. The "specific time" should be as short as possible in case some indicator changes during the survey period. "Specific scope" can include collectives, cities, provinces or even the whole country. It is mainly used for: (1) early detection of patients in the population, such as cervical cancer screening; (2) Describe the basic distribution of health conditions or diseases, such as the investigation of growth and nutritional status indicators of children or the distribution of tuberculosis.

指根据一定目的，在特定时间内对特定范围内所有对象进行调查或检查。"特定时间"应该尽可能短，以防某些指标在调查期间发生变化。"特定范围"可以包括集体单位、全市、全省甚至全国。主要用于：(1)在人群中早期发现病人，例如开展子宫颈癌普查；(2)描述健康状况或疾病的基本分布情况，例如儿童的生长发育及营养状况指标的调查或结核病的分布等。

1.1.2 Sampling Survey(抽样调查)

According to a certain purpose, in a specific period of time to a certain population, according to the method of sampling a part of the object as a sample for investigation and analysis, and its results to deduce the situation of the population of a survey method. In practical work, if the purpose is not to find out all patients in the population, but to reveal the distribution law or prevalence level of a certain event, the method of sampling survey can be used. According to the different purposes of the survey, reasonable sampling methods should be selected, sufficient sample size should be selected, and the principle of randomization should be followed.

指根据一定目的，在特定时间内对特定范围内某人群总体中，按照方法抽取一部分对象作为样本进行调查分析，并用其结果来推论该人群状况的一种调查方法。在实际工作中，如果不是为了查出人群中全部患者，而是为了揭示某种事件的分布规律或流行水平，就可以采用抽样调查的方法。根据调查的不同目的，调查需选择合理的抽样方法，要有足够的样本量，遵循随机化原则。

1.2 Longitudinal Study(纵向研究)

Regular follow-up of diseases, health conditions and certain factors in the same population at different points in time to understand the dynamic changes of these factors over time, namely, a comprehensive study of multiple cross-sectional studies of this population at different times, is a prospective study.

指在不同时点对同一人群的疾病、健康状况和某些因素进行定期随访，了解这些因素随时间的动态变化情况，即在不同时间对这一人群进行多次横断面研究的综合研究，是前瞻性研究。

2. Correlational Research(相关性研究)

When researchers study the effect of a potential cause that they cannot manipulate, they use correlational designs to examine relationships between variables. A correlation is a relationship or association between two variables, that is, a tendency for variation in one variable to be related to variation in another. For example, in human adults, height and weight are correlated because there is a tendency for taller people to weigh more than shorter people.

当研究人员研究一个他们无法操纵的潜在原因的影响时，他们使用相关设计来检查变量之间的关系。相关是两个变量之间的一种关系或关联，也就是说，一个变量的变化与另一个变量的变化相关联的趋势。例如，在成年人中，身高和体重是相关的，因为个子高的人比个子矮的人体重更重。

As mentioned earlier, one criterion for causality is that an empirical relationship (correlation) between variables must be demonstrated. It is risky, however, to infer causal relationships in correlational research. A famous research dictum is relevant: Correlation does not prove causation. The mere existence of a relationship between variables is not enough to warrant the conclusion that one variable caused the other, even if the relationship is strong. In experiments, researchers have direct control over the independent variable; the experimental treatment can be administered to some and withheld from others, and the two groups can be equalized with respect to everything except the independent variable through randomization. In correlational research, on the other hand, investigators do not control the independent variable, which often has already occurred. Groups being compared can differ in ways that affect outcomes of interest—that is, there are usually confounding variables. Although correlational studies are inherently weaker than experimental studies in elucidating causal relationships, different designs offer different degrees of supportive evidence.

如前所述，因果关系的一个标准是必须证明变量之间的经验关系(相关性)。然而，在相关研究中推断因果关系是有风险的。一个著名的研究格言是：相关性不能证明因果关系。仅仅存在变量之间的关系，并不足以证明一个变量导致另一个变量的结论，即使这种关系很强。在实验中，研究者可以直接控制自变量，可以对一些患者进行实验性治疗，而对另一些患者则不进行治疗。另一方面，在相关研究中，研究者不控制自变量，这往往是已经发生的。被比较的群体可能在影响利益结果的方式上有所不同——也就是说，通常存在混杂变量。虽然相关性研究在阐明因果关系方面天生就比实验研究弱，但不同的设计提供不同程度的支持证据。

3. Analytical Research(分析性研究)

The study of similarities and differences between two or more different things, phenomena, behaviors, or people in a state of nature. As an observation method, exposure is not artificial intervention or random assignment, but objective existence before the study, which is an important difference from experimental study. An important difference between analytical research and descriptive research is that a control group must be established.

在自然状态下，对两种或两种以上不同的事物、现象、行为或人群的异同进行比较的研究方法，属于观察法，暴露不是人为干预或随机分配，而是研究前已客观存在的，这是与实验性研究的重要区别；分析性研究必须设立对照组，这是与描述性研究的重要区别。

3.1 Cohort Study(队列研究)

It is a prospective study that divides a group of subjects (cohort) into the exposed group and the non-exposed group (control group) according to whether they are exposed to a certain factor or not, and follows up for an appropriate period of time to compare the relationship between the studied events (or diseases) and exposure factors between the two groups. The direction of cohort study is longitudinal and prospective, that is, from cause to effect. In other words, at the beginning of the study, "cause" exists, and no "effect" (outcome) occurs. Under the effect of "cause", the occurrence of "effect" is directly observed. Exposure factors are objective rather than human intervention. The classification of groups was determined by the presence or absence of exposure factors, which could not be randomly assigned. Cohort studies provide a direct calculation of morbidity and allow evaluation of the association of exposure factors with disease.

队列研究,亦称定群研究,属于前瞻性研究,是将一群研究对象(队列),按是否暴露于某因素分为暴露组与非暴露组(对照组),并随访适当一段时间,比较两组之间所研究事件(或疾病)与暴露因素之间的关系。队列研究的方向是纵向的、前瞻性的,即由因到果的研究方向,也就是说在研究开始时有"因"存在,并无"果"(结局)发生,在"因"的作用下,直接观察"果"的发生;暴露因素是客观存在,而不是人为干预的;群组的划分是根据暴露因素的有无来确定的,研究者不能将其随机化分配;队列研究可直接计算发病率,并借此评价暴露因素与疾病的联系。

3.2 Case-control Study(病例对照研究)

Case-control study is a retrospective study. From the perspective of the chronological order of causality, the research method of "effect" and "cause" is to look for factors that may be related to the disease in the past starting from the cases that have been affected. It is based on the basic theory of cohort research, but it greatly simplifies its implementation process, so it has more extensive application value. Case-control studies are conducted after the onset of a disease (event) to investigate exposure to study factors. Only the exposure rate or exposure level of the two study factors could be known, and incidence could not be calculated.

病例对照研究是一种回顾性研究,从因果关系的时间顺序来看是从"果"查"因"的研究方法,也就是从已患病的病例出发,去寻找过去可能与疾病有关的因素。它以队列研究的基本理论为基础,但又极大地简化了其实施过程,因而其更具有广泛的使用价值。病例对照研究在疾病(事件)发生后进行，调查研究因素的暴露情况；仅能了解两组研究因素的暴露率或暴露水平，不能计算发病率。

4. The Delphi Method(德尔菲法)

The Delphi Method also known as expert consultation method or expert scoring method, the questionnaire is prepared by the investigator, and the expert panel members are consulted by back-to-back communication in accordance with established procedures, and the expert panel members submit their opinions anonymously (by letter). After several times of repeated consultation and feedback, the opinions of expert group members gradually tend to be concentrated, and finally according to the comprehensive opinions of experts, the evaluation of the research object is a method.

德尔菲法又称专家咨询法或专家评分法，是由调查者拟定调查问卷，按照既定程序采用背对背的通信方式向专家组成员进行征询，而专家组成员又以匿名的方式(函件)提交意见。经过几次反复征询和反馈，专家组成员的意见逐步趋于集中，最后根据专家的综合意见，对研究对象做出评价的一种方法。

Delphi method is to sort out, summarize, and make statistics on the problems to be studied after obtaining the opinions of experts, and then feedback anonymously to the experts, and solicit opinions again, and then concentrate, and then feedback until unanimous opinions are obtained. The process mainly includes three stages: preparation stage, round consultation stage and data processing stage (Figure 8.4.1). Delphi method generally includes four rounds of consultation and investigation, and the feedback between each round is included in the investigation process:

德尔菲法是在对所要研究的问题征得专家的意见之后，进行整理、归纳、统计，再匿名反馈给各专家，再次征求意见，再集中，再反馈，直至得到一致的意见。其过程主要包括三个阶段：准备阶段、轮番征询阶段与数据处理阶段(见图8.4.1)。德尔菲法一般包括四轮征询调查，且在调查过程中包含着每轮间的反馈：

Round 1: the first round of questionnaire, sent to experts by the organizers, is open-ended, with no strings attached, and only presents topics. Ask experts to present relevant events around the topic. Then the organizer summarized the questionnaire completed by the experts, merged similar events, excluded minor events, put forward a list of events with accurate terms, and sent it to the experts as a second round of questionnaire.

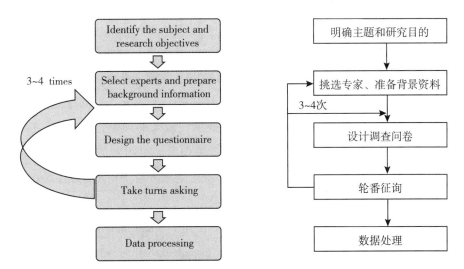

Figure 8. 4. 1　Design principle of Delphi method(德尔菲法的设计原理)

第一轮：由组织者发给专家的第一轮调查表是开放式的，不带任何附加条件，只提出主题。请专家围绕主题提出相关事件。然后组织者对专家填好的调查表进行汇总整理，归并同类事件，排除次要事件，用准确术语提出一个事件的一览表，并作为第二轮调查表发给专家。

Round 2: experts evaluate each event listed in the second round questionnaire. For example, stating when the event occurred, stating the reasons why the event occurred late or early. The organizer counted and processed the expert opinions in the questionnaire, calculated the probability distribution of the overall expert opinions, and sorted out the third questionnaire. The third questionnaire included events, the median and upper and lower quartiles, and reasons for events occurring outside the quartile.

第二轮：专家对第二轮调查表所列的每个事件做出评价。例如，说明事件发生的时间、叙述事件或迟或早发生的理由。组织者统计处理调查表中的专家意见，统计出专家总体意见的概率分布，整理出第三张调查表。第三张调查表包括事件、事件发生的中位数和上下四分点，以及事件发生时间在四分点外侧的理由。

Round 3: after the third questionnaire is handed out, experts are invited to do the following things: review the reasons; Make an evaluation of the opposing opinions outside the upper and lower quadrants; Give your own new evaluation (especially for experts outside the upper and lower quartiles, you should restate your reasons); If you revise your opinion, please also state why it changed, where the original reason was wrong, or where it was incomplete. When the experts' new comments and reasons were returned to the organizers, their work was much like the second round: counting the median and upper and lower quartiles; Summarize the opinions of experts, focus on both sides of the controversial opinions, form the fourth questionnaire.

第三轮：把第三张调查表发下去后，请专家做以下事情：重审理由；对上下四分点外的对立意见作一个评价；给出自己新的评价（尤其是在上下四分点外的专家，应重述自己的理由）；如果修正自己的观点，也请叙述为何改变，原来的理由错在哪里，或者说明哪里不完善。专家们的新评论和新理由返回组织者手中后，组织者的工作与第二轮十分类似：统计中位数和上下四分点；总结专家观点，重点是双方有争论的意见，形成第四张调查表。

Round 4: the fourth questionnaire invites experts to evaluate and weigh again, and make detailed and sufficient arguments if necessary. The organizers still need to collect the collected questionnaires, conduct statistical analysis and prediction, and find out the expert opinions with high convergence degree.

第四轮：第四张调查表请专家再次评价和权衡，并在必要时做出详细、充分的论证。组织者依然要将回收的调查表进行汇总整理、统计分析与预测，并寻找出收敛程度较高的专家意见。

The above four rounds of surveys are not simply repeated, but a spiraling process, with each cycle and feedback, the experts absorb new information, gain a deeper and more comprehensive understanding of the research content, and improve the accuracy of the results each round. After the end of the fourth step, experts may not reach a consensus on all events. If they do not reach a consensus, they can also use the median and upper and lower quartiles to draw conclusions. Not all predicted events take four steps. Possible events reach unity in round 2 that need not occur in round 3.

上述四轮调查不是简单的重复，而是一种螺旋上升的过程，每循环和反馈一次，专家都吸收了新的信息，并对研究内容有了更深刻、更全面的认识，结果的精确性也逐轮提高。在第四步结束后，专家对各事件也不一定都达到统一，不统一时也可以用中位数和上下四分点来做结论。不是所有被预测的事件都要经过四步。可能有的事件在第二步就达到统一，而不必在第三步中出现。

📖 Studies Cited in Chapter 8（第八章参考文献）

Lazarsfeld, P. Survey design and analysis[M]. New York：The Free Press, 1955.

Chapter 9: Rigor and Validity in Quantitative Research
第九章 量性研究的严谨性和有效性

When conducting quantitative research, it is very important to ensure its rigor and validity, which is an important factor in ensuring the successful conduct of research. Therefore, this chapter will discuss how to measure validity in quantitative research and its influencing factors.

在进行量性研究时，确保其严谨性和有效性十分重要，是确保研究成功进行的一大重要因素。因此，本章节将探讨量性研究中如何测定效度以及其影响因素。

Section Ⅰ Validity and Inference
第一节 有效性及推论

Validity refers to the accuracy of responses on self-report, norm-referenced measures of attitudes and behaviors. Validity representing the degree of authenticity and validity of research conclusions is the core indicator to measure the success or failure of an experiment.

效度是指对自我报告、以规范为参照的态度和行为测量的反应的准确性。效度代表研究结论的真实性程度和有效性程度，是衡量实验成败优劣的核心指标。

1. Types of Validity(效度的类型)

Validity is used by researchers to prove the effectiveness of the design from different aspects. It is an overall investigation. Usually we refer to Shadish et al. (2002) to divide the validity into four types: statistical conclusion validity, internal validity, construct validity, and external validity.

效度是研究者从不同方面用于证明设计的有效性，是一个整体的考察，通常我们参考 Shadish 等(2002)将效度分为四种类型：统计结论效度、内部效度、结构效度和外部效度。

1.1 Statistical Conclusion Validity(统计结论效度)

The validity of statistical conclusions is to detect the relationship between variables. In short, it is to judge "Is there a correlation between these two variables? What kind of relationship is it? (Such as causality, etc.)"

统计结论的有效性是检测变量与变量之间的关系。简而言之,就是判断"这两个变量之间是否存在相关性?这是一种什么样的关系(例如因果关系等)?"

1.2 Internal Validity(内部效度)

Internal validity refers to the effectiveness of the causal relationship between the independent variable and the dependent variable in the study. When considering the relationship between the independent variable and the dependent variable, factors other than the independent variable that may affect the dependent variable should be removed. For example, to study the impact of smoking on the prevalence of lung cancer, we must first exclude family genetic factors, physical and chemical factors, air pollution and other factors that may affect the prevalence. This exclusion can be achieved by statistical methods such as multi-factor regression.

内部效度是指研究中自变量和因变量之间因果关系的有效程度。在考虑自变量和因变量之间关系时要去除自变量以外可能会影响因变量的因素。比如,如果要研究吸烟对肺癌患病率的影响,首先要排除家庭遗传因素、理化因素、空气污染及其他可能影响患病率的因素。这种排除可以用多因素回归等统计方法实现。

1.3 Construct Validity(结构效度)

Construct validity refers to the degree to which the actual results measured in research can reflect the theoretical structure and characteristics to be measured. The higher the construct validity, the better the research can reflect the theory, and the more consistent the two are. There is no single quantitative indicator to describe construct validity.

结构效度是指研究中测量的实际结果能够反映被测量的理论结构和特征的程度。结构效度越高,说明研究越能反映理论,两者的一致性越高。没有单一的定量指标来描述结构效度。

1.4 External Validity(外部效度)

External validity refers to the suitability of the results and conclusions of the study for other groups of people or the general environment, which is the universality of the study conclusions. If a research conclusion can be realized at any time, in any population, and in any environment, it shows that it has high external validity.

外部效度是指研究得出的结果及结论对其他人群或一般环境的适合性，即研究结论推广的普遍性。如果一个研究结论可以在任意时间、任意人群、任意环境中实现就说明该研究的外部效度高。

2. Controlling Confounding Participant Characteristics
（控制参与者特征的混杂影响）

This part describes five ways to control the characteristics of participants in order to control the resulting confounding effects.

以下部分讲述五种控制参与者特征的方法，以控制其产生的混杂效应。

2.1　Randomization(随机化)

Randomization is the most effective method of controlling individual characteristics. The function of randomization is to ensure the accuracy of grouping and to avoid grouping moving with subjective wishes. Randomization can reduce errors caused by inaccurate sampling methods and improper allocation methods, etc., and significantly improve the credibility of research. Randomization can control all possible confounding factors, but it cannot subjectively control a single factor.

随机化是控制个体特征的最有效方法。随机化的作用是保证分组的准确性，避免分组随主观意愿移动。随机化可以减少抽样方法不准确和分配方法不当等造成的误差，显著提高研究的可信度。随机化可以控制所有可能的混杂因素，但不能主观控制单一因素。

2.2　Crossover(交叉)

Crossover design can effectively control the confounding effects of participant characteristics. Crossover means that participants use two relative interventions in pre-and post-study phases, so that they can form their own control in pre-and post-study phases. Using an example to understand the crossover design looks like this: A study exploring the effectiveness of a newly developed drug had 50 participants. They are divided into two groups by randomization, and 25 people used the newly developed drug in the first half of the study, then used an effective drug in the second half of the study; the other 25 people did the opposite, which played a self-control effect. However, the crossover design also has limitations. Firstly, it is only suitable for research with small sample size, and secondly, it cannot eliminate the possible error of the first half of the study on the second half of the study.

交叉设计可以有效地控制参与者特征产生的混杂影响。交叉是指参与者研究前后阶段使用两种相对的干预，从而达到自身在研究前后阶段能形成自身对照。用一个例子来理解交叉设计：一个探索新研发的药物有效程度的研究有 50 个参与者，随机分为两组，有 25 人在研究前半段时间使用新研发的药物，在研究后半段时间使用已知有效的药物；另外 25 个人则相反，这样起到了自身对照的效果。不过交叉设计也有局限性，首先它仅适用于样本量小的研究，其次它无法消除研究前半段对后半段可能产生的误差。

2.3　Stratification/Blocking（分层）

Stratification/Blocking designs are commonly used type of experimental design. The characteristic of blocking design is that the variables used to divide the level and the level of division are closely related to the dependent variable of the study, so this method is used to reduce the error variation. Stratifying participants according to certain characteristics, and then applying different interventions to different groups of participants. In the actual research, the confounding variable is used as the stratification basis of the stratification design, and the gap between the levels becomes smaller, which can reduce the amount of error variation, so that the influence of the variable on the result can be eliminated.

分层设计是一种常用的实验设计类型。分层设计的特点在于用于划分层级的变量和划分的层级与研究的因变量有密切的关系，所以用这种方法降低误差变异。根据参与者的某些特征进行分层，然后对不同组别的参与者实行不同的干预。在实际研究中将混杂变量作为分层设计的分层依据，层级间的差距变小，可以使误差变异量减小，这样就可以消除该变量对结果的影响。

2.4　Matching（匹配）

Matching refers to the selection of participants who are basically the same in certain characteristics for pairing to eliminate the interference of the characteristics. Such characteristics are generally demographic characteristics such as age, gender, education level, marriage and childbirth. But matching also has shortcomings. First, you need to know the relevant confounding factors in advance, otherwise it is difficult to eliminate the impact. Secondly, the use of matching to eliminate the interference of confounding factors can only eliminate the influence of one variable. So matching is not the preferred method of controlling variables.

匹配是指选择在某些特征上基本一致的参与者进行配对，以消除该特征的干扰。这种特征一般为年龄、性别、教育程度、婚育情况等人口学特征。但匹配也有缺点，首先需要提前知道相关的混杂因素，否则难以消除影响。其次使用匹配消除混杂因素的干扰只能消除一个变量的影响。所以匹配不作为首选的控制变量的方法。

2.5　Statistical Control(统计学方法控制)

Statistical analysis is another way to control confounding variables. This method does not change the research design, but processes the data so as to reduce the interference of confounding variables and obtain better results.

统计分析是另一种控制混杂变量的方法。这种方法没有改变研究设计，而是对数据进行处理从而达到削弱混杂变量的干扰，得到较理想的结果。

Section Ⅱ　Statistical Conclusion Validity
第二节　统计结论的有效性

The validity of statistical conclusions is to detect the relationship between variables. In short, it is to judge "Is there a correlation between these two variables? What kind of relationship is it? (Such as causality, etc.)" Researchers can make better research designs and prevent erroneous statistical conclusions from being drawn by improving the validity of statistical conclusions. Shadish et al. (2002) discussed nine threats to statistical conclusion validity.

统计结论效度检测两个变量之间的关系。简而言之，就是判断"这两个变量之间是否存在相关性？这是一种什么样的关系(例如因果关系等)？"研究人员通过提高统计结论效度，可以做出更好的研究设计，防止得出错误的统计结论。Shadish 等(2002)提出了统计结论效度的九大威胁。

1. Reliability of Measures(测量方法的信度)

Reliability is a prerequisite for maintaining high efficiency. If reliability cannot be guaranteed, validity cannot be maintained. One of the methods to maintain validity is to ensure the reliability of the measures.

信度是保持高效度的前提，如果无法保证信度，就无法保持效度。保证效度的方法之一就是确保测量方法的信度。

2. Reliability of Intervention Implementation(干预实施的信度)

One of the other methods to maintain reliability is to ensure the reliability of intervention implementation. If the same implementation process is implemented by different experimenters in different environments, the results are different, which will affect the data analysis and the process of the conclusion. Therefore, it is very important to maintain the reliability of the intervention implementation.

保持可靠性的其他方法之一是确保干预实施的可靠性。如果同样的实施过程在不同环境中被不同实验者进行实施，结果有差异，这会影响数据分析与结论的提出，因此，维持干预实施的信度非常重要。

3. Inaccurate Effect Size Estimates(不精确的效应量估计)

One of the main reasons for the inaccurate estimation of the effect size is the existence of outliers in the data, and data errors may affect the overall effect. There is also an incorrect use of the effect size estimation method, which will also cause the inaccurate effect size.

效应量的估计不准确的主要原因之一是数据中有异常值，数据的错误可能会影响到总体效应。还有错误使用效应量的估计方法，也会导致效应量不准确。

4. Violated Assumptions of Statistical Tests(违背统计检验假设)

Statistical hypotheses are hypotheses about the attributes of the research population. Corty (2007) and Grove (2007) all mentioned that most statistical tests have assumptions about the data collected, such as the following: (1) the data are at least at the interval level; (2) the sample is randomly obtained; and (3) the distribution of scores is normal. Violation of statistical assumptions may cause different results.

统计假设就是关于研究总体属性的假设。Corty(2007)和Grove(2007)都提到大多数统计检验对收集的数据都有假设，例如：(1)数据至少处于区间水平；(2)样本是随机获得的；(3)分数分布正常。违反统计假设可能会得到不同的结果。

5. Fishing and the Error Rate Problem(捕捉和错误率问题)

In research, it is difficult to include everyone in the research population. Different sampling methods are used in order to develop the research. However, this may be a high probability that the results and the hypothesis do not match, and even prove a causal relationship that does not exist in the research population. Type Ⅰ errors are the wrong conclusion that non-existent relationships or differences exist, which means the rejection of a true null. When fishing is used, the part of the analysis accidentally shows a significant relationship or difference, which increases the error rate. Goodwin (1984) has developed a multivariate statistical technique to deal with this error rate problem.

在研究中因很难包含研究人群中的所有人，为了研究的开展会选用不同的抽样方法，但这样可能就会有大概率出现结果和假设不符，甚至证明出一个在研究总体中不存在的因果关系。Ⅰ类错误就是错误地得出不存在的关系或差异存在的结论，即拒绝真正的空值。当使用钓鱼时，分析的部分总体偶然地显示出显著的关系或差异，这就是增加了错误率。Goodwin(1984)已经开发了多变量统计技术来处理这个错误率问题。

6. Low Statistical Power(低统计功效)

Statistical power is the ability to detect the true relationship between variables. A sufficient sample of research is the most direct way to ensure statistical power. Low statistical power means that there is a greater possibility of obtaining results that are directly insignificant in the samples. Aberson (2010) mentioned that Type Ⅱ errors are most likely to occur when the sample size is small or the power of the statistical test to determine the difference is low. Type Ⅱ errors are difficult to reject a false null.

统计功效是检测变量之间真实关系的能力。研究有足够的样本是保证统计功效最直接的方法。统计功效低意味着有更大的可能性得出样本直接没有显著性差异的结果。Aberson(2010)提到当样本量较小或确定差异的统计检验功效较低时，最有可能发生Ⅱ类错误。Ⅱ类错误是指难以拒绝错误的零值。

7. Restriction of Range(范围限制)

Range restrictions affect the relationship between two variables. When the variable range of the independent variable is small, it will be threatened by range restriction. If the measurement of the dependent variable is affected by the ceiling or floor effect, it will also be threatened. Therefore, while controlling the influence of confounding factors, it is also necessary to leave variable space for the measured variables to avoid changing or even disappearing causality.

范围限制会影响两个变量之间的关系。当自变量的变化范围很小，就会受到范围限制的威胁。如果因变量的测量受到天花板或地板效应的影响，同样也会受到其威胁。因此在控制混杂因素影响的同时，也要给所测变量留有可变空间，避免导致因果关系的变化或消失。

8. Random Irrelevancies in the Experimental Setting (实验环境中的随机不相关性)

The environment is the largest and most uncertain influencing variable. As it changes, the measurement and results of the dependent variable will also be affected. Even a slight change in the environment may result in no causal relationship between the independent variable and the dependent variable. Therefore, it is necessary to maintain the consistency of the environment during the research process and reduce interference.

环境作为最大最具不确定性的影响变量，随着它的改变，因变量的测定和结果也会受到影响，甚至稍微改变一下环境，都可能导致自变量和因变量之间不存在因果关系。所以要在研究过程中尽量维持开展时环境的一致性，降低干扰。

9. Random Heterogeneity of Respondents(参与者的随机异质性)

Random heterogeneity refers to the way that participants in the intervention group and the control group are related to the dependent variable in a different way. This is because there is a difference between each individual, which affects the relationship between the independent variable and the dependent variable, and may affect the results of the study.

随机异质性是指干预组和对照组之间的参与者与因变量相关的方式是不一样。这是因为每个个体之间均有差异，会影响自变量和因变量之间的关系，并可能会影响研究的结果。

Section Ⅲ Internal Validity
第三节 内部效度

Internal validity refers to the effectiveness of the causal relationship between the independent variable and the dependent variable in the study, which can represent the authenticity of the research. We infer from an effect to a cause by eliminating or controlling other potential causes.

内部效度是指研究中自变量和因变量之间因果关系的有效程度，可以代表研究的真实程度。我们通过消除或者控制其他潜在原因从结果推断原因。

1. Internal Validity and Research Design(内部效度和研究设计)

Internal validity is very important for research. When conducting experimental research, quasi-experimental research and other related research, it is extremely important to maintain its internal validity, because the internal validity of the studies is very susceptible to the influence of confounding factors.

内部效度对研究来说非常重要。当开展实验性研究、准实验性研究等相关研究时，维持其内部效度极其重要，因为研究的内部效度易受到混杂因素的影响。

The feasibility of each research design will be affected by confounding factors. Due to different research designs, confounding factors also have different influence. For example, the internal validity of the pretest-posttest research design is more sensitive to factors such as instrumentation and history, while factors such as selection and temporal ambiguity have small impact.

研究设计的可行性都会受到混杂因素的影响。由于研究设计的不同，混杂因素对其产生的影响也不同。如前测-后测研究设计的内部效度就对工具和历史等因素较为敏感，而选择和时间模糊等因素就对其影响不大。

When conducting research design, we can improve internal validity by randomly selecting samples, eliminating the influence of confounding factors, repeating measurement data, and choosing appropriate statistical analysis methods, etc.

在进行研究设计时，我们可以通过随机抽取样本，排除混杂因素的影响，重复测量数据，选择合适的统计分析方法等提高内部效度。

2. Internal Validity and Data Analysis(内部效度和数据分析)

The use of appropriate research design can ensure better internal validity. At the same time, appropriate statistical analysis methods are used to control deviations, thereby improving internal validity. In the research process, researchers need to constantly look for variables that may cause bias, and can focus on variables that vary greatly, such as personal characteristics and environmental variables. During data analysis, regression analysis and other methods can be used to reduce the influence of deviation on dependent variables.

使用合适的研究设计可以确保较好的内部效度。同时通过合适的统计分析方法来控制偏差，可以提高内部效度。在研究过程中，研究者就需不断寻找可能会导致偏差的变量，可以重点关注个人特征和环境变量这种变化较大的变量。在进行数据分析时可以通过回归分析及其他方法减弱偏差对因变量的影响。

3. Influencing Factors of Internal Validity(内部效度的影响因素)

3.1 Selection Bias(选择偏差)

Selection bias refers to the deviation in sampling and grouping, because individuals in the population will inevitably have differences. Randomization can significantly weaken the threat of selection (Kerlinger & Lee, 2000; Thompson, 2002). Selection bias is the most problematic and frequent threats to the internal validity of studies not using an experimental design.

选择是指总体和样本难免会有差异，因为总体中的个体不可避免地会有差异。随机化可以明显削弱选择这一方面的威胁(Kerlinger 和 Lee, 2000; Thompson 2002)。选择偏差是对不使用实验设计的研究的内部有效性的最大问题和最常见的威胁。

3.2 Temporal Ambiguity(时间模糊)

Causality means that an event is considered to be the result of the previous event. When measuring variables, it should also be noted that the measurement of processing variables must be before the measurement result variables, otherwise there will be time ambiguity, which will threaten internal validity.

因果关系是指一个事件被认为是前一个事件的结果。测量变量时也要注意，处理变量的测量必然是在测量结果变量之前的，否则就会出现时间模糊，而对内部效度产生威胁。

3.3　Instrumentation(工具)

The choice of research instruments also affects internal validity. For example, questionnaires with reliability and validity can be used after obtaining the consent of the original author, which has no effect at all. However, a self-made questionnaire may have certain risks, so it is necessary to conduct a pre-test to measure its reliability and validity. For tools that cannot be measured for reliability and validity, such as thermometers and sphygmomanometers, though we cannot avoid errors, we must do a good job in the calibration of the tools and maintain a good internal validity of the research.

研究工具的选择也会影响内部效度。例如，在获取原作者的同意后，可以使用已经有信效度的问卷，这种完全没有影响。但自制的问卷可能就会有一定的风险，所以必须要进行前测，测量其信效度。对于无法测量信效度的工具，如温度计和血压计，我们虽然难以避免误差，但必须做好工具的校准工作，维持良好的研究内部效度。

3.4　Testing Effect(测试效应)

The test effect refers to the influence of the pretest on the posttest. This threat has the greatest impact on research designs that requiring repeated testing. If there is a short interval between two tests, participants remember uncontrollable factors such as the last answer, which may affect the measurement of the results and the internal validity.

测试效应是指前测对后测造成的影响。这种威胁对需要反复进行测试的研究设计影响最大。如果出现两次测试时间之间相隔时间短，参与者记得上次的答案等不可控因素，可能就会影响结果的测量，影响内部效度。

3.5　History(历史)

External events unrelated to the research that have not been controlled and processed affect the measurement of the dependent variable, which is the historical effect. For example, we want to study the awareness of the elderly people in the community about senile diseases, but during the investigation process, suddenly a medical school volunteer come to preach knowledge about hypertension and diabetes, and the elderly in the community may learn more about hypertension and diabetes, which will affect our research results

没有进行控制处理的与研究无关的外部事件会影响因变量的测量，这就是历史效应。

例如，我们要研究社区内老人对老年病的认知情况，但在调查过程中，突然有医学院的志愿者来宣讲关于高血压、糖尿病的知识，社区内的老人对高血压、糖尿病有更多的了解，这会影响我们的研究结果。

3.6 Maturation(成熟)

"Maturation" in research means that the physical and psychological changes of participants over time, and such changes, whether positive or negative, will threaten internal validity.

"成熟"在研究中意味着随着时间的推移，参与者的生理和心理发生了变化，这种变化无论是正向还是负向的都会对内部效度产生威胁。

3.7 Mortality/Attrition(死亡率/流失)

The loss and death of participants is unavoidable in the research process. For example, long-term follow-up in a cohort study cannot guarantee the loss of sample size caused by the cooperation of participants, or researches on cancer patients cannot be sure that that they will not encounter the death of the participant during the research process. However, as long as the loss rate is within the normal range and the loss of the population is random, it can be guaranteed that the research will not be biased.

在研究过程中，参与者的损失和死亡是不可避免的。例如，在队列研究中的长期随访难以保证因参与者的配合度导致的样本量流失，又或是针对癌症患者的研究不能确定在研究过程中不会遇到参与者的死亡。不过只要流失率在正常范围内，流失的人群是随机的，就可以保证研究不会有偏差。

Section Ⅳ Construct Validity
第四节 结构效度

Construct Validity is an indicator that reflects whether the experiment actually measures the hypothesis or construction. Construct validity is determined by adding up variables that need to be measured and variables that do not need to be measured, so a single quantitative index cannot be used to describe it.

结构效度是反映实验是否真正测量了假设或者构造的指标。结构效度是通过需要测量的变量和不需要测量的变量累加起来给予确定的，所以不可以用单一的数量指标来描述结构效度。

1. Enhancing Construct Validity(增强结构效度)

Shadish et al. (2002) have broadened the concept of construct validity, which covered persons, settings, outcomes and treatments. Qualitative description is often a powerful means of enhancing the construct validity.

Shadish 等(2002)拓宽了结构效度的概念,它涵盖了人、环境、结果和治疗。定性描述通常是增强结构效度的有力手段。

If you want to improve the construct validity, pay attention to the issues related to the results. Whether the selected intervention or treatment can be fed back by measuring the independent variable, and whether the selected dependent variable can provide true feedback of the results. Besides, the selected research population needs to meet the requirements. For example, a certain study is for perinatal women, and the research population we need is maternal women from 28 weeks of pregnancy to one week after delivery. In non-experimental studies, the independent variable (intervention or treatment) is difficultly predicted and intervened, so the construct validity should be more controlled.

如果你想要提高结构效度,就要关注与结果相关的问题:选择的干预或治疗是否可以通过测量自变量反馈;选择的因变量是否可以真实地反馈结果;选择的研究人群需要符合要求。例如,某一研究是针对围产期女性,我们需要的研究人群是怀孕 28 周到产后一周的孕产妇。在非实验性研究中,自变量(干预或治疗)难以预测和干预,所以结构效度更需要控制。

2. Influencing Factors of Construct Validity(结构效度的影响因素)

2.1 Inadequate Clarification of Constructs(构造的不充分说明)

Inaccurate or inappropriate definitions and main characteristics of constructs will cause changes in the relationship between variables and constructs, resulting in low construct validity.

构造的定义和主要特征的不准确或不恰当会引起变量和构造之间的关系发生变化,导致低结构效度。

2.2 Mono-operation Bias(单操作偏差)

Mono-operation bias occurs when only one questionnaire or instrument is used to measure the dependent variable. The measured structural dimensions are less. If researchers use more than one instrument, the construct validity will be greatly improved (Waltz 等, 2010). Using multiple tools can not only ensure construct validity, but also avoid research hindrance caused by unsatisfactory measures of outcome indicators.

当测量因变量仅使用一种问卷或工具时就会出现单一操作误差。测量的构造维度较少。如果研究人员使用一种以上的工具，则结构效度会很大提高（Waltz 等, 2010）。使用多种工具不仅可以确保结构效度，还可以避免结局指标测量不理想而导致的研究阻碍。

2.3 Monomethod Bias(单方法偏差)

Monomethod bias refers to the threat caused by using only one processing or measurement method. For example, the measure of tension cannot only be measured by questionnaires, but can also be measured by physical signs such as heart rate and blood pressure, and the construct validity will be consolidated.

单方法偏差是指只用一种处理或测量方法而导致的威胁。例如紧张感的测试并不能只通过问卷，同时可以通过心率、血压等体征来衡量，结构效度就会有所巩固。

2.4 Reactivity to the Study Situation(对研究情况的反应性)

Participants may behave in a specific way, because they are aware of their role in the research. For example, at the time of the questionnaire, the participants may fill in the direction that is beneficial to them. Subjective measurement methods are easily affected by this factor.

参与者可能会以特定的方式行事，因为他们意识到自己在研究中的角色。例如，问卷调查时，参与者可能会向有利于他们的方向填写。主观性强的测量方式易受到该因素的影响。

2.5 Experimenter Expectancies(实验者期望)

Every experimenter hopes that the research can produce a satisfactory result. Therefore, during the research process, the experimenter will reveal this expectation to participants intentionally or unintentionally, and the final result of the research will be passively changed. In experimental studies, double-blind experiments can well avoid this threat. No matter in what kind of research, the experimenter must control himself and not subjectively influence the participants.

　　每个实验者都希望研究能得出一个满意的结果，所以在研究过程中，实验者会有意无意地向参与者透露这种期望，研究的最终结果就会被动地改变。在实验性研究中，双盲实验可以很好地避免这一威胁。无论在哪种研究中实验者都要去控制自己，不去主观地影响参与者。

2.6　Novelty Effects(新奇效应)

When an intervention or treatment is novel, participants will be either full of interest or full of suspicion, and this will affect the results of the research. This new treatment method may have disruptive effects when it affects the participants' routine lives. The research result may reflect the effect of the new treatment method due to novelty, not its own effect.

　　当一个干预或治疗是很新颖的，参与者就会充满兴趣或者充满怀疑，这都会影响到研究的结果。当这种新处理方法影响到参与者的常规生活时可能就会出现扰乱效应。研究结果可能反映的是新处理方法因新奇产生的效应，并不是其本身的效应。

Section Ⅴ　External Validity
第五节　外部效度

External validity refers to the suitability of the results and conclusions of the study for other groups of people or the general environment.

　　外部效度是指研究结果及结论对其他人群或一般环境的适合性。

1. Enhancements to External Validity(增强外部效度)

External validity mainly needs to consider the validity of two aspects, on the one hand, whether the sample can effectively represent the whole, on the other hand, whether the research results can be effectively applied in reality.

　　外部效度主要需要考虑两方面的有效性，一方面是样本是否能有效地代表整体，另一方面是研究结果是否能有效地应用于现实中。

The research sample is only a part of the whole, and it is hard to say that it can completely represent the whole, but we can get more similar answers through different sampling methods and repeated experiments. A single study is difficult to generalize to the population, but it is more convincing if the same results are obtained from repeated studies of different samples.

研究样本只是总体的一部分，难以说能完全代表总体，但我们可以通过不同的抽样方法和反复实验得到更相近的答案。单一的研究难以推广到总体中，但如果针对不同样本的重复多次研究都得出相同结果的话就能更让人信服。

The environment is the most difficult to predict influencing factor, and the variability is much stronger than other factors. Therefore, in the research process, we cannot blindly eliminate confounding factors and create an ideal environment. The results obtained in this way may be difficult to generalize to "real life".

环境是最难预测的影响因素，可变性相对于其他因素来说要强很多。所以在研究过程中不能一味地剔除混杂因素，营造理想化的环境，这样得出来的结果可能难以推广到"现实"中。

2. Influencing Factors of External Validity(外部效度的影响因素)

2.1　Interaction Between Relationship and People(关系和人群的交互作用)

The relationship between the independent variable and the dependent variable can be reflected in this special population, but it has no relationship in another population with different characteristics. Similarly, although the research sample is part of the overall relationship, sometimes the relationship obtained is difficult to generalize, so we should try to randomize as much as possible when conducting research.

自变量和因变量之间的关系在这一特殊人群中能体现，然而在另一不同特征的人群中却没有关系。同样地，虽然研究样本为总体的一部分，但是有时得出的关系也难以进行推广，所以我们进行研究时要做到尽可能地随机化。

2.2　Interaction Between Causal Effects and Treatment Variation(因果效应和处理变异的交互作用)

This refers to the impact on causality when dealing with variables. How to deal with the influence of confounding variables on independent and dependent variables and the mutual influence between confounding variables is the key to controlling this big threat.

这是指在处理变量时对因果关系造成的影响。如何处理混杂变量对自变量和因变量的影响以及处理混杂变量之间的相互影响是控制这一大威胁的关键。

2.3 Interaction Between Relationship and Results(关系和结果的交互作用)

The causality depends on how the dependent variable is measured in the research. For example, if we want to measure the postpartum depression of parturient, we can choose different scales such as Edinburgh Postpartum Depression Scale (EPDS), Hamilton Depression Scale (HAMD), etc. The measured values and results will be different, which may affect the final conclusions.

因果关系取决于研究中如何测量因变量。例如，如果我们要测产妇产后抑郁的情况，我们可以选择不同的量表，如爱丁堡产后抑郁量表(EPDS)和汉密顿抑郁量表(HAMD)等。测出来的数值和结果会有不同，可能会影响最后的结论。

2.4 Interaction Between Relationship and Setting(关系和环境的交互作用)

The environment as an uncertain factor has a great influence on variables. The causal relationship between the independent variable and the dependent variable may change due to changes in the environment. If there is an intermediary variable between the causality between the two, this intermediary variable may also change due to changes in the environment.

环境作为一个不确定因素对变量有极大的影响。自变量和因变量之间的因果关系可能会因为环境的改变而变化。如果两者的因果关系之间有中介变量，这个中介变量可能也会因为环境的改变而变化。

Section Ⅵ Critiquing Guidelines for Study Validity
第六节 研究效度的评判指引

Ensuring the validity of research is the way for the research processed smoothly. Focus on issues related to validity to further help to criticize the quantitative research design. The following are some guidelines mentioned by D. F. Polit et al. (2012) to evaluate the validity of research in quantitative research:

确保研究的有效性是研究顺利进行的必经之路。关注效度相关的问题，进一步帮助批评定量研究设计。下面是 D. F. Polit 等(2012)提到的一些在定量研究中评估研究有效性的指南：

（1）Was there adequate statistical power? Was precision enhanced by controlling confounding variables? What evidence did the report provide that selection biases were eliminated or minimized?

是否有足够的统计功效？是否通过控制混杂变量提高了精确度？报告提供了哪些证据表明选择偏差已被消除或最小化？

（2）What extent did the study design rule out other threats to internal validity? What are your overall conclusions about the internal validity of the study?

研究设计在多大程度上排除了对内部效度的其他威胁？您对研究内部效度的总体结论是什么？

（3）Were there any major threats to the construct validity of the study?

研究的结构效度是否存在重大威胁？

（4）Was the context of the study sufficiently described to enhance its external validity? Were there other factors that threaten external validity?

是否充分描述了研究背景以增强其外部效度？是否还存在其他威胁外部效度的因素？

（5）Did the researcher appropriately balance validity concerns?

研究人员是否适当地平衡了效度问题？

Overall, statistical conclusion validity, internal validity, construct validity, and external validity all need to be considered. There may be a restraining relationship between them, and how to balance them well is the key to the problem.

总体而言，统计结论效度、内部效度、结构效度和外部效度都需要考虑到。它们之间可能存在着一种制约关系，如何平衡好它们才是问题的关键。

📖 Studies Cited in Chapter 9（第九章参考文献）

［1］Shadish, W., Cook, T., Campbell, D. Experimental and Quasi-Experimental Designs For Generalized Causal Inference［M］. Boston: Houghton Mifflin, 2002.

［2］Waltz, C. F., Strickland, O. L., Lenz, E. R. Measurement in nursing and health research ［M］. 4th ed. New York, NY: Springer Publishing Company, 2010.

［3］Corty, E. W. Using and interpreting statistics: A practical text for the health, behavioral, and social sciences［M］. St. Louis, MO: Mosby Elsevier, 2007.

［4］Grove, S. K. Statistics for health care research: A practical workbook［M］. Philadelphia, PA: Saunders Elsevier, 2007.

［5］Aberson, C. L. Applied power analysis for the behavioral sciences［M］. New York, NY:

Routledge Taylor & Francis Group，2010.

［6］Kerlinger，F. N.，Lee，H. B. Foundations of behavioral research （4th ed.）［M］. Fort Worth，TX：Harcourt College Publishers，2000.

［7］Thompson，S. K. Sampling［M］. 2nd ed. New York：John Wiley & Sons，2002.

［8］Polit，D. F.，Tatano Beck，C. Nursing Research Generating and Assessing Evidence for Nursing Practice［M］. London：Wolters Kluwer，2012.

Chapter 10: Sampling in Quantitative Research
第十章 量性研究的抽样

Section Ⅰ Basic Sampling Concepts
第一节 抽样基本概念

1. Populations(总体)

Population (the "P" of PICO questions) is the entire aggregation of cases that the researcher is interested. For instance, if we were studying American nurses with doctoral degrees, the population could be defined as all U. S. citizens who are registered nurses (RNs) and have a PhD, DNSc, DNP, or other doctoral degrees. Other possible population might be all patients who had cardiac surgery in Hospital in 2015, all women with irritable bowel syndrome in Beijing, or all children in China with cystic fibrosis. Population is not restricted to humans. Population might consist of all hospital records in a particular hospital or all blood samples at a particular laboratory. Whatever the basic unit, the population comprises the aggregate of elements in which the researcher is interested.

总体(PICO 问题的"P")是研究人员感兴趣的所有案例的集合。例如，如果我们研究的是拥有博士学位的美国护士，那么总体可以定义为拥有 PhD、DNSc、DNP 或其他博士学位的注册护士的所有美国公民。其他潜在的人群可能是 2015 年在医院接受心脏手术的所有患者、北京所有患有肠易激综合征的女性，或者中国所有患有囊性纤维化的儿童。总体并不局限于人类，可以由某家医院的所有医院记录或者某个实验室的所有血液样本组成。无论基本单位是什么，总体都是由研究者感兴趣的元素的总和组成的。

2. Samples and Sampling(样本和抽样)

Sampling is the process of selecting cases to represent an entire population to permit inferences about the population. The sample is a subset of population elements, which is the most basic unit of data collection. In nursing research, the most common elements are humans.

抽样是选择代表整个总体的案例,以便对总体进行推断的过程。样本是总体元素的子集,是收集数据的最基本单位。在护理研究中,最常见的因素是人。

Sample and sampling plans vary in quality. Two key considerations in assessing a sample in a quantitative study are its representativeness and size. A representative sample is one whose key characteristics closely approximate those of the population. If the population in a study of patients who fall is 50% male and 50% female, then a representative sample would have a similar gender distribution. If the sample is not representative of the population, the study's external validity and construct validity are at risk.

样本和抽样计划的质量各不相同。在定量研究中评估样本的两个关键考虑因素是其代表性和规模。具有代表性的样本是其关键特征接近于总体特征的样本。如果在一项跌倒患者的研究中,50%的男性和50%的女性,那么具有代表性的样本将具有类似的性别分布。如果样本不能代表总体,那么研究的外部效度和结构效度就有风险。

Certain sampling methods are less likely to produce biased samples than others, but a representative sample can never be guaranteed. Researchers work under conditions where errors are likely to occur. Quantitative researchers strive to minimize errors and estimate the magnitude of error where possible.

某些抽样方法比其他方法产生有偏差的样本的可能性更低,但一个具有代表性的样本是无法得到保证的。研究人员在可能出现错误的条件下工作。定量研究人员努力减少误差,并在可能的情况下估计误差的大小。

Sampling designs can be divided into probability sampling and nonprobability sampling. Probability sampling involves the random selection of elements. In probability sampling, researchers can specify the probability that an element of the population will be included in the sample.

抽样设计可分为概率抽样和非概率抽样。概率抽样涉及元素的随机选择。在概率抽样中,研究人员可以指定总体中的一个元素将被包括在样本中的概率。

3. Strata(分层)

Sometimes, it is useful to think of populations as consisting of sub-populations or strata. A stratum is a mutually exclusive part of population, defined by one or more characteristics. For instance, assume that the population of the United Kingdom is all registered nurses. This population could be divided into two strata based on gender. Alternatively, we could divide nurses into three groups: those younger than 30 years old, those aged 30 to 45 years, and those 46 years or older. Stratification is often used in sample selection to improve the sample's representativeness.

有时，把总体看作由亚总体或阶层组成是有用的。一个阶层是一个总体中相互排斥的部分，由一个或多个特征来定义。例如，假设英国的人口都是注册护士。这个总体可以根据性别分为两个阶层。或者，我们可以把护士分为三组：30 岁以下的护士，30~45 岁的护士，以及 46 岁以上的护士。为了提高样本的代表性，在样本选择中经常使用分层。

4. Staged Sampling(分段抽样)

Sampling is sometimes carried out in several stages, known as multi-stage sampling. In the first stage, large units (such as hospitals or nursing homes) are selected. Then, in the next stage, individuals are sampled. In staged sampling, it is possible to combine probability and nonprobability sampling. For example, the first stage can include the deliberate (nonrandom) selection of study sites. Then, people within the selected sites can be selected through random procedures.

抽样有时要分多个阶段进行，即所谓的多阶段采样。在第一阶段，选择大的单位(如医院或疗养院)。然后，在下一阶段，对个体进行抽样。在分阶段抽样中，概率抽样和非概率抽样可以结合使用。例如，第一阶段可以包括有意(非随机)选择研究地点。然后，可以通过随机程序选择被选地点内的人。

5. Sampling Bias(抽样偏差)

Researchers work with samples rather than with populations because it is cost-effective to do so. Researchers seldom have the resources to study all members of the population. It may be possible to obtain reasonably accurate information from a sample, but data from samples can be erroneous. Finding 100 people willing to participate in a study may be easy, but it is usually difficult to select 100 people who are an unbiased subset of the population. Sampling bias refers to the systematic over-or underrepresentation of the population segment on a characteristic relevant to the research question.

研究人员使用的是样本而不是总体，因为这样做具有成本效益。研究人员很少有资源来研究一个总体的所有成员。从样本中获得的信息可能是合理准确的，但从样本中获得的数据可能有错误。找到 100 个愿意参与一项研究的人可能很容易，但通常很难选出 100 个不带偏见的人。抽样偏差指的是与研究问题相关的某一特征的总体部分具有系统性的过多或过少的代表性。

As an example of consciously biased selection, suppose we were investigating patients' responsiveness to nurses' touch and decide to recruit the first 50 patients meeting eligibility criteria. We decide, however, to omit Mr. Z from the sample because he has been hostile to nursing staff. Mrs. X, who has just lost a spouse, is also bypassed. These decisions to exclude certain people do not reflect bona fide eligibility criteria. This can lead to bias because responsiveness to nurses' touch (the outcome variable) may be affected by patients' feelings about nurses or their emotional state.

作为有意识偏向选择的一个例子，假设我们正在调查病人对护士触摸的反应性，并决定招募前 50 名符合资格标准的病人。然而，我们决定将 Z 先生从样本中删除，因为他对护理人员怀有敌意。刚刚失去配偶的 X 夫人也被忽略了。这些排除某些人的决定并不反映真实的资格标准。这可能会导致偏见，因为对护士触摸的反应性(结果变量)可能会受到患者对护士的感觉或他们的情绪的影响。

However, sampling bias often occurs unconsciously. If we were studying nursing students and systematically interviewed every 10th student who entered the nursing school library, the sample would be biased towards library enthusiasts, even if we do not consider age, gender or other characteristics.

然而，抽样偏差往往是无意识地产生的。如果我们以护理专业的学生为研究对象，系统地采访每 10 个中第 10 个进入学校图书馆的学生，即使我们不考虑年龄、性别或其他特征，样本也会偏向于喜欢待在图书馆的学生。

Section Ⅱ　Principles of Sampling and Grouping
第二节　抽样和分组原则

Randomization is the basic principle of sampling and grouping. Random sampling means that in the process of sampling, whether each individual in the population will be selected or not is not determined subjectively by the researcher, but according to the principle of randomness. To ensure that each object in the population has a known probability of being selected as the object of study, so as to ensure the representativeness of the sample. Random grouping means that each observation unit of the whole population has the same chance to be selected into the sample and divided into groups. The purpose is to make the experimental group and the control group comparable through randomness and balance the influence of interference factors, so as to avoid bias caused by subjective arrangements.

随机化是抽样和分组的基本原则。随机抽样是指在进行抽样时，总体中每一个体是否被抽取，并不由研究者主观决定，而是按照随机的原则。保证总体中每一个对象都有已知的一定概率被选入作为研究的对象，从而保证样本的代表性。随机分组是指总体的每一个观察单位都有同等的机会被选入样本中来，并有同等的机会进行分组。目的是通过随机，均衡干扰因素的影响，使试验组和对照组具有可比性，避免主观安排带来的偏性。

Section Ⅲ　Nonprobability Sampling
第三节　非概率抽样

1. Convenience Sampling(便利抽样)

Convenience sampling entails using the most conveniently available people as participants. For example, a nurse who conducts a study of adolescent risk-taking at a local senior high school is relying on a convenience sample. The problem with convenience sampling is that those who are available might be atypical of the population with regard to critical variables.

方便抽样要求使用最方便的人作为参与者。例如，一名护士对当地一所高中的青少年冒险行为进行了一项研究，研究依据的是便利样本。便利抽样的问题是，那些可用的人在关键变量方面可能是非典型的人群。

Sometimes, researchers look for people with certain characteristics place an advertisement in newspapers, put up signs in clinics, or post messages on online social media. These "convenient" approaches are subject to bias because people select themselves as volunteers in response to posted notices and likely differ from those who do not volunteer.

有时，研究人员通过在报纸上登广告、在诊所张贴标语、在线上社交媒体上发布消息的方式寻找具有某些特征的人。这些"方便"的方法容易受到偏见的影响，因为人们选择自己作为志愿者来响应张贴的通知，很可能不同于那些不做志愿者的人。

Snowball sampling (also called network sampling or chain sampling) is a variant of convenience sampling. With this approach, early sample members (called seeds) are asked to refer other people who meet the eligibility criteria. This approach is often used when the population involves people who might be difficult to identify (e. g., people who are afraid of hospitals).

滚雪球抽样(又称网络抽样或链式抽样)是方便抽样的一种变体。通过这种方法,早期的样本成员(称为种子)被要求推荐其他符合资格标准的人。当人群中包括那些可能难以确定的人(例如,害怕去医院的人)时,通常使用这种方法。

Convenience sampling is the weakest form of sampling. In heterogeneous populations, there is no other sampling approach in which the risk of sampling bias is greater. However, convenience sampling is the most commonly used method in many disciplines.

方便抽样是抽样的最弱形式。在异质群体中,没有其他抽样方法存在更大的抽样偏差风险。然而,便利抽样是许多学科中最常用的方法。

2. Quota Sampling(配额抽样)

A quota sample is one in which the researcher identifies population strata and determines how many participants are needed from each strata. By using information about population characteristics, researchers can ensure that diverse segments are represented in the sample, and in the proportion in which they occur in the population.

配额样本是研究者确定人口阶层并确定每个阶层需要多少参与者的样本。通过使用有关总体特征的信息,研究人员可以确保在样本中代表总体的不同部分,以及他们在总体中的比例。

Suppose we were interested in studying nursing students' attitude toward working with AIDS patients. The accessible population is a school of nursing with 500 undergraduate students; a sample of 100 students is desired. The simplest procedure would be to distribute questionnaires in classrooms through convenience sampling. However, suppose we suspect that male and female students have different attitudes. A convenience sample might result in too males or females.

假设我们有兴趣研究护理学生对与艾滋病患者打交道的态度。可获取人群是一所有 500 名本科生的护理学院;要求以 100 名学生为样本。最简单的方法是通过方便抽样在教室里分发问卷。然而,假设我们怀疑男女学生有不同的态度,便利样本可能会导致过多的男性或女性。

Quota sampling does not require complex techniques or a lot of effort. Many researchers who use convenience samples could profitably use quota sampling. Stratification should be based on variables that would reflect important differences in the dependent variable. Variables such as gender, ethnicity, education, and medical diagnosis may be good stratifying variables.

配额抽样不需要复杂的技术或大量的努力。许多使用方便样本的研究人员可以有益地使用配额抽样。分层应以反映因变量中重要差异的变量为基础。性别、种族、教育和医疗诊断等变量可能是很好的分层变量。

Procedurally, quota sampling is similar to convenience sampling. People in any subgroup are a convenience sample from that population strata. Quota sampling can share similar weaknesses as convenience sampling. For instance, if a researcher needs to interview 10 men between the ages of 65 and 80 years under a quota sampling plan, a visit to a nursing home might be the most convenient method of obtaining participants. Yet this approach would fail to represent the many older men living independently in the community. Despite its limitations, quota sampling is a major improvement over convenience sampling.

从程序上讲，配额抽样类似于方便抽样。任何子群体中的人都是来自该群体阶层的便利样本。配额抽样与方便抽样有相似的缺点。例如，如果一名研究人员根据配额抽样计划需要采访 10 名年龄为 65 岁的男性，那么去养老院可能是获得参与者的最方便的方法。然而，这种方法不能代表社区中许多独立生活的老年人。尽管有局限性，但配额抽样相对于方便抽样是一个重大改进。

3. Purposive Sampling(目的抽样)

Purposive sampling uses researchers' knowledge about the population to make selections. Researchers might purposefully select people who are judged to be particularly knowledgeable about the issues under study, for example, in the case of a Delphi survey. A drawback is that this approach seldom results in a typical or representative sample. Purposive sampling is sometimes superior in two-staged sampling. That is, a purposive sample of locations can be taken first, followed by a sample of people in other ways.

目的抽样利用研究者对总体的了解来进行选择。研究人员可能会有目的地选择那些被认为对所研究问题特别了解的人，例如，在德尔菲调查的情况下。缺点是这种方法很少产生典型或有代表性的样本。在两阶段抽样中，目的抽样有时具有很强的优越性。也就是说，可以先对地点进行有目的的抽样，然后再以其他方式对人进行抽样。

4. Evaluation of Nonprobability Sampling(评估非概率抽样)

Except for some consecutive samples, nonprobability samples are rarely representative of the population. When every element in the population does not have a chance of being included in the sample, it is likely that some segment of it will be systematically underrepresented. Results could be misleading when there is sampling bias, and efforts to generalize to a broader population could be misguided.

除了一些连续的样本外，非概率样本很少能代表总体。当总体中的每个元素都没有机会被纳入样本时，样本中的某些部分很可能会被系统地低估。当存在抽样偏差时，结果可能会产生误导，而将结果推广到更广泛的人群时会产生误导。

However, non-probability samples will continue to predominate because of their practicality. Probability sampling requires skills and resources, so there may be no option but to use a nonprobability approach. However, strict convenience sampling should be avoided in the absence of to improve representativeness. Indeed, it has been argued that quantitative researchers would likely do better at achieving representative samples for generalizing to the population if they have a more purposive approach.

然而，由于其实用性，非概率抽样将继续占主导地位。概率抽样需要技能和资源，所以除了使用非概率方法外可能没有其他选择。但是，在没有明确努力提高代表性的情况下，应该避免严格的便利抽样。事实上，有人认为，如果定量研究人员有一种更有目的性的方法，他们可能会更好地获得具有代表性的样本，以推广到总体。

Quota sampling is a semi-purposive sampling strategy that is far superior to convenience sampling because it seeks to ensure sufficient representation within key strata of the population. Another purposive strategy for enhancing generalizability is deliberate multi-site sampling. For instance, a convenience sample could be obtained from two communities known to differ socio-economically, so that the sample would reflect the experiences of both lower and middle-class participants. In other words, if the population is known to be heterogeneous, then this step should be taken to capture significant variation in the sample.

配额抽样是一种半目的抽样策略，它远优于方便抽样，因为它寻求确保在总体的关键阶层中有足够的代表性。另一个增强可泛化性的目的策略是有意地多地点抽样。例如，可以从已知的社会经济上不同的两个社区获得便利样本，以便该样本反映低收入和中产阶级参与者的经验。换句话说，如果已知总体是异质性的，那么应该采取此步骤来捕获样本中的重要变异。

Even in one-site studies in which convenience sampling is used, researchers can make an effort to explicitly add cases to correspond more closely to population characteristics. For example, if half the population is known to be male, then the researcher can check to see if approximately half the sample is male and use outreach to recruit more males if necessary.

即使在使用方便抽样的单点研究中，研究人员也可以努力明确地增加案例，以更接近于总体特征。例如，如果已知总体的一半是男性，那么研究人员可以检查是否大约样本的一半是男性，如果必要的话，扩大招募更多的男性。

Quantitative researchers using non-probability samples must be cautious about the inferences they make. When there are efforts to deliberately improve representativeness and to interpret results conservatively, non-probability sampling may work quite well when the study is repeated with a new sample.

使用非概率抽样的定量研究人员必须对他们做出的推论保持谨慎。当有刻意提高代表性和保守地解释结果时，当用新的样本重复这项研究时，非概率抽样可能会发挥相当好的作用。

Section IV　Probability Sampling
第四节　概率抽样/随机抽样

1. Simple Random Sampling(简单随机抽样)

Simple random sampling is the most basic probability sampling design. In simple random sampling, researchers establish a sampling frame, the technical name for the list of elements from which the sample will be selected. If nursing students at the University of Connecticut are the accessible population, then a roster of those students would be the sampling frame. If the sampling unit were 300-bed or larger hospitals in Taiwan, then a list of all such hospitals would be the sampling frame. Sometimes, a population is defined in terms of an existing sampling frame. For example, if we wanted to use a voter registration list as a sampling frame, we would have to define the community population as residents who had registered to vote.

简单随机抽样是最基本的概率抽样设计。在简单随机抽样中，研究人员建立一个抽样框架，将从中选择样本的元素列表的名称。如果康涅狄格大学的护理学生是可获取的人群，那么这些学生的花名册将是抽样框架。若抽样单位为中国台湾地区拥有 300 个病床及以上的医院，则以所有此类医院的名称列表为抽样框架。有时，总体是根据现有的抽样框架来定义的。例如，如果我们想使用选民登记列表作为抽样框架，我们必须将社区总体定义为已登记投票的居民。

A sample selected randomly in this way is unbiased. Although there is no guarantee that a random sample will be representative, random selection ensures that differences in the attributes of the sample and the population are purely a function of chance. The probability of selecting an unrepresentative sample decrease as the sample size increases.

以这种方式随机选取的样本是无偏的。虽然不能保证一个随机样本具有代表性，但随机选择可以确保样本和总体属性的差异纯粹是一个概率函数。选择非代表性样本的概率随着样本大小的增加而降低。

Simple random sampling tends to be laborious. Developing a sampling frame, numbering all elements, and selecting elements are time-consuming chores, particularly if the population is large. In practice, simple random sampling is used infrequently because it is relatively inefficient. Furthermore, it is not always possible to obtain a listing of every element in the population, so other methods may be required.

简单的随机抽样往往是费力的。开发一个采样框架、对所有元素进行编号和选择元素都是非常耗时的工作，特别是在数量很大的情况下。在实际应用中，由于简单随机抽样的效率相对较低，所以很少使用。此外，并不总是可能获得一个列表包含总体中的每个元素，因此可能需要其他方法。

2. Stratified Random Sampling(分层随机抽样)

In stratified random sampling, the population is first divided into two or more strata, with the goal of improving representativeness. Researchers using stratified random sampling subdivide the population into homogeneous subsets (e. g., based on gender or illness severity), from which elements are selected at random.

在分层随机抽样中，首先将总体分为两个或两个以上的阶层，目的是提高代表性。研究人员使用分层随机抽样将总体细分为均匀的子集(例如，根据性别或疾病严重程度)，从这些子集中随机选择元素。

In stratified sampling, a person's status in a stratum must be known before random selection, which can be problematic. Patient listings or organizational directories may contain information for meaningful stratification (e. g., about a person's gender), but many lists do not.

Quota sampling does not have the same problem because researchers can ask people questions that determine their eligibility for a particular stratum.

在分层抽样中，一个人在一个阶层中的状态必须在随机选择之前知道，这可能是有问题的。病人列表或组织目录可能包含有意义的分层信息（例如，关于一个人的性别），但许多列表没有。配额抽样不存在同样的问题，因为研究人员可以问人们一些问题，来确定他们是否有资格进入某个特定阶层。

Stratification usually divides the population into unequal subpopulations. For example, if the person's race were used to stratify the population of U. S. citizens, the subpopulation of white people would be larger than that of nonwhite people. In proportionate stratified sampling, participants are selected in proportion to the size of the population stratum. If the population is students in a nursing school with 10% African American, 10% Hispanic, 10% Asian, and 70% white students, then a proportionate stratified sample of 100 students, with race/ethnicity as the stratify, will be drawn 10, 10, 10, and 70 students from the respective strata.

分层化通常把总体分成不相等的亚总体。例如，如果一个人的种族被用来对美国公民的总体进行分层，那么白人的亚总体就会比非白人的亚总体大。在比例分层抽样中，参与者是按人口阶层的大小比例选择的。如果人群是一所护理学校的学生，其中有10%的非裔美国人、10%的西班牙裔、10%的亚洲裔和70%的白种人学生，然后按比例分层抽样100名学生，以种族/族裔为分层，将从各自的阶层中抽取10名、10名、10名和70名学生。

Proportionate sampling may result in insufficient numbers for making comparisons among strata. In our example, it would be risky to draw conclusions about Hispanic nursing students based on only 10 cases. For this reason, researchers may use disproportionate sampling when comparisons are sought between strata of greatly unequal size. In the example, the sampling proportions might be altered to select 20 African American, 20 Hispanic, 20 Asian, and 40 white students. This design would ensure a more adequate representation of the three racial/ethnic minorities. When disproportionate sampling is used, however, it is necessary to make an adjustment to arrive at the best estimate of overall population values. This adjustment is known as weighting and is a simple mathematic computation described in sampling textbooks.

比例抽样可能会导致在阶层间进行比较时数量不足。在我们的例子中，仅根据10个案例就得出关于西班牙裔护生的结论是有风险的。由于这个原因，研究人员在对大小极不相同的阶层进行比较时，可以使用不成比例的抽样。在这个例子中，可以改变抽样比例，选择 20 名非洲裔美国人、20 名西班牙裔、20 名亚裔和 40 名白种人学生。这一设计将确保更充分地代表三个种族/族裔少数群体。然而，当使用不成比例的抽样时，就有必要进行调整，以达到总体值的最佳估计。这种调整被称为加权，是抽样教科书中描述的一种简单的数学计算。

Stratified random sampling enables researchers to sharpen a sample's representativeness. Stratified sampling, however, may be impossible if information on the critical variables is unavailable. Furthermore, stratified sampling requires even more labor and effort than simple random sampling because the sample must be drawn from multiple enumerated lists.

分层随机抽样可以提高样本的代表性。然而，如果无法获得关键变量的信息，分层抽样或许是不可能的。此外，分层抽样比简单随机抽样需要更多的精力，因为样本必须从多个枚举列表中提取。

3. Multistage Cluster Sampling（群集抽样）

For many populations, it is impossible to obtain a listing of all elements. For example, the population of full-time nursing students in Canada would be difficult to list and enumerate for the purpose of drawing random sample. Large-scale surveys almost never use simple or stratified random sampling; they usually rely on multistage sampling, beginning with clusters.

对于许多总体来说，获取所有元素的列表是不可能的。例如，加拿大的全日制护理学生的人数很难列出和枚举，以抽取随机样本。大规模调查几乎从不使用简单或分层随机抽样，他们通常依靠多阶段抽样，从集群开始。

Multistage cluster sampling involves selecting broad groups (clusters) rather than selecting individuals—typically the first stage of a multistage approach. For a sample of nursing students, we might first draw a random sample of nursing schools and then draw a sample of students from the selected schools. The usual procedure for selecting samples from a general population in the United States is to sample successively such administrative units as census tracts, then households, and then household members. The resulting design can be described in terms of the number of stages (e. g., three-stage sampling). Clusters can be selected by simple or stratified methods. For instance, in selecting nursing schools, one could stratify on geographic region.

群集抽样涉及选择广泛的群体(集群)，而不是选择个体——通常是多阶段方法的第一阶段。对于护理学生的样本，我们可以先从护理学校中随机抽取一个样本，然后从所选学校中抽取一个学生样本。在美国，从一般人口中选择样本的通常程序是依次对人口普查区、家庭、家庭成员等行政单位进行抽样。最终的设计可以用阶段的数量来描述（例如，三阶段抽样）。可以通过简单或分层的方法来选择聚类。例如，在选择护理学校时，可以按地理区域进行分层。

For a specified number of cases, multistage sampling tends to be less accurate than simple or stratified random sampling. However, multistage sampling is more practical than other types of probability sampling, particularly when the population is large and widely distributed.

在一定数量的情况下，多阶段抽样往往不如简单或分层随机抽样准确。然而，多阶段抽样比其他类型的概率抽样更实用，特别是当总体较大且分布广泛时。

4. Systematic Sampling(系统抽样)

Systematic sampling involves selecting every kth case from a list, such as every 10th person on a patient list or every 25th person on a student roster. When this sampling method is applied to a sampling frame, an essentially random sample can be drawn, using the following procedure.

系统抽样涉及从名单中选择第 k 个病例，例如病人名单上的每第 10 人或学生名单上的每第 25 人。当将这种抽样方法应用于抽样帧时，可以使用下列程序绘制一个基本上是随机的抽样。

The required sample size is established at some number (n). The size of the population must be known or estimated (N). A sampling interval (k) can be obtained by dividing N by n. The sampling interval is the standard distance between sampled elements. For instance, if we wanted a sample of 200 from the population of 40,000, then our sampling interval would be as follows:

所需的样本量确定为某个数字(n)。总体的大小必须是已知的或估计的(N)。通过 N 除以 n，可以得到一个采样区间(k)。采样区间是被采样元素之间的标准距离。例如，如果我们想从 40000 个总体中抽取 200 个样本，那么我们的抽样区间将如下所示：

In other words, every 200th element on the list would be sampled. The first element should be selected randomly. Suppose that we randomly selected number 73 from a random number table. People corresponding to numbers 73, 273, 473, etc. would be sampled.

换句话说，将对列表中的第 200 个元素进行采样。第一个元素应该随机选择。假设我们从一个随机数表中随机选择了 73。与 73、273、473 等数字对应的人将被抽样。

Systematic sampling yields essentially the same results as simple random sampling but involves less work. Problems can arise if a list is arranged in such a way that a certain type of element is listed at intervals coinciding with the sampling interval. For instance, if every 10th nurse listed in a nursing staff roster was a head nurse and the sampling interval was 10, then head nurses would either always or never be included in the sample. Fortunately, problems of this type are rare. Systematic sampling can also be applied to lists that have been stratified.

系统抽样的结果与简单随机抽样的结果基本相同，但工作量较小。如果一个列表以这样一种方式排列，即某种类型的元素在与采样区间相一致的区间上排列，那么就会出现问题。例如，如果护士名册上的每第 10 名护士是护士长，采样间隔为 10，那么护士长将总是包括或永远不包括在样本中。幸运的是，这类问题很少见。系统抽样也可以应用于分层的列表。

5. Evaluation of Probability Sampling(评估概率抽样)

Probability sampling is the best method of obtaining representative samples. If all elements in the population have an equal probability of being selected, then the resulting sample is likely to do a good job of representing the population. Another advantage is that probability sampling allows researchers to estimate the magnitude of sampling error. Sampling error refers to differences between sample values (e. g., the average age of the sample) and population values (the average age of the population).

概率抽样是获得代表性样本的最佳方法。如果总体中的所有元素被选中的概率相等，那么结果样本很可能很好地代表总体。概率抽样的另一个优点是，研究人员可以估计抽样误差的大小。抽样误差是指样本值(例如样本的平均年龄)与总体值(总体的平均年龄)之间的差异。

The disadvantage of probability sampling is its impracticality. It is beyond the scope of most studies to draw a probability sample, unless the population is narrowly defined—and if it is narrowly defined, probability sampling might be "overkill." Probability sampling is the preferred and most respected method of obtaining sample elements, but it is often unfeasible.

概率抽样的缺点是它的不切实际。绘制一个概率样本超出了大多数研究的范围，除非人口被狭义地定义——如果它被狭义地定义，概率抽样可能是"多余的"。概率抽样是获得样本元素的首选和最受尊重的方法，但通常是不可行的。

Section V Sample Size in Quantitative Studies
第五节 量性研究中的样本量的确定

1. Sample Size Basics(样本量基础知识)

There are no simple formulas that can tell you how large a sample you will need in a given study, but as a general recommendation, you should use as large a sample as possible. The larger the sample, the more representative of the population it is likely to be. Every time researchers calculate a percentage or an average based on sample data, they are estimating the population value. The larger the sample, the smaller the sampling error.

没有简单的公式可以告诉你在特定研究中需要多大的样本，但作为一般建议，应该使用尽可能大的样本。样本越大，它可能就越具有代表性。每次研究人员根据样本数据计算一个百分比或平均值时，他们都在估计一个总体值。样本越大，采样误差越小。

Many nursing studies are based on relatively small samples due to practical constraints such as time and resources often limit sample size. Most nursing studies use convenience samples, and many are based on samples that are too small to provide adequate test of research hypotheses. Quantitative studies typically are based on samples of fewer than 200 participants, and many have fewer than 100 participants. Power analysis is not routinely used by nurse researchers, and research reports often offer no justification for sample size. When samples are too small, quantitative researchers run the risk of gathering data that will not support their hypotheses, even when their hypotheses are correct, thereby undermining statistical conclusion validity.

由于时间和资源等实际限制经常限制样本量，许多护理研究是基于相对较小的样本。大多数护理研究使用方便的样本，许多基于的样本太小，无法提供足够的研究假设的测试。定量研究通常是基于少于 200 名参与者的样本，许多研究的参与者少于 100 人。护士研究人员通常不使用效力分析，而且研究报告经常没有提供样本量的理由。当样本太小时，定量研究人员就会面临收集不支持其假设的数据的风险，即使他们的假设是正确的，从而削弱统计结论的有效性。

2. Factors Affecting Sample Size Requirements in Quantitative Research(影响量性研究中样本量需求的因素)

Sample size requirements are affected by various factors, some of which we discuss in this section.

样本量的需求受到各种因素的影响，其中一些因素我们将在本节中讨论。

2.1 Effect Size(效应量)

Power analysis builds on the concept of an effect size, which expresses the strength of relationships among research variables. If there is reason to expect that there is a strong correlation between the independent and dependent variables, then a relatively small sample may be adequate to reveal the relationship statistically. For example, if we were testing a powerful new drug, it might be possible to demonstrate its effectiveness with a small sample. However, nursing interventions have small to moderate effects. When there is no a priori reason for believing that relationships will be strong, then small samples are risky.

效力分析建立在效应大小的概念上，它表达了研究变量之间的关系强度。如果有理由认为自变量和因变量之间存在很强的相关性，那么一个相对较小的样本就足以在统计学上揭示这种关系。例如，如果我们正在测试一种功效强大的新药，也许可以用少量样本来证明它的有效性。然而，护理干预通常有小到中度的效果。当没有一个先验的理由来相信关系会很牢固时，那么小的样本是有风险的。

2.2 Homogeneity of the Population(人口的同质性)

If the population is relatively homogeneous, a small sample may be adequate. The greater the variability, the greater is the risk that a small sample will not adequately capture the full range of variation. For most nursing studies, it is probably best to assume a fair degree of heterogeneity, unless there is evidence from prior research to the contrary.

如果总体是相对均匀的，一个小的样本可能就足够了。可变性越大，小样本不能充分捕获全部变异范围的风险就越大。对于大多数护理研究来说，最好假设有相当程度的异质性，除非以前的研究有相反的证据。

2.3 Cooperation and Attrition(合作与失访)

In most studies, not everyone invited to participate in a study agrees to do so. Therefore, when developing a sampling plan, it is best to begin with a realistic, evidence-based estimate of the percentage of people likely to cooperate. Thus, if your targeted sample size is 200 but you expect a 50% refusal rate, you would have to recruit about 400 eligible people.

在大多数研究中，并不是每个被邀请参加研究的人都同意这样做。因此，在制定抽样计划时，最好从基于现实和证据的评估为百分百合作的人开始。因此，如果你的目标样本量是 200，但你预期 50% 的拒绝率，那么你将不得不招募大约 400 名合适的人。

In studies with multiple points of data collection, the number of participants usually declines over time. Attrition is most likely to occur if the time lag between data collection points is great, if the population is mobile, or if the population is at risk of death or disability. If the researcher has an ongoing relationship with participants, then attrition might be low—but it is rarely 0%. Therefore, when estimating sample size needs, researchers should factor in anticipated loss of participants over time.

在有多个数据收集点的研究中，参与者的数量通常会随着时间的推移而下降。如果数据收集点之间的时间差很大，如果人口是流动的，或者人口面临死亡或残疾的风险，则最可能出现人员流失。如果研究人员与参与者有持续的关系，那么人员流失率可能很低——但很少是 0%。因此，在估计样本量需求时，研究人员应该考虑到随着时间的推移参与者的预期损失。

The problem of staff attrition is not restricted to longitudinal studies. People who initially agree to cooperate in a study may be subsequently unable or unwilling to participate for various reasons, such as death, deteriorating health, early discharge, discontinued need for an intervention, or simply changing their minds. Researchers should expect participant loss and recruit accordingly.

人员流失问题并不局限于纵向研究。最初同意合作研究的人可能随后因各种原因无法或不愿意参与研究，如死亡、健康状况恶化、提前出院、不再需要干预或只是改变了主意。研究人员应该预料到参与者的流失，并相应地招募参与者。

2.4 Subgroup Analysis(亚组分析)

Researchers sometimes wish to test hypotheses not only for an entire population but also for subgroups. For example, suppose we were interested in assessing whether a structured exercise

Chapter 10：Sampling in Quantitative Research

第十章　量性研究的抽样

program is effective in improving infants' motor skills. We might also want to test whether the intervention is more effective for certain infants（e. g., low birth weight versus normal birth weight infants）. When a sample is divided to test for subgroup effects, the sample must be large enough to support analyses with subsets of the sample.

研究人员有时希望测试假设，不仅针对整个总体，也针对子群总体。例如，假设我们感兴趣的是评估一个结构化的锻炼计划是否能有效地提高婴儿的运动技能。我们可能还想测试这种干预对某些婴儿是否更有效(例如，低出生体重婴儿与正常出生体重婴儿)。当一个样本被划分为测试子组效应时，样本必须足够大，以支持样本子集的分析。

3. Methods of Calculating Sample Size(常用样本量估算方法)

There are three common methods for sample size estimation：table lookup, formula calculation and software calculation. Table lookup method is to directly check the sample scale according to the research conditions to obtain the sample size, but its scope is limited by the table. A sample size table is a data table compiled by statisticians according to specific formulas and different conditions such as α, $1-β$ for convenience. In addition, table lookup is not suitable for dissertation design and research proposal. Formula calculation method is to use the calculation formula of sample size to estimate the sample size, the formula is often based on the formula of test statistics backward to calculate the sample size. Software calculation is the use of computer software to assist the calculation of the method, still based on statistical calculation formula.

样本量估算常用的方法有查表法、公式计算法和软件计算法3种。查表法是按照研究条件直接查样本量表来获得样本量，但其范围受到表的限制。样本量表是统计学家为方便使用，根据特定的公式，按不同α，1-β等条件编制的数据表。此外，查表法也不适合在学位论文设计和研究计划书中使用。公式计算法是使用样本量的计算公式来估算样本量，其公式往往是根据检验统计量的公式反推过来求样本量。软件计算法是利用计算机软件协助计算的方法，其依据仍然是统计学计算公式。

The estimation formulas of sample size are numerous and the calculation is complicated. The estimation results are often different due to different research purposes, data properties, number of treatment groups and types of comparison parameters.

样本量的估计公式众多，计算也较为复杂。估算结果常因研究目的、资料性质、处理组数、比较的参数种类不同而异。

Section Ⅵ Implementing a Quantitative Sampling Plan
第六节 实施量性研究中的抽样计划

This section provides some practical guidance about implementing a sampling plan.

本节提供一些关于实现抽样计划的实用指南。

Steps in Sampling in Quantitative Studies:

定量研究中抽样的步骤：

The steps to be undertaken sample vary somewhat from one sampling design to the next, but a general outline of procedures can be described.

在抽样时所采取的步骤因抽样设计的不同而有所不同，但可以描述出大致的程序大纲。

(1)Identify the population. You should begin with a clear idea about the target population to which you would like to generalize your results. Unless you have extensive resources, you are unlikely to have access to the full target population, so you will also need to identify the population that is accessible to you. Researchers sometimes begin with identifying an accessible population and then decide how best to characterize the target population.

识别总体。首先，你应该清楚你想要推广你的结果的目标总体。除非你拥有广泛的资源，否则你不太可能接触到完整的目标总体，因此你还需要确定你可以接触到的总体。研究人员有时首先确定一个可获取的人群，然后决定如何最好地描述目标总体。

(2)Specify the eligibility criteria. The criteria for eligibility in the sample should then be spelled out. The criteria should be as specific as possible with regard to characteristics that might exclude potential participants (e.g., extremes of poor health, inability to read English). The criteria might lead you to redefine the target population.

指定资格标准。然后应该详细说明样本的资格标准。对于可能排除的潜在参与者的特征，标准应尽可能具体（例如，健康状况极差、无法阅读英语）。这些标准可能会引导你重新定义目标总体。

(3)Specify the sampling plan. Next, you must decide the method of sampling and sample size. If you can perform power analysis to estimate the needed number of participants, we highly recommend that you do so. Similarly, if probability sampling is a viable option, that option should be exercised. If you are not in a position to do either, we recommend using as large a sample as possible and taking steps to build representativeness into the design (e.g., by using quota or consecutive sampling).

指定抽样计划。接下来，你必须决定抽取样本的方法和样本的大小。如果你可以执行效力分析来估计所需的参与者数量，我们强烈建议使用效力分析来估计所需的参与者数量。类似地，如果概率抽样是可行的选项，则应该执行该选项。如果你不能做到这两个，我们建议使用尽可能大的样本，并采取措施设计中建立代表性（例如，通过使用配额或连续抽样）。

（4）Recruit the sample. The next step is to recruit prospective participants (after any needed institutional permissions have been obtained) and ask for their cooperation. Issues relating to participant recruitment are discussed next.

招募样本。下一步是招募潜在参与者（在获得任何必要的机构许可之后），并请求他们的合作。下面将讨论有关招募参与者的问题。

1. Sample Recruitment(样本招募)

Recruiting people to participate in a study involves two major tasks: identifying eligible candidates and persuading them to participate. Researchers must consider the best sources for recruiting potential participants. Researchers must ask questions such as, where do large numbers of people matching my population construct live or obtain care? Will I have direct access, or will I need to work through gatekeepers? Will there be sufficiently large numbers in one location, or will multiple sites be necessary? During the recruitment phase, it may be necessary to create a screening instrument, which is a brief form that allows researchers to determine whether prospective participants meets the study's eligibility criteria.

招募人们参加一项研究涉及两个主要任务：确定合格的候选人和说服他们参加。研究人员必须考虑招募潜在参与者的最佳来源。研究人员必须问这样的问题：大量的与我的人群相匹配的人在哪里居住或获得照顾？我是否有直接访问权限，或者我的工作是否需要通过信息传递者？一个地点是否有足够多的人，还是需要多个地点？在招募阶段，可能需要创建一个筛选工具，它是一个简短的表格，允许研究人员确定未来的参与者是否符合研究的资格标准。

The next task involves gaining the cooperation of people who have been deemed eligible. There is considerable evidence that the percentage of people willing to cooperate in clinical trials and investigations is declining, and so it is critical to have an effective recruitment strategy.

下一个任务是争取那些被认为有资格的人的合作。有相当多的证据表明，愿意在临床试验和调查中合作的人的百分比正在下降，因此有一个有效的招募策略是至关重要的。

In recent years, much methodologic research in health fields has focused on strategies for effective recruitment. Researchers have found that rates of cooperation can often be enhanced by means of the following: face-to-face recruitment, multiple contacts and requests, monetary and nonmonetary incentives, brief data collection, inclusion of questions perceived as having high relevance to participants, assurances of anonymity, and endorsement of the study by a respected person or institution.

近年来，卫生领域的许多方法学研究都集中在有效招聘的策略上。研究人员发现，合作率通常可以通过以下方法来提高：面对面招聘，多次联系和请求，金钱和非金钱激励，简要的数据收集，包含被认为与参与者有高度相关性的问题，保证匿名，以及受尊敬的人或机构对研究的认可。

2. Generalizing from Samples(从样本进行推广)

Ideally, the sample is representative of the accessible population, and the accessible population is representative of the target population. By using an appropriate sampling plan, researchers can be reasonably confident that the first part of this ideal has been realized. The second part of the ideal entails greater risk. Are diabetic patients in Boston representative of diabetic patients in the United States? Researchers must exercise judgment in assessing the degree of similarity.

理想情况下，样本代表可获得的人群，可获得人群代表目标总体。通过使用适当的抽样计划，研究人员可以有理由相信理想的第一部分已经实现。理想的第二部分需要更大的风险。波士顿的糖尿病患者是否代表美国的糖尿病患者？研究人员在评估相似程度时必须进行判断。

The best advice is to be realistic and conservative and to ask challenging questions: Is it reasonable to assume that the accessible population is representative of the target population? In what ways might they differ? How would such differences affect the conclusions? If differences are great, it would be prudent to specify a more restricted target population to which the findings could be meaningfully generalized.

最好的建议是采取现实和保守的态度，并提出具有挑战性的问题：假设可获取的人群代表目标总体是否合理？他们在哪些方面可能不同？这种差异会如何影响结论？如果差异很大，审慎的做法是指定一个更严格的目标人群，以便研究结果能够有意义地推广。

Where possible，interpretations about the generalizability of findings can be enhanced by comparing sample characteristics with population characteristics. Published information about the characteristics of many populations may be available to help in evaluating sampling bias. For example，if you were studying low-income children in Chicago，you could obtain information on the Internet about salient characteristics（e. g.，race/ethnicity，age distribution）of low-income American children from the U. S. Census Bureau. Population characteristics could then be compared with sample characteristics and differences taken into account in interpreting the findings.

在可能的情况下，通过比较样本特征和总体特征，可以增强对研究结果的概括性的解释。已发表的关于许多总体特征的信息可能有助于评估抽样偏差。例如，如果你正在研究芝加哥低收入家庭的孩子，你可以在互联网上从美国人口普查局获得低收入美国孩子的显著特征(例如，种族/民族，年龄分布)的信息。然后可以将总体特征和样本的特征及差异进行比较，以解释研究结果。

Section Ⅶ　Critiquing Sampling Plans
第七节　评判抽样计划

In coming to conclusions about the quality of evidence that a study yields，you should carefully scrutinize the sampling plan. If the sample is seriously biased or too small，the findings may be misleading or just plain wrong.

在得出关于一项研究产生的证据质量的结论时，应该仔细审查抽样计划。如果样本有严重的偏见或太少，那么结果可能具有误导性或完全错误。

You should consider two issues in your critique of a study's sampling plan. The first is whether the researcher adequately described the sampling strategy. Ideally，research reports should include a description of the following：

在你对研究抽样计划的评论中，你应该考虑两个问题。第一，研究者是否充分描述了抽样策略。理想情况下，研究报告应该包括以下描述：

（1）The type of sampling approach used（e. g.，convenience，simple random）.

抽样方法的类型(例如，方便，简单随机)。

（2）The study population and eligibility criteria for sample selection.

研究总体和样本选择的资格标准。

（3）The number of participants and a rationale for the sample size，including whether a power analysis was performed.

参与者的数量和样本大小的基本原理，包括是否进行了效力分析。

（4）A description of the main characteristics of sample members（e. g., age, gender, medical condition, etc.）and, ideally, of the population.

对抽样成员的主要特征（如年龄、性别、健康状况等）的描述，最好是对整个总体的描述。

（5）The number and characteristics of potential participants who declined to participate in the study.

拒绝参与研究的潜在参与者的数量和特征。

If the description of the sample is inadequate, you may not be able to come to conclusions about whether the researcher made good sampling decisions. And, if the description is incomplete, it will be difficult to know whether the evidence can be applied in your clinical practice.

如果对样本的描述不充分，可能无法得出结论，研究人员是否做出了良好的抽样决策。而且，如果描述不完整，就很难知道这些证据是否能应用到临床实践中。

Sampling plans should consider their effects on the construct, internal, external, and statistical conclusion validity of the study. If the sample size is small, statistical conclusion validity will likely be undermined. If the eligibility criteria are restrictive, this could benefit internal validity—but possibly to the detriment of construct and external validity.

抽样计划应考虑其对研究结构、内部、外部和统计结论效度的影响。如果样本太小，统计结论的有效性很可能会受到影响。如果资格标准是限制性的，这可能有利于内部效度，但可能会损害结构和外部效度。

We have stressed that a key criterion for assessing the adequacy of a sampling plan in quantitative research is whether the sample is representative of the population. You will never be sure, but if the sampling strategy is weak or if the sample size is small, it is reasonable to suspect some bias. When researchers adopt a sampling plan with a high risk of bias, they should take steps to estimate the direction and degree of this bias so that readers can draw some informed conclusions.

我们已经强调，在定量研究中，评估抽样计划是否充分的一个关键标准是该抽样是否具有总体代表性。你永远无法确定，但如果抽样策略较弱或样本容量较小，就有理由怀疑存在一些偏差。当研究人员采用偏差风险高的抽样计划时，他们应该采取措施估计这种偏差的方向和程度，以便读者可以得出一些有根据的结论。

Even with a rigorous sampling plan, the sample may be biased if not all people invited to participate in a study agree to do so—which is almost always the case. If certain segments of the population refuse to participate, then a biased sample can result, even when probability sampling is used. Research reports should provide information about response rates (i. e., the number of people participating in a study relative to the number of people in the sample) and about possible nonresponse bias—differences between participants and those who declined to participate (also sometimes referred to as response bias). In longitudinal studies, attrition bias should be reported.

即使有严格的抽样计划，如果不是所有被邀请参加研究的人都同意这样做的话，样本可能会有偏差——几乎总是如此。如果总体中的某些部分拒绝参与，那么即使使用概率抽样，也会产生一个有偏差的样本。研究报告应提供答复率的信息(即，参与研究的人数相对于抽样的人数)和可能的无反应偏差——参与者和拒绝参与的人之间的差异(有时也被称为反应偏差)。在纵向研究中，应报告失访偏倚。

Quantitative researchers make decisions about the specification of the population as well as the selection of the sample. If the target population is defined broadly, researchers may have missed opportunities to control confounding variables, and the gap between the accessible and the target population may be too great. One of your jobs as reviewer is to come to conclusions about the reasonableness of generalizing the findings from the researcher's sample to the accessible population and from the accessible population to a target population. If the sampling plan is seriously flawed, it may be risky to generalize the findings at all without replicating the study with another sample.

定量研究人员决定总体的规格和样本的选择。如果目标总体的定义过于宽泛，研究人员可能会错过控制混杂变量的机会，而且可获得人群与目标总体之间的差距可能太大。作为审查员，工作之一是得出结论，从研究人员的样本到可获得人群和从可获得人群到目标总体的结论的合理性。如果抽样计划有严重的缺陷，在不使用其他样本重复研究的情况下推广研究结果可能是有风险的。

Chapter 11: Data Collection in Quantitative Research
第十一章　量性研究中的数据收集

Data collection is a process of obtaining data and information from research subjects through different methods, which is a scientific and rigorous process and an important part of scientific research.

数据收集是通过不同方法从研究对象处获取数据和资料的过程，是一个科学严谨的过程，是科学研究中的重要环节。

Section Ⅰ　Developing a Data Collection Plan
第一节　制订数据收集计划

1. Determining Who, When and Where the Data Will Be Collected
（确定数据收集的对象、时间和地点）

The selection of appropriate subjects, time and place is an important part of the data collection process. In terms of the study subjects, the appropriate inclusion and exclusion criteria should be developed according to the purpose of the study, and the calculation of the sample size has been described in Chapter 10. There are various factors that affect the time of data collection, such as the cooperation of the study subjects, the attrition rate of the study subjects, and the accessibility of the study subjects, etc. Therefore, researchers should consider various factors when determining the time of data collection, and in addition, it is important to choose an appropriate time point, for example, people with depression have serious sickness in the morning and mild sickness at night, thus if a study wants to understand the improvement in mood of depressed patients by a particular intervention, the results obtained may vary depending on the time point of data collection. As far as the location of data collection is concerned, it should be considered according to the purpose of the study, the characteristics of the study subjects and the cost. For example, studies about maternity are generally conducted in obstetric clinics or wards for the first data collection, which can shorten the time of data collection and also obtain sufficient sample size.

选择合适的对象、时间和地点是数据收集过程中的重要环节。就研究对象而言，要根据研究目的制定相应的纳入和排除标准，关于样本量的计算已经在第十章有所介绍。影响数据收集时间的因素有很多，如研究对象的配合度、研究对象的流失率和研究对象的可及性，等等，因此，研究者在确定数据收集时间时要考虑多方面因素，此外，选择一个合适的时间点也非常重要，如抑郁症患者临床症状有晨重夜轻的特点，因此如果一个研究想要了解某项干预措施对抑郁症患者情绪的改善情况，其结果可能会受数据收集时间的影响而有所不同。就数据收集的地点而言，要根据研究目的、研究对象的特点和成本考虑，如有关产妇的研究一般在产科门诊或病房进行首次数据收集，既可以缩短数据收集的时间，又可以获得足够的样本量。

2. Determining the Needed Data(确定需要的数据及类型)

Determining the information to be collected for the study according to the purpose and problem of the study is a prerequisite for obtaining valid data, and the results of the study are derived by analyzing the characteristics of these data and the relationships between them, therefore, it is important to determine the variables and types of data needed for the study.

根据研究目的和研究问题确定研究所需要收集的资料是获得有效数据的前提，研究结果就是通过分析这些数据的特点以及数据之间的关系得出的，因此，确定研究所需要的变量及类型十分重要。

3. Selecting Appropriate Data Collection Methods(选择合适的数据收集方法)

After determining the types of data needed for study, the next step is to select an appropriate measurement method. Data such as weight, height and blood pressure are usually measured by biomedical methods, and behavioral modalities are measured by observation and questionnaire methods. The measurement methods commonly used in quantitative research mainly include structured observation, structured self-report, biomedical measurement and secondary data collection methods, which are described in detail in this chapter.

确定了所需要的数据和类型后，下一步就要选择合适的测量方法，如体重、身高和血压等数据通常采用生物医学法测量，行为方式采用观察法和问卷法测量。量性研究中常用的测量方法主要包括结构化观察法、结构化自我报告法、生物医学测量法和二手资料收集法，在本章节中会详细介绍。

4. Selecting and Developing Instruments(选择和开发工具)

After determining the method of data collection, the researchers must first consider the availability of a research instrument to measure the study variables, and then consider the applicability, reliability and validity of the measurement instrument (see Chapter 12), accessibility and cost of the tools. If a suitable measurement instrument is not available, the researchers may get a new scale by developing or modifying (see Chapter 13).

确定了数据的收集方法之后，研究者首先要考虑是否有测量研究变量的研究工具，其次考虑测量工具的适用性、信效度(见第十二章)、可及性和成本。如果没有合适的测量工具，研究者可能需要通过开发或修改形成一个新的量表(见第十三章)。

5. Developing Data Collection Forms(制定数据收集表格)

Data collection forms should be simple, aesthetic and readable, sometimes confidentiality is also required. Forms include mainly general demographic information, scales or questionnaires selected or self-administered according to the purpose of the study and informed consent forms. Developing a rigorous data collection form can also help reduce errors of quantitative study data (Schneider & Deenan, 2004).

数据收集表格要具有简洁性、美观性和易读性，有时还需要注意保密性。表格主要包括一般人口学资料，根据研究目的选择或自设量表、问卷和知情同意书。制定一个严谨的数据收集表格也有助于减少量性研究数据的错误(Schneider 和 Deenan, 2004)。

6. Pilot Study(预实验)

Before formally conducting the study, the researchers may conduct a pilot study according to the research plan, usually selecting 10-20 study subjects who meet the inclusion and exclusion criteria. Pilot testing can help researchers identify possible problems in the data collection process and develop solutions to potential problems.

在正式开展研究之前，研究者可以根据研究计划进行一个预实验，通常选择符合纳入和排除标准的10~20个研究对象进行实验。预实验可以帮助研究者识别数据收集过程中可能存在的问题，并制定解决潜在问题的方案。

Section Ⅱ Structured Self-Report Instruments
第二节 结构化的自我报告工具

1. Types of Structured Questions(结构化问题的类型)

1.1 Open-ended Questions(开放式问题)

The application of open-ended questions in quantitative research is rare. Open-ended questions usually only set up questions with no fixed answers, and the research subjects can answer the questions in their own words, but in quantitative research the researcher usually limits what the research subjects answer. For example：

Please list three factors that you believe most influence changes in blood pressure?

开放式问题在量性研究中的应用很少。开放式问题通常只设立问题，没有固定的答案，研究对象可以用自己的语言回答问题，但在量性研究中研究者通常会限定研究对象所回答的内容。例如：

请列出三个你认为最影响血压改变的因素？

（1）_____

（2）_____

（3）_____

1.2 Closed-ended Questions(闭合式问题)

Closed-ended questions are the most structured, setting up not only questions but also fixed answers, and the research subjects can only make choices based on the given answers. Closed-ended questions can be divided into dichotomous questions, single-choice questions, multiple-choice questions, rank-order questions, rating scale questions, forced-choice questions and so on, depending on the form of the answer set(see Table 11.2.1).

闭合式问题的结构性最强，不仅设立问题，还设立了固定的答案，研究对象只能根据给出的答案做出选择。闭合式问题根据答案设置的形式不同又可以分为两分制问题、单选题、多选题、排序题、等级量表式问题和强迫选择性问题等(见表11.2.1)。

（1）Dichotomous questions contain two response options and are primarily used to gather factual information.

两分制问题包含两个回答选项，主要用于收集事实性信息。

（2）Single-choice questions are usually set with 3-5 response options, but with one and only one appropriate answer.

单选题通常设置3~5个回答选项，但有且只有一个合适的答案。

（3）Multiple-choice questions usually set 3-8 response options with at least two appropriate answers. The answer options for multiple-choice questions should be comprehensive and often have "other" options.

多选题通常设置3~8个回答选项，至少有两个合适的答案。多选题的回答选项应考虑全面，经常会设置"其他"选项。

（4）Ranking questions usually have 10 or fewer response options and ask the respondent to rank the listed options in some way, either by selecting the first few or by ranking all of the listed options.

排序题通常设置10个及以下的回答选项，要求受访者按照某种程度对所列出的选项进行排序，可以是选出前面几个，也可以是对列出的全部选项进行排序。

（5）Rating scale questions ask respondents to rate something or a phenomenon in terms of degree, and answers can be presented in the form of words, numbers, straight lines, and expressions.

等级量表式问题要求回答者对某一事物或现象进行程度上的评价，答案可以通过文字、数字、直线和表情等形式展现。

（6）Forced-choice questions contain two response options that hold completely opposite views.

强迫选择性问题包含两个持完全相反观点的回答选项。

Table 11.2.1   **Example of closed questions（闭合式问题示例）**

Question type（问题类型）	Example（示例）
Dichotomous question （两分制问题）	Have you experienced a miscarriage? （　　） A Yes　　B No 您是否经历过流产? （　　） A 是　　　B 否
Single-choice question （单选题）	How many times does the infant wake up at night? （　　） A =1 time　B 2-3 times　C 4-5 times　D =6 times 婴儿的夜醒次数? （　　） A =1次　　B 2~3次　　C 4~5次　　D =6次

续表

Question type(问题类型)	Example(示例)
Multiple-choice question (多选题)	What do you think are the benefits of breastfeeding? ( ) (A) Promote baby's intellectual development (B) Save family expenses (C) Enhance baby's immunity (D) Promote mother and baby's emotional communication (E) Promote mother's physical health 您觉得母乳喂养有哪些好处? ( ) (A) 促进宝宝智力发育　(B) 节约家庭开销　　(C) 增强婴儿免疫力 (D) 促进母婴情感交流　(E) 促进母亲身体健康
Rank-order question (排序题)	Below is a list of relevant factors that affect nurses' motivation. Please rank them according to your situation, from 1 (least impact) to 7 (most impact). 下面列出了影响护士工作积极性的相关因素, 请您根据自身情况进行排序, 从1(影响最小)到7(影响最大)。 ( ) nurse-patient relationship 护患关系 ( ) salary and remuneration 工资待遇 ( ) work tasks 工作任务 ( ) family reasons 家庭原因 ( ) social status 社会地位 ( ) departmental atmosphere 科室氛围 ( ) own personality 自身性格
Question type(问题类型)	Example(示例)
Rating scale question (等级量表式问题)	I can be sure that the baby is getting enough breast milk ( ) 1 Not at all confident　　2 Slightly confident　　3 Confident 4 More confident　　　　5 Always very confident 我能确定婴儿母乳充足( ) 1 完全没有信心　　2 略有信心　　3 有信心 4 较有信心　　　　5 总是很有信心
Forced-choice question (强迫选择性问题)	Your attitude toward the legalization of euthanasia is ( ) A Supportive, individuals should have the right to choose euthanasia under the condition that it is not against the law of the country, the will of individuals and the interests of others. B Opposed, it is a waste of life, and it may easily lead to criminal behavior. 对于安乐死合法化, 您的态度是( ) A 支持, 在不违背国家法律、个人意愿和他人利益下的情况下, 个人应该有权选择安乐死。 B 反对, 这是在浪费生命, 而且容易引发犯罪行为。

2. Composite Scales and Other Structured Self-Reports
（综合量表及其他结构化的自我报告工具）

2.1 Likert-type Summated Rating Scales（李克特量表）

The Likert scale is one of the most commonly used scales in nursing research, usually to measure attitudes, and was developed and refined by the American social psychologist Likert. The scale's questions often consist of several declarative sentences expressing the same topic, most often on a 5-point scale, i. e., the options are divided into five levels, with 1, 2, 3, 4, and 5 representing strongly disagree, disagree, neither agree nor disagree, agree and strongly agree, respectively, and respondents are asked to choose their attitude toward each topic stated, allowing for a detailed division of respondents who hold different views.

李克特量表是护理研究中最常用的一种量表，通常用来测量态度，由美国社会心理学家李克特开发和改进。该量表的题目往往由几个陈述句构成，表达同一个主题，最常采用的是 5 级评分法，即将选项分为 5 个层次，1、2、3、4、5 分别代表着强烈反对、不同意、既不同意也不反对、同意和坚决同意，要求受访者选择他们对每个题目所陈述的态度，可以将持有不同观点的受访者进行详细划分。

2.2 Cognitive and Neuropsychological Tests（认知和神经心理测试）

Cognition is a complex concept that includes abilities in perception, discrimination, memory, learning, attention, comprehension, reasoning, and judgment, and nursing researchers often assess the cognitive functioning of study subjects by asking questions. In nursing research, cognitive function tests are mostly administered to older adults. There are many types of cognitive tests, and some cognitive tests are designed to assess neuropsychological functioning in people with potential cognitive impairment, such as the Mini-mental State Examination (MMSE) and the Montreal Cognitive Assessment (MoCA).

认知是一个复杂的概念，包括感知、辨别、记忆、学习、注意、理解、推理和判断方面的能力，护理研究者通常通过提问题来评估研究对象的认知功能。在护理研究中，认知功能测试的研究对象多为老年人。认知测试的类型有很多，一些认知测试的目的是评估潜在认知障碍人群的神经心理功能，如简易精神状态检查和蒙特利尔认知评估。

2.3 Other Types of Structured Self-reports(其他类型的结构化自我报告工具)

There are other types of structured self-reporting tools in nursing research. The following are examples:

在护理研究中还存在其他类型的结构化自我报告工具，下面简单地举例介绍:

2.3.1 Q Sorts(Q 分类法)

A set of pictures or cards is given to the research subject, the content of which is a statement with value judgments formed by the researcher about the research variables according to the purpose of the study, and the research subject classifies these pictures or cards according to a specific dimension.

给研究对象一组图片或卡片，内容为研究者根据研究目的对研究变量形成的有价值判断的陈述语句，研究对象按照特定的维度对这些图片或卡片进行分类。

2.3.2 Semantic Difference Scale(语义差异量表)

This scale consists of a series of bipolar adjectives (e. g., good/bad and positive/negative) that require the subject of the study to state an evaluation of a concept and its related problematic nature or attribute aspects.

这种量表由一系列两极性形容词组成(如好的/坏的和积极的/消极的)，要求研究对象对某一概念及其相关问题性质或属性方面做出评价。

3. Questionnaires Versus Interviews(问卷与访谈)

Both the questionnaire and interview methods are commonly used in the data collection process, and each has its own advantages.

问卷法和访谈法都是数据收集过程中常用的方法，各有优势。

3.1 Advantages of Questionnaires(问卷的优点)

(1) Compared with the interview method, the questionnaire method saves more time, money and manpower, and the questionnaire method can obtain a larger sample size, which is suitable for large-scale surveys.

与访谈法相比，问卷法更节省时间、经费和人力，而且问卷法可以获得更大的样本量，适用于大规模调查。

（2）The interview process is a process of communication and interaction between the interviewer and the interviewee, in which the interviewer may have questions to guide the answers, which may easily cause interviewer bias and affect the validity of the information, while the questionnaire method without the presence of the interviewer can effectively avoid interviewer bias.

访谈的过程是访谈者和受访者交流互动的过程。在这个过程中，访谈者可能会提出问题来引导回答，容易造成访谈者偏见，影响资料的效度，而问卷法没有采访者在场可以有效避免访谈者偏差。

（3）The findings of the questionnaire method are easy to quantify, which is convenient for statistics and analyses.

问卷法的调查结果容易量化，便于统计和分析。

3.2 Advantages of Interviews（访谈的优点）

（1）Most of the questions in the questionnaire are structured questions, which are more superficial and can obtain less information compared to the questions in the interview, while the face-to-face interview can obtain more comprehensive, detailed and deeper information from the interviewees.

问卷中的问题大多是结构化问题，相对访谈中的问题较为表浅，可获得的信息量较少，面对面的访谈可以获得受访者更全面、更详细和更深层次的信息。

（2）The questionnaire method suffers from low recall rate and incomplete or inaccurate information filling, while in the process of interview, respondents generally do not reject the questions asked by the interviewer, and the interviewer can probe some incomplete, ambiguous and confusing answers.

问卷法存在回收率低、信息填写不完善或不准确的问题，而在访谈的过程中，受访者一般不会拒绝访谈者提出的问题，而且访谈者可以对一些不完整的、模棱两可的和令人困惑的回答进行探究。

（3）The interview method has a wider audience than the questionnaire method, e. g., the interview method is also applicable to children, illiterates, the blind, and the elderly.

访谈法比问卷法的受众面更广，如访谈法也适用于儿童、文盲、视障人士和老人。

4. Administering Structured Self-report Instruments
（结构化自我报告工具的应用）

The administration of the structured self-reporting tool included the administration of interviews and questionnaires.

结构化自我报告工具的管理包括访谈的管理和问卷的管理。

4.1 Collecting Interview Data（收集访谈数据）

In the interview, firstly, the interviewer should create a relaxed atmosphere for the interviewee and establish a good trusting relationship with the interviewee, which will help the interviewee to answer the questions sincerely; secondly, the interviewer should remain neutral during the interview, on the one hand, he/she should maintain a neutral attitude towards all the answers of the interviewee, and on the other hand, the interviewer should also maintain a neutral attitude when asking questions; in addition, the interviewer should neither mechanically asking questions, nor interpreting the meaning of questions as they see fit, nor guiding, interpreting, and summarizing respondents' responses. Interviewers often use probing methods to obtain complete and accurate data, and probing takes a variety of forms, including long pauses to suggest that respondents continue to answer, repeating questions, and asking additional questions, etc. The development of probing skills is important for interviewers, and interviewers need to know when and how to probe. More information about the principles of interviewing can be found in Fowler (2014).

在访谈中，首先，访谈者要给受访者创造一个放松的氛围，与受访者建立良好的信任关系，这样有助于受访者真诚地回答问题；其次，访谈者在访谈过程中要保持中立，一方面对受访者的所有回答要保持中立的态度，另一方面，访谈者在提问时也要保持中立的态度；此外，访谈者既不能机械地提问问题，也不能按自己的理解随意解释问题的含义，更不能引导、解释和总结受访者的回答。访谈者经常使用探究的方法以获得完整和准确的数据，探究的形式是多种多样的，包括长时间的停顿暗示受访者继续回答，重复提问和补充提问等。探究能力的培养对访谈者来说是很重要的，访谈者需要知道什么时候探究以及如何探究。更多有关访谈的原则可以在 Fowler（2014）的研究中找到。

4.2 Collecting Questionnaire Data(收集问卷数据)

4.2.1 Collecting Questionnaire Data through In-Person Distribution (通过当面发放问卷收集数据)

Data collectors can distribute the questionnaire to a group of study participants or to individual study participants in person; the former is the most convenient method and allows for a larger number of questionnaires, both are highly feasible in both educational and clinical settings, and both facilitate communication between the investigator and the respondent, which facilitates higher return rates and valid completion rates.

数据收集者可以向一组研究对象或个别研究对象当面发放问卷，前者是最方便的方法，并且可以获得较多的问卷数量，两者在教育环境和临床环境中的可行性很大，而且两者都方便调查者和受访者间的交流，利于提高问卷的回收率和有效填写率。

4.2.2 Collecting Questionnaire Data via the Internet(通过互联网收集问卷数据)

Due to its affordability, convenience, and quickness, questionnaire collection via the Internet is widely used in nursing research, mainly in the form of E-mails, codes, and links to questionnaires, which researchers can place in dedicated questionnaire websites or in websites related to the survey topic. However, Internet questionnaires have a low recall rate and there are network issues (e. g., study participants will not use the Internet for questionnaire completion) and questionnaire reception issues (e. g., questionnaires are blocked by security software) to consider. More information on conducting Internet surveys can be found in Dillman et al. (2014), Tourangeau et al. (2013), and Fitzpatrick and Montgomery (2004).

由于经济性、方便性和快捷性，通过互联网收集问卷的方法在护理研究中被广泛使用，主要形式包括电子邮件、二维码和问卷链接，研究人员可以将问卷放置在专门的调查问卷网站中，也可以放在与调查主题相关的网站中。但是互联网问卷的回收率很低，而且要考虑网络问题(如研究对象不会使用互联网进行问卷填写)和问卷接收问题(如问卷被安全软件拦截)。有关开展互联网调查的更多信息可以在 Dillman 等 (2014)，Tourangeau 等 (2013)，Fitzpatrick 和 Montgomery (2004)的研究中找到。

5. Evaluation of Structured Self-reports(结构化自我报告的评估)

The structured self-report method is an easy-to-use and efficient method of data collection, and the results obtained are more easily quantifiable for statistical and analytical purposes.

结构化自我报告法是一种易操作和高效率的数据收集方法，获得的结果也更容易量化，便于统计和分析。

Structured self-reports also have some limitations. Compared to unstructured interviews, structured self-report questions are usually closed-ended questions and are more superficial. Response bias is also a frequent problem in structured self-reports and is unavoidable in unstructured self-report methods, such as social desirability response bias, which refers to the tendency of subjects to respond in a manner consistent with social values, which is often difficult to eliminate and can be reduced by indirect questioning, appropriate wording, creating a nonjudgmental atmosphere, and anonymous responses, and some response biases are known as response sets, often found in composite scales, such as extreme response sets, where subjects choose consistent extreme options such as strongly agree, and default response sets, where subjects choose to agree with all of the questions regardless of their content, and the opposite but less common case, where subjects choose to disagree with all of them.

结构化自我报告也存在一些局限性，与非结构访谈相比，结构化自我报告的问题通常是闭合式问题，问题比较表浅。反应偏差也是经常出现在结构化自我报告中的问题，非结构化自我报告法也不可避免，如社会期许性反应偏差，指受试者会倾向于做出符合社会价值观的回答，这种偏差通常很难消除，可以通过间接的提问、合适的措辞、创造非批判性的氛围、匿名回答等方式减少这种偏差，还有一些反应偏差被称为反应集，经常在复合量表中出现，如极端反应集，指的是受试者选择了一致的极端选项，如强烈同意，以及默认反应集，指不论题目内容是什么，受试者全部选择认同，还有一种与之相反但不常见的情况，即受试者全部选择反对。

Section Ⅲ　Structured Observation
第三节　结构化观察法

1. Methods of Recording Structured Observations(结构化观察的记录方法)

Methods of recording structured observations typically include classification systems, checklists and rating scales.

结构化观察的记录方法通常包括分类系统，清单和等级量表。

1.1　Category Systems and Checklists(分类系统和清单)

Observed behaviors or events are diverse, and to facilitate the collection, recording, and management of observed information, researchers usually create a systematic classification system that can be divided into exhaustive and non-exhaustive categories depending on the recorded categories, including temporal and content categories. The categories in the classification system should be mutually exclusive, otherwise the accuracy of the information will be compromised. To ensure consistent data collection, classification systems usually require clear definitions and detailed explanations for each category, and even then, observers are often faced with the task of making on-the-spot inferences. The degree of on-the-spot inference required in different classification systems varies, and in general, the greater the degree of inference required, the more difficult the category system is to use.

观察到的行为或事件是多种多样的，为了方便收集、记录和管理观察到的信息，研究人员通常会建立一个系统的分类系统，根据记录的范畴不同，包括时间范畴和内容范畴，可以将分类系统分为详尽分类和非详尽分类。分类系统中的类别应该是相互排斥的，否则会影响信息的准确性。为了保证数据收集的一致性，分类系统通常要求对每一类别进行清晰的定义和详细的解释，即使如此，观察者也会经常面临着现场推断的任务，不同分类系统中所需要的现场推断度有所不同，一般来说，需要的推理程度越大，类别系统使用就越困难。

A checklist is a tool used by the observer to record whether and how many times and when the behaviors or events under study occurred, and the researchers will list the behaviors or events in the category system used on the checklist.

清单是观察者用来记录的一种工具，记录的内容通常包括研究的行为或事件是否发生，以及发生的次数和时间，研究者会在清单上列出使用的分类系统中的行为或事件。

1.2　Rating Scales(等级量表)

The observer can rate the continuous variables in the observed behaviors or events on a rating scale, either during the course of the observation or at the end of the observation to rate the whole, but the evaluation at the end of the observation is more demanding and requires the observer to evaluate all behaviors or events in the context of the whole observation.

观察者可以通过评级量表对观察到的行为或事件中的连续变量进行等级评价，可以在观察的过程中进行评价，也可以在观察结束后对整体进行等级评价，但观察结束后的评价对观察者的要求较高，需要观察者结合整个观察过程中的所有行为或事件进行评价。

2. Sampling for Structured Observations(结构化观察法的采样)

In order to observe representative examples of behaviors or events in a short period of time, the observer needs to perform appropriate sampling, and two sampling methods for structured observation are described below.

为了在短时间内观察到具有代表性的行为或事件例子，观察者需要进行合适的抽样，下面介绍了两种结构化观察的抽样方法。

2.1 Time Sampling(时间抽样)

When the behaviors or events of interest occur frequently, researchers often use time sampling, where the researchers systematically or randomly select the time intervals at which observations are made, finding a representative sample by choosing different time intervals, usually requiring several different sampling plans.

当感兴趣的行为或事件发生频繁时，研究者常常采用时间抽样，时间抽样即研究者系统地或随机地选择进行观察的时间间隔，通过选择不同的时间间隔来寻找有代表性的样本，通常需要多个不同的抽样计划。

2.2 Event Sampling(事件抽样)

When the behaviors or events of interest occur infrequently, researchers often use event sampling, in which the observer predetermines the categories to be observed and observes behaviors or events that fit within the categories in a natural setting.

当感兴趣的行为或事件发生不频繁时，研究者常常采用事件抽样，事件抽样即观察者预先设定观察的类别，在自然环境下观察符合类别中的行为或事件。

3. Technical Aids in Observations(结构化观察的技巧)

The most commonly used devices for recording and analyzing structured observations are video and audio recording devices, which allow the observer to notice small details that are overlooked during the observation process and facilitate the recording and analysis of the data afterwards with the aid of the devices. Nowadays, there are more and more advanced technologies applied in the recording and analysis of structured observation, which make the quality, function, sensitivity and concealment of recording devices improved. More information on ways to improve the quality of data observed in video recordings can be found in Haidet et al. (2009).

结构化观察的记录和分析最常用的是录像和录音设备，观察者通过设备的辅助可以注意到观察过程中被忽视的小细节，也方便之后数据的记录和分析。现在有越来越多的先进技术应用于结构化观察的记录和分析中，使得记录设备的质量、功能、灵敏度和隐蔽性都有所提高。更多有关提高视频录像观察的数据质量的方法可以在 Haidet 等（2009）的研究中找到。

4. Evaluation of Structured Observation(结构化观察法的评估)

The structured self-observation method is a very common method when reliable data cannot be obtained through self-report methods and when the study variables are difficult to be measured accurately. However, the structured observation method is highly influenced by subjective factors (including study subjects and observers) and therefore requires attention in its use for the presence of the following biases:

当不能通过自我报告法获得可靠的数据时，以及研究变量很难被准确地测量时，结构化自我观察法是一种很常用的方法。但结构化观察法受主观因素的影响较大（包括研究对象和观察者），在使用过程中需要注意是否有以下偏差的存在：

4.1 Hawthorne Effect(霍桑效应)

That is, the research subject will unconsciously change his or her original behavior and performance when he or she realizes that he or she is being observed, and tends to change in the direction desired by the observer or in line with social expectations.

霍桑效应指研究对象意识到自己正在被观察时会不自觉地改变自己原本的行为和表现，且往往朝着观察者希望的方向或符合社会期望的方向去改变。

4.2 Halo Effect(光环效应)

It is a phenomenon of generalization. In the rating scale, the observer may be influenced by a prominent outstanding characteristic of the research subject and make positive comments on other unrelated characteristics of the person, such as the observer's overall impression of a person as positive, he may think he is also smart and brave, the devil effect is the opposite.

光环效应是一种以偏概全的现象。在等级量表中，观察者可能会受研究对象某一突出的优秀品质的影响而对这个人其他不相关的品质也做出积极的评价，如观察者对一个人的总体印象是积极向上的，就会认为他也是聪明勇敢的，恶魔效应则与之相反。

4.3 Observer Consistency(观察者一致性)

This includes interobserver consistency (consistency of observations of the same study subject by different observers) and intraobserver consistency (consistency of observations of the same study subject by the same observer under different conditions). This is described in detail in Chapter 12.

观察者一致性包括观察者间一致性(不同观察者对同一研究对象的观察结果的一致性)和观察者内一致性(同一观察者在不同条件下对同一研究对象的观察结果的一致性)，第十二章会详细介绍。

Section Ⅳ Biophysiologic Measures
第四节 生物医学测量法

1. Types of Biophysiologic Measures(生物医学测量法的类型)

1.1 Classification by Measurement Objects(按照测量对象分类)

1.1.1 In Vivo Measurements(在体测量)

Measurements taken on or in living organisms (e. g., blood pressure, body temperature, and body weight).

在生物体活体上或生物体活体内进行的测量(如血压、体温和体重)。

1.1.2 Ex Vivo Measurements(离体测量)

Measurements performed outside the living organism (e. g., blood specimens, urine specimens, and pathology section specimens).

在生物体活体外进行的测量(如血液标本、尿液标本和病理切片标本)。

1.2　Classification by Measurement Indexes（按照测量指标分类）

1.2.1　Physiological Index Measurements（生理学指标测量）

Measurements concerning the functional activity of living organisms, such as cardiac activity, blood pressure, and pulse rate.

有关生物体活体功能活动的测量，如心电活动、血压和脉搏等。

1.2.2　Biochemical Index Measurements（生化学指标测量）

Measurements concerning the chemical structure, substance content, and substance metabolism of living organisms, such as sodium ion content in serum, coagulation factors, and blood lipids, etc.

有关生物体活体化学结构、物质含量、物质代谢等指标的测量，如血清中的钠离子含量、凝血因子和血脂等。

1.2.3　Morphological Index Measurements（形态学指标测量）

Measurements of the structure and morphological position of organs, tissues and cells of living organisms. For example, pathological section examination, MRI examination, etc.

对生物体活体的器官、组织和细胞的结构、形态位置等进行的测量。如病理切片检查、核磁共振检查等。

2. Selecting a Biophysiologic Measure（生物医学测量法的选择）

There are several factors to consider when choosing a biomedical measurement method：

在选择生物医学测量法时要考虑以下几个因素：

（1）Are there other more suitable alternative measures?

是否有其他更适合的替代测量方法？

（2）Is there available instrumentation or technology and what is their reliability and validity?

是否有可用的仪器设备或技术，以及它们的信效度如何？

（3）Can the budget cover the cost of measurement（e. g., instrumentation and training of measurement personnel）?

预算是否能负担测量成本（如仪器的使用和测量人员的培训）？

(4)Will it cause harm to the study population? What is the severity of the harm?

是否会给研究对象造成伤害？伤害的严重程度如何？

(5)Is professional measurement staff needdcd? Does the researcher need training? Are there resources available to help the researcher with operation and interpretation?

是否需要专业的测量人员？研究人员是否需要培训？是否有资源帮助研究者的操作和解释？

(6) Does the study need to be approved by some appropriate committee (e. g., ethics review board)?

是否需要获得一些相应的委员会的认可(如伦理审查委员会)？

3. Evaluation of Biophysiologic Measures(评价生物医学测量法)

3.1 Advantages of Biomedical Measurement Method(生物医学测量法的优点)

(1)The biomedical measurement method uses sophisticated instrumentation and advanced technology for measurement, obtaining more objective and accurate results and minimizing the influence of subjective factors.

生物医学测量法采用精密的仪器设备和先进的技术进行测量，获得的结果更加客观和准确，最大程度减少主观因素的影响。

(2)Biomedical measurements are more specific for measuring study variables, such as blood pressure by sphygmomanometer and body temperature by thermometer.

生物医学测量法测量研究变量更具有针对性，如血压计测量血压、体温计测量体温等。

3.2 Disadvantages of Biomedical Measurement Method(生物医学测量法的缺点)

(1)The sophisticated instrumentation, advanced technology, and specialized measurement staff required for biomedical measurement methods can increase the cost of research, and therefore the method is sometimes limited by funding and technology and cannot be implemented.

生物医学测量法所需的精密的仪器设备、先进的技术和专业的测量人员会提高研究的成本，因此该方法有时会受到经费和技术的限制而无法实施。

(2)Biomedical measurements sometimes require invasive methods of specimen collection that may cause pain or injury to the study subject, such as blood specimen collection and invasive arterial pressure monitoring.

生物医学测量法有时需要采用有创的方法采集标本，可能会给研究对象带来痛苦或伤害，如血液标本的采集、有创动脉压监测等。

Section V Second-hand Data Collection
第五节 二手资料的收集

Depending on the source of the data, the data can be divided into primary and secondary data. Secondary data are those existed before the study and were not collected for the purpose of this study.

根据资料来源的不同，可以将资料分为一手资料和二手资料。二手资料是指在研究前已经存在的，并非出于本研究目的而收集的资料。

1. Sources, Advantages and Disadvantages of Second-hand Data （二手资料的来源与优缺点）

1.1 Sources（来源）

1.1.1 Internal Sources（内部来源）

Information derived from clinical institutions that are non-public in nature, such as patient medical records and videos of treatment.

来源于临床机构中的资料，具有非公开性质，如患者病历和治疗的录像。

1.1.2 External Sources（外部来源）

Information from government agencies, Internet platforms, international organizations, etc., with public nature, such as data obtained from census and epidemiological surveys.

来源于政府机构、互联网平台、国际组织等的资料，具有公开性质，如人口普查和流行病学调查所获得的数据。

1.2 Advantages （优点）

（1）Secondary data existed prior to the study, greatly saving the cost and time of the study. 二手资料在研究前已经存在，大大地节约了研究的成本和时间。

（2）Secondary sources often come from authoritative institutions, specialized databases and experts and are highly reliable.

二手资料常常来自权威机构、专业数据库和专家，可靠性强。

(3) Secondary sources from authoritative institutions, specialized databases and experts are in a constant state of renewal, and secondary sources are not limited to the field of nursing research, therefore, secondary sources are widely available.

来自权威机构、专业数据库和专家的二手资料处于不断更新中，且二手资料不局限于护理研究领域，二手资料的来源广泛。

1.3　Disadvantages(缺点)

(1) Since secondary sources are not collected for the purposes of the secondary source analyst, the secondary source analyst has limited usable information from the secondary sources, and in addition, some of the study variables and terms in the secondary sources may be defined and classified differently from the secondary source analyst.

由于二手资料不是出于二手资料分析者的目的而收集的，因此二手资料分析者从二手资料中获得的可用的信息有限，此外，二手资料中的一些研究变量和术语的定义和分类可能与二手资料分析者的不同。

(2) The analyst of secondary data has no access to every aspect of data collection, much less control over it, so the quality of secondary data is difficult to judge.

二手资料的分析者无法了解到资料收集的每一环节，更无法控制，因此二手资料的质量难以判断。

(3) There is a time lag between the collection of primary data and the analysis of secondary data because of the multiple steps of sample determination, data collection and data entry.

从原始数据的收集到二手资料的分析中间要经历确定样本、数据收集和数据录入等多个步骤，因此二手资料存在时间滞后性。

2. Collection and Analysis of Second-hand Data(二手资料的收集与分析)

2.1　Collection and Analysis of Secondary Data from the Research Problem
(从研究问题开始二手资料的收集与分析)

2.1.1　Formulate Research Questions and Develop Theoretical or Conceptual Frameworks(提出研究问题，建立理论框架或概念框架)

The research begins with the formulation of the research question, clarifies the research question and purpose, and searches for existing research or theories related to the research question, on the basis of which the theoretical or conceptual framework of this study is formed, which also provides the basis for the selection of the research variables that follow.

从提出研究问题开始进行研究，明确研究问题和目的，寻找与研究问题相关的现有的研究或理论，在此基础上，形成本研究的理论框架或概念框架，也为之后的研究变量的选择提供了依据。

2.1.2　Identify the Research Subject（明确研究对象）

The researcher needs to describe the study population (e. g., the scope of the sample and the sample population) in detail to facilitate subsequent database selection and evaluation as well as to determine the secondary sources needed for the study.

研究者需要详细地描述研究对象（如样本的范围和研究的人群），便于之后数据库的选择和评价，以及确定研究需要的二手资料。

2.1.3　Identify Study Variables（明确研究变量）

Databases contain a wide variety of variables, and different studies may have different interpretations and definitions of the same variable. In addition, the inclusion of too many relevant study variables or the inclusion of irrelevant study variables can increase the burden of researchers, and the inclusion of too few relevant study variables tends to lose useful variables; therefore, clarifying the study variables is a very important aspect, and the theoretical or conceptual framework of the study can guide the selection of study variables.

数据库中包含各种各样的变量，而且对同一变量，不同的研究可能有不同的解释和定义。此外，纳入相关的研究变量过多或纳入不相关的研究变量会加重研究者的负担，纳入相关的研究变量过少容易丢失有用的变量。因此，明确研究变量是一个很重要的环节，研究的理论或概念框架可以指导研究变量的选择。

2.1.4　Identify Data Information and Types（明确数据信息和类型）

After identifying the study variables, it is important to identify the information and types of data that are most helpful and relevant to the study.

二手资料提供的数据信息和类型种类很多，确定研究变量之后，要明确对研究最有帮助、与研究最相关的数据信息和类型。

2.1.5 Select and Evaluate Database(选择和评价数据库)

Databases relevant to the research questions are selected by reviewing relevant literature, searching websites, and seeking advice from professional researchers, Liu, Z. C. and Zhang, X. J. (2011) provided a method for secondary data collection using the Internet. Relevant information about the databases (e.g., purpose, content, measurement time, etc.) can be obtained from documents such as their accompanying coding manuals, resource guides, and instructions for use, and secondary data analysts later screen relevant databases according to the specific requirements of the study. Once a database is selected, the secondary data analyst searches for as much information as possible about the data collection and data analysis, and evaluates the quality of the data related to the study variables.

通过查阅相关文献、网站搜索和寻求专业研究人员的建议等方法来选择与研究问题相关的数据库,刘志超和张小娟(2011)提供了用互联网进行二手数据收集的方法。数据库的相关信息(如目的、内容、测量时间等)可以从其附带的编码手册、资源指南和使用说明等文件中获取,二手资料分析者之后根据研究的具体要求对相关的数据库进行筛选。一旦选择了数据库,二手资料分析者就要尽可能地搜寻数据收集和数据分析的有关信息,对研究变量相关的数据的质量进行评价。

2.1.6 Collection and Organization of Secondary Data(二手资料的收集与整理)

Generally speaking, secondary data are characterized by a wide range of sources, extensive coverage and large amount of information, and secondary data analysts need to select data information in the database according to the needs of the research problem. The secondary data are mainly organized by merging data and cleaning data. The researcher can merge the database or research variables according to the research needs, and cleaning data mainly includes data conversion, logical error checking of data values, finding outliers and dealing with missing values(Xi X. & Guo G. F., 2014). A detailed method for handling missing values is presented by Tang J. Y. et al. (2011).

一般而言,二手资料具有来源广泛、涉及面广且信息量大的特点,二手资料分析者需要根据研究问题的需求来选择数据库中的数据信息。对二手资料的整理主要包括合并数据和清理数据。研究者根据研究需要可以对数据库或研究变量进行合并,清理数据主要包括数据的转换、数据值的逻辑检错、查找异常值和处理缺失值。(奚兴、郭桂芳,2014)唐健元等(2011)介绍了处理缺失值的详细方法。

2.1.7　Analysis of Secondary Information(二手资料的分析)

The analysis of secondary data is similar to that of primary research, with the difference that secondary data need to describe the characteristics of the primary data, the reliability and validity of the data, and the problems that exist (Doolan & Froelicher, 2009).

二手资料的分析与原始研究相似，不同点在于二手资料需要说明原始资料的特征、资料的信效度和存在的问题(Doolan 和 Froelicher, 2009)。

2.2　Collection and Analysis of Secondary Data from the Database
(从数据库开始二手资料的收集与分析)

The researcher first selects a database of interest and then thinks about the problems that can be solved with this database, similar to the steps of collecting and analyzing secondary data starting with the research question, but in a changed order.

研究者先选择一个数据库，然后思考用这个数据库可以解决的问题，和从研究问题开始的二手资料的收集与分析步骤是相似的，但顺序有所改变。

Section Ⅵ　Implementing a Data Collection Plan
第六节　实施数据收集计划

1. Selecting Research Personnel(选择研究人员)

The selection of data collectors is an important decision in the data collection process. There are several aspects to consider in selecting the appropriate data collector:

选择数据收集人员是数据收集过程中的一个重要决定。选择合适的数据收集人员要考虑以下几个方面：

(1)Is the personality suitable? For example, positive but not overly enthusiastic, sociable but not overly talkative.

性格是否合适？如积极但不过分热情，善于交际但不过分健谈。

(2)Is there any political or social bias?

是否有政治或社会偏见？

(3)Any experience with data collection? What is the potential for data collection? What is the experience with data collection?

有无数据收集的经验？数据收集的潜力如何？数据收集的经验如何？

(4) Can the researcher remain neutral on the research question?

研究人员能否对研究问题保持中立？

2. Training Data Collectors(培训数据收集人员)

Training of data collectors is usually the responsibility of the principal investigator, and the materials used in the training are usually developed by the principal investigator, such as presentations, video materials, and training manuals, which typically include background materials, general instructions, specific instructions, and all data collection forms used in the study, and the length of the training varies depending on the complexity of the study. The training is divided into two main sections, one for general procedures training (e. g., communication skills in interviews) and one for specific procedures training (i. e., training specific to the content of the study).

数据收集人员的培训通常由首席研究员负责，培训中用到的资料也通常由首席研究员开发，如演示文稿、录像资料和培训手册，培训手册一般包括背景材料、一般说明、具体说明和研究中使用的所有数据收集表格，培训的时长因研究的复杂程度而定。培训的内容主要分为两个部分，一个是一般程序培训(如访谈中的沟通技巧)，一个是特殊程序培训(即特定于研究内容的培训)。

Section Ⅶ   Critiquing Methods of Data Collection
第七节   评判数据收集方法

Each decision in data collection methods affects the accuracy, validity, and veracity of the data, and more importantly, the quality of the study as a whole. This section provides guidelines for critiquing data collection methods for researchers.

数据收集方法中的每个决定都影响着数据的准确性、有效性和真实性，更影响着整个研究的质量。这个章节提供了评判量性数据收集方法的指导供研究者参考。

(1) Did the information and type of data collected meet the purpose and needs of the study?

收集的数据信息和类型是否符合研究目的和需求？

(2) Was the location of data collection appropriate?

数据收集的地点是否合适？

（3）Were the correct data collection methods used? Was the data collection instrument used appropriate? Was it necessary for the researcher to develop new measurement instruments, and if so, did the development process meet the requirements of standard procedures? Were the data collection forms developed in a way that meets the needs of the study and was simple and straightforward without burdening the participants?

是否采用了正确的数据收集方法？采用的数据收集工具是否合适？研究者是否有必要开发新的测量工具，如果有，开发过程是否符合标准程序的要求？数据收集表格的制定是否既符合研究需求，又简单明了不会加重参与者负担？

（4）Was the amount of data collected appropriate (i. e., was the amount of data sufficient without overburdening the participants)?

收集的数据量是否合适(即数据量既充足又不会太多而导致参与者负担)？

（5）Was there adequate pre-experimentation of the data collection process?

是否对数据收集过程进行了充分的预实验？

（6）Did the study provide sufficient information about the data collection process?

研究是否提供了有关数据收集过程的充分的信息？

（7）Were data collectors selected for characteristics consistent with the collection of high-quality data? Were the data collectors trained? What were the results of the training?

是否选择了符合收集高质量数据的特征数据收集人员？是否对数据收集人员进行了培训？培训结果如何？

（8）Were there any biases in the data collection process such as Hawthorne effect, halo effect, social desirability response bias, etc.? If so, what was the impact on study quality?

数据收集过程中是否存在霍桑效应、光环效应、社会期许性反应偏差等偏倚的存在？如果存在，对研究质量的影响如何？

📖 Studies Cited in Chapter 11(第十一章参考文献)

[1]Schneider, J. K., Deenan, A. Reducing quantitative data errors: tips for clinical researchers [J]. Applied nursing research: ANR, 2004, 17(2): 125-129.

[2]Fowler, F. J. Survey research methods[M]. 5th ed. Thousand Oaks: Sage Publications, 2014.

[3]Dillman, D., Smyth, J., Christian, L. M. Internet, phone, mail, and mixed-mode surveys: The tailored design method[M]. 4th ed. New York: Wiley, 2014.

［4］Tourangeau，R.，Conrad，F.，Couper，M. The science of web surveys［M］. New York：Oxford University Press，2013.

［5］Fitzpatrick，J. J.，Montgomery，K. S. Internet for nursing research：A guide to strategies，skills，and resources［M］. New York：Springer，2004.

［6］Haidet，K. K.，Tate，J.，Divirgilio-Thomas，D.，et al. Methods to improve reliability of video-recorded behavioral data［J］. Research in Nursing & Health，2009，32：465-474.

［7］刘志超，张小娟. 基于互联网的二手资料收集方法研究［J］. 科技管理研究，2011（03），187-190.

［8］奚兴，郭桂芳. 如何利用二手资料进行护理研究［J］. 中国护理管理，2014(3)，334-336.

［9］唐健元，杨志敏，杨进波，等. 临床研究中缺失值的类型和处理方法研究［J］. 中国卫生统计，2011(3)，338-341，343.

［10］Doolan，D. M.，Froelicher，E. S. Using an existing data set to answer new research questions：a methodological review［J］. Research and theory for nursing practice，2009，23(3)：203-215.

Chapter 12: Measurement and Data Quality
第十二章 测量及数据质量

Section Ⅰ Measurement
第一节 测量

1. Measurement(测量)

Measurement is the process of assigning numbers to objects, events, or situations in accord with some rule (Kaplan, 1963). Measurements produce some values that indicate whether and to what extent attributes exist, and rules are necessary to promote consistency and interpretability. Measurement requires first clarifying the objects, attributes and elements to be measured, and then identifying or developing strategies and methods suitable for measuring it based on these. When the measurements are objective, specific and direct, such as height, weight, temperature, heart rate and respiration, as well as in laboratory values and measures of demographic variables such as age, gender, race, diagnosis, marital status, income and education, they can be measured directly using rules that are familiar to us. However, the characteristics usually measured in nursing are abstract, such as pain, stress, depression, anxiety, coping, or quality of life, and abstract concepts cannot be measured directly and are usually represented by indicators or attributes of the concept, thus selecting or developing appropriate methods for measuring the concept, which is called indirect measurement. For measuring psychosocial phenomena, physical measurements are more accurate than instruments via self-report or observation, but few measurements are error-free.

测量是指根据某些规则为对象、事件或者情况分配数字的过程（Kaplan，1963）。测量会产生表示属性是否存在以及存在程度的数值，而规则对于促进一致性和可解释性是必要的。测量首先需要明确测量的对象、属性和要素，然后根据这些确定或者开发出适合衡量它的策略和方法。当测量的对象是客观的、具体的、直接的，例如身高、体重、温度、心率和呼吸，以及实验室检查和社会人口学测量中的如年龄、性别、种族、诊断、婚姻状况、收入和教育，可以用我们所熟悉的工具直接测量。然而，在护理中，通常测量的特征是抽象的，例如疼痛、压力、抑郁、焦虑、应对或生活质量，抽象概念不能被直接测量，通常用概念的指标或者属性来表示，从而选择或发展适当的测量概念的方法，称之为间接测量。对于测量社会心理现象来说，物理测量的仪器比通过自我报告或观察更准确，但几乎没有任何一种测量方式是无错误的。

2. Advantages of Measurement(测量的优点)

Measurement is very important in health care. The main advantage of measurement is that it gives objective information about the results, eliminates subjective guesswork, and its results can be independently verified. For example, two people using the same scale to measure the weight of the same person may get the same result.

在医疗卫生保健中，测量是极其重要的。测量主要的优点就是它得到的结果信息是客观的，消除了主观臆测，并且它的结果可以被独立验证。例如，两个人用同一个体重秤先后测量同一个人的体重，得到的结果可能是相同的。

In addition, measurement may also yield accurate information. By taking measurements, we can describe Yao Ming's height as 226cm, rather than generalizing "how come he is so tall". Measurements can also help researchers distinguish between people with different degrees of attributes.

另外，测量还可能获得准确的信息。通过测量，我们可以描述姚明的身高为226cm，而不是笼统地表达"他怎么这么高"。测量也可以帮助研究人员区分具有不同程度属性的人。

Finally, measurement is a language of communication. Numbers express more clearly than words.

最后，测量是一种沟通的语言。比起文字，数字表达得更加清晰。

3. Theories of Measurement(测量理论)

Psychometrics is a branch of psychology that focuses on the theory and methods of psychological measurement. There are three influential theories in psychometrics (health measurement). The dominant position is occupied by classical test theory (CTT), a psychometric theory that is easily understood, well-structured and has been used as a basis for the development of multi-item measures of health constructs and is also applicable to conceptualize all types of measures (e.g., bio physiological measures). The other is Item Response Theory (IRT), which is only applicable to multi-item scales. Item response theory integrates information from various item analyses through item response curves, allowing us to visualize the characteristics of item analysis such as item difficulty and discrimination, and thus serves as a guide for item selection and preparation of test comparison scores. The last theory is the generalization theory (GT), which mainly addresses the problem of measurement error and can estimate multiple sources of measurement error for different measurement contexts, providing useful information for improving measurement and improving measurement quality. Researchers need to understand the logic in measurement theory so that they can select and use existing instruments or develop new quality measurements for their studies.

　　心理测量学是心理学的一个分支，主要研究心理测量的理论和方法。在心理测量学（健康测量）中有三个具有影响力的理论。占据主导位置的是经典测试理论（CTT），经典测试理论是一种心理测量理论，容易理解、体系完整，已被用作发展健康结构的多项目测量的基础，也适用于概念化所有类型的测量（例如，生物生理测量）。另外一种是项目反应理论（IRT），只适用于多项目量表。项目反应理论通过项目反应曲线综合各种项目分析的资料，使我们综合直观地看出项目难度、鉴别度等项目分析的特征，从而起到指导项目筛选和编制测验比较分数等作用。最后一个理论是概化理论（GT），概化理论主要解决测量误差的问题，它能针对不同测量情境估计测量误差的多种来源，为改善测量，提高测量质量提供有用的信息。研究人员需要理解测量理论中的逻辑，以便他们可以为他们的研究选择和使用现有的仪器或开发新的质量测量方法。

4. Errors of Measurement(测量误差)

Errors are present in all measurement strategies. Measurement error is the difference between what is actually present and what is measured with an instrument. Measurement errors can occur in both direct and indirect measurements. For example, in direct measurement, the scale may not be accurate, the equipment inside the laboratory may be accurately calibrated but may change as it is used more often, and the tape measure used to measure an object may not be placed in the same position every time. In indirect measurement, the metric describing a concept may be only a part of the concept or the measured metric contains parts that are not part of the concept, resulting in measurement error. Measurement error contains random error and systematic error. According to measurement theory, we can learn that the measurement results consist of three parts: true score, observed score and error score. The true score (T) is the result of the measurement we obtained without error. The true score is assumed and cannot be known because the measurement method is not absolutely reliable and there will always be some measurement error. The observation score (O) is the result of the measurement for the subject using the selected instrument during the study, and the error score (E) is the random error in the measurement process. The theoretical equations for these three components are as folows:

$$\text{Observed score}(O) = \text{true score}(T) + \text{random error}(E)$$

所有的测量策略都会存在一定的误差。测量误差是指实际存在的与用仪器测量出来的之间的差异。无论是直接测量还是间接测量都可能产生测量误差。例如在直接测量中，体重秤可能不是精确的，实验室里面的设备虽然被精确校准，但是随着使用次数的增加，精确度可能会降低，测量物体的卷尺不是每次都放在相同的位置。在间接测量中，描述概念的指标可能只是概念的一部分或者测量的指标包含了不属于概念的部分，从而造成了测量误差。测量误差包含随机误差和系统误差。根据测量理论，我们可以得知测量结果由真实得分、观察得分和错误得分三部分组成。真实得分(T)是指我们在没有误差的情况下得到的测量结果，真正的分数是假设的，不可能被知道的，因为测量方法不是绝对可靠的，总会有一些测量误差。观察得分(O)是在研究过程中，使用选定的仪器为受试者测量的结果，错误得分(E)为测量过程中的随机误差。这三个组成部分的理论方程如下：

$$\text{观察得分}(O) = \text{真实得分}(T) + \text{随机误差}(E)$$

Theoretically, the smaller the error score, the more the observed score reflects the true situation. Therefore, using instruments that reduce the error can improve the accuracy of the measurement (Waltz et al., 2010).

理论上，误差得分越小，观察到的分数越能反应真实情况。因此，使用能够减小误差的仪器可以提高测量的精度（Waltz 等，2010）。

There are many factors that add to the error in measurement, and they can be random or systematic. Random errors cause an individual's observed score to vary in no particular direction around the true score, and non-random measurement errors are called systematic errors, such as a scale that weighs 1 kg more than the subject's weight. The following are common sources of measurement error:

在测量的过程中，有很多因素会增加测量的误差，它们可以是随机的或者系统的。随机误差导致个体的观察分数在真实分数周围没有特定的方向变化，非随机的测量误差称为系统误差，例如一个比受试者的体重多 1 公斤的体重秤。下面是测量误差的常见来源：

（1）Personal factors：such as fatigue，hunger，attention span，emotion，etc. Personal factors can act directly on the measurement results，for example，heart rate increases when people are stressed and anxious，and can also affect the measurement results by influencing people's behavior，etc.

个人因素：例如疲劳、饥饿、注意力持续时间、情绪等。个人因素可以直接作用于测量结果，例如人在紧张焦虑时，心率会增加，也可以通过影响人们的行为等影响测量结果。

（2）Environmental factors：scores are influenced by the surrounding conditions at the time they are generated，such as temperature，relationship to the researcher，quiet or noise，other distracting things for the subject，etc.

环境因素：得分会受到他们周围情况的影响，例如温度、与研究者的关系、安静或嘈杂、其他使受试者分心的事情等。

（3）Variations in the administration of measurement procedures：such as changes in the order or phrasing of questions during the interview may produce errors，or physiological measurements some taken before eating and some after eating may also produce measurement errors.

测量程序管理的变化：如在访谈中问题的顺序或语序的变化可能会产生误差，或者在进食前后进行生理测量，也可能会产生测量误差。

（4）The process of data processing：such as errors when entering data，errors when coding data or errors when calculating instrument scores，etc.

数据处理的过程：例如输入数据时发生错误，数据编码时发生错误或计算量表分数时发生错误等。

（5）Perception of the instrument：If there is a bias in the perceived understanding of the instrument，the results obtained may be inaccurate，and different subjects may have a different understanding of the self-report instrument，which may also lead to measurement error.

对工具的认知：如果对工具的认知理解有偏差，得到的结果就可能有误差，不同的受试者可能对自我报告工具的理解不同，也会导致测量误差。

5. Major Types of Measures(测量的主要类型)

Measures can be divided into self-report and observation，depending on the source of the information; simple visual analogue scales or multidimensional scales containing dozens of items, depending on their complexity; and continuity scores and categorical scores, depending on the score produced by the measure.

测量可以根据信息的来源不同分为自我报告和观察等；根据复杂程度不同可分为简单的视觉模拟量表或者包含几十个条目的多维量表；根据测量产生的得分不同而分为连续性得分和分类得分。

In addition, there are some measures that are generic and can be used in a wide range of clinical and non-clinical patients, while there are some measures that are specific and can only be used for certain specific populations. For example, there are generic self-efficacy scales in research and there are self-efficacy scales specific to people with Alzheimer's disease.

另外，有一些测量是通用的，可以广泛地运用于临床和非临床的病人，而有一些测量是特定的，只能用于某些特定的人群。例如，研究中有通用的自我效能量表，也有专门针对阿尔兹海默病的人群的自我效能量表。

6. Measurement and Statistics(测量与统计)

Assessing the properties of a measurement requires some knowledge of statistics. In this section, we mainly describe the principles of statistics rather than the details or calculations of statistics, because usually the estimation of measurement parameters is done with software. Since the calculation of the correlation coefficient of a statistical indicator is extremely important for the properties of a measurement, we need to know what is the correlation coefficient.

评估测量的属性需要一些统计学的知识。在这部分，我们主要描述的是统计的原则，而不是统计的细节或者计算，因为通常情况下测量参数估计都是用软件来完成的。由于统计指标相关系数的计算对测量的属性极为重要，所以我们需要知道相关系数是什么。

The correlation coefficient is an important statistical tool when assessing the quality of an instrument. In general, the larger the absolute value of the correlation coefficient, the higher the correlation between the two variables. However, the correlation coefficient has only a relative meaning, not an absolute meaning, which is related to the size of the sample space, different sample space sizes correspond to a critical correlation coefficient, if the actual value of the correlation coefficient is higher than it means that the relationship is significant, otherwise, it is not significant.

在评估工具的质量时，相关系数是重要的统计学工具。一般情况下，相关系数的绝对值越大，表明两变量的相关程度越高。但是相关系数只有相对意义，没有绝对意义，这与样本含量的大小有关，不同样本含量大小对应一个临界相关系数，若实际相关系数的值高于它就代表关系显著，否则，则为不显著。

Section Ⅱ　Reliability
第二节　信度

Reliability refers to the ability of a measurement instrument to measure an attribute, entry or situation consistently in research or clinical practice. The higher the agreement of the results obtained, the higher the reliability, i. e. the lower the random error in the measurement method. In order to increase the credibility of a study, researchers need to select instruments with high reliability. In addition, before conducting other statistical analyses, researchers need to test the reliability of the measurement instruments used in their studies and reflect the reliability of the measurement instruments in the published studies.

信度是指在研究或者临床实践中，测量工具、测量属性、条目或者情况一致的能力。当所得结果的一致性越高，它的信度就越高，也就是说测量方法中的随机误差越小。为了增加研究的可信度，研究人员需要选择信度较高的工具。另外，在进行其他统计分析之前，研究人员需要对他们研究中所使用的测量工具进行可靠性测试，并在发表的研究报告中体现测量工具的信度。

1. Reliability(信度)

The reliability of quantitative measurements is the main criterion for evaluating their quality. Reliability testing is a test of the measurement error of the instrument used in a study. All measurement techniques contain some random errors that may be caused by the measurement method, the study participants, or the researcher collecting the data. The degree of confidence present is usually expressed in the form of a correlation coefficient, with 1. 00 indicating perfect reliability and 0. 00 indicating unreliability (Bialocerkowski et al., 2010). This chapter describes four different methods of assessing reliability, including retest reliability, inter-rater reliability, intra-rater reliability and parallel test reliability.

定量测量的信度是评价其质量的主要标准。可靠性测试是对用于研究的工具的测量误差进行检测。所有的测量技术都包含一些随机误差，这些误差可能是由测量方法、研究参与者或收集数据的研究人员造成的。信度的存在程度通常以相关系数的形式表示，1.00 表示完全可靠，0.00 表示不可靠（Bialocerkowski 等，2010）。本章将介绍 4 种不同评估信度的方法，包括重测信度、评定者间信、评定者内部信度和平行测试信度。

1.1　Test-Retest Reliability（重测信度）

Test-retested reliability, also known as the stability coefficient, is the correlation coefficient between the scores obtained from two successive measurements of the same subject using the same measurement instrument. The higher the degree of consistency, the closer the correlation coefficient is to 1.00, indicating that the higher the retested reliability of the research instrument, the more reliable the results will be.

重测信度也称稳定系数，是指用同一测量工具对同一对象进行先后两次的测量，然后计算测量所得的分数的相关系数。一致程度越高，相关系数就越趋近于1.00，说明研究工具的重测信度越高，测得的结果就越可靠。

Ideally, if a research instrument gives a good estimate of the true score for an attribute, it will give the same result in a different situation, but an assumption is needed when retesting reliability that the factor being measured remains constant between tests and that any change in value or score is the result of random error. Therefore, the following issues need to be kept in mind when retesting reliability: many phenomena in nursing research change over a short period of time, such as hopes, coping, anxiety, attitudes, knowledge, skills, etc., when the measure cannot be used to measure reliability, and the variable being measured must be stable, such as self-esteem, personality, values, etc. Furthermore, if researchers are to test the reliability of an instrument through retest reliability, they need to determine the optimal time period for the instrument to be used. The optimal time period for retest reliability depends on the variability of the variables being measured, the complexity of the measurement process and the characteristics of the participants, and for some scales, retest reliability is not as effective as expected, possibly because subjects remember their responses when they were first tested, (Bialocerkowski et, al., 2010). Therefore, the interval is appropriate so that the first measurement does not have an effect on the results of the second measurement, usually 2-4 weeks. Another issue is the change in people's psychology; they will not be as careful and cautious on the second measurement as they were on the first, and may find the test boring and respond more casually, leading to a false estimate of reliability.

在理想的情况下，如果一个研究工具能很好地评估出某种属性的真实得分，那么它在不同的情况下也能得到同样的结果，但是在重测信度时需要一个假设，被测量的因素在两次测试时保持不变，值或分数的任何变化都是随机误差的结果。因此，在重测信度时需要注意以下问题：护理研究中的许多现象都会在短时间内发生变化，例如希望、应对、焦虑、态度、知识、技能等，这时测量就不能用来衡量信度，所测量的变量必须是稳定的，例如自尊、个性、价值观等。另外，如果研究人员要通过重测信度检验工具的可靠性，则需要确定工具使用的最佳时间，重测信度的最佳时间周期取决于被测量变量的可变性，测量过程的复杂性以及参与者的特性，对于一些量表，重测信度并没有预期的那么有效，原因可能是被试者记得他们第一次测试时的反应（Bialocerkowski 等，2010）。因此，间隔的时间以第一次测量不会对第二次测量的结果产生影响为宜，一般为 2~4 周。另一个问题是人们心理的变化，在第二次测量时他们不会像第一次一样谨慎小心，可能觉得测试很无聊，就会更加随意地作出反应，从而导致对信度的错误估计。

1.2　Inter-rater and Intra-rater Reliability(评定者间信度和评定者内部信度)

Inter-rater reliability refers to the consistency of results obtained by different raters using the same instrument to measure the same object. Inter-rater reliability is not necessary when the measurement is objective, such as measuring scales, skinfold thickness and head circumference, but is assessed when the measurement is subjective, such as in interviews, personality tests or when clinicians want to know whether they or their staff can apply a measure reliably.

评定者间信度是指不同的评定者使用相同的工具测量相同的对象所得到的结果的一致性。当测量是客观的时候，例如测量尺度、测量皮褶厚度以及头围等，主要评估的是被测者属性的可靠性，不必考虑评定者间信度，但是当测量是主观的，例如面试、人格测试或者临床医生想知道他们自己或者他们的员工是否能够可靠地应用某种测量方法时，则需要评估评定者间信度。

Intra-rater reliability refers to the consistency of results obtained by the same rater using the same instrument in different situations. Intra-rater reliability is an indicator of self-consistency and is similar to re-test reliability in that it requires careful selection of the time interval between tests, except that re-test reliability focuses on respondent consistency whereas intra-rater reliability focuses on rater consistency.

评定者内部信度是指同一评定者在不同的情况下使用相同的工具测量所得到的结果的一致性。评定者内部信度是自我一致性的一个指标，它与重测信度相似，都需要仔细选择测试之间的时间间隔，不同的是重测信度重点在于被测者的一致性，而评定者内部信度在于评定者的一致性。

Inter-rater reliability and intra-rater reliability can be estimated by calculating the correlation coefficients between the raters' measurements if the results are expressed numerically, and in other cases by calculating the proportion of agreement using the following formula.

如果测量结果是用数字表示的，则可以计算评定者们测量结果之间的相关系数来估计评定者间信度及评定者内部信度，而在其他情况下，则需要使用下列公式计算一致的比例：

number of agreements/(number of agreements+disagreements)

一致的数目/(一致的数目+不一致的数目)

However, this formula tends to overestimate agreement and does not take into account the probability of agreeing by chance. If the rater only had to judge whether or not the observed behavior was present, then there would be a 50% probability that the rater would be consistent by chance. Cohen's Kappa coefficient, adjusted for chance agreement, is more appropriate for this situation. Kappa values usually range from 0.00 to 1.00, with no less than 0.60 being acceptable and greater than or equal to 0.75 indicating a high degree of confidence. If more than two raters are involved, statistical methods can be used to calculate alpha coefficients. Alternatively, analysis of variance can be used to test for differences between raters.

但是，这个公式往往高估了一致性，没有考虑到偶然达成一致的概率。假如评定者只需要判断被观察的行为是否存在，那么评定者就有50%的概率是偶然一致的。科恩的Kappa系数根据机会的一致性进行了调整，更加适合这种情况。Kappa值通常为0.00~1.00，而不小于0.60是可以接受的，大于等于0.75则表示信度较高。如果涉及两个以上的评定者，可以使用统计方法来计算alpha系数。另外，方差分析也可用来检验评定者之间的差异。

1.3 Parallel Test Reliability(平行测试信度)

Parallel test reliability refers to the degree of agreement in the results obtained when two similar research instruments are used to measure the same group of subjects. And proving that a person is actually testing the same content in two tests is very complex, i.e., designing instruments that can be substituted for each other is difficult and therefore rarely used in clinical studies. When the same group of subjects completes both instruments, the mean and standard deviation obtained should also be approximately equal. If two instruments are developed to measure pain, patients can be asked to answer both instruments consecutively and the correlation coefficient of the scores can be calculated to determine whether the two research instruments are equivalent, with a coefficient greater than or equal to 0.80 indicating good equivalence (Waltz et al., 2010).

平行测试信度是指利用两个类似的研究工具对同一组研究对象进行测量，所得结果的一致性程度。而证明一个人在两个测试中，实际上测试的是相同的内容是非常复杂的，即设计出可以互相替代的工具是困难的，因此在临床的研究中很少使用。当同一组研究对象完成这两种研究工具时，得到的平均值和标准差应该也大致相等。如果开发了两种测量疼痛的工具，可以让病人连续应用这两种工具，计算出得分的相关系数来确定两种研究工具是否等价，系数大于等于 0.80 表示等价性较好 (Waltz 等，2010)。

1.4 Interpretation of Reliability Coefficients(信度系数的解释)

The reliability coefficient is an important indicator for judging the quality of an instrument, and a low reliability of a measurement instrument not only reduces statistical efficacy but also affects the validity of the conclusions. For intergroup comparisons of studies, the reliability coefficient needs to be greater than or equal to 0.80, while for group comparisons, such as youth and elderly groups, and men and women, the reliability coefficient needs to be greater than or equal to 0.90.

信度系数是判断工具质量的重要指标，测量工具的信度较低不仅会降低统计功效，而且会影响结论的有效性。对于研究的组间比较，信度系数需要大于等于 0.80，而对于群体的比较，比如青年群体和老年群体，男性和女性，信度系数则需要大于等于 0.90。

If we give 50 cancer patients a scale to measure their hope, the scores will vary from person to person, and some of the variance in the scores is true variance reflecting differences in their hope, but some of the variance is due to measurement error. If V_O is used to denote the total variation in observed scores, V_T denotes true variation, and V_E denotes variation due to measurement error, then

$$V_O = V_T + V_E$$

假如我们给 50 个癌症患者做一个量表来衡量他们的希望，得分会因人而异，有些得分的变异是真实的变异，反应了他们在希望上的差异，但是有些变异是由测量误差引起的。若用 V_O 表示观察到的得分的总变异，V_T 表示真实变异，V_E 表示由测量误差引起的变异，则

$$V_O = V_T + V_E$$

And reliability is the proportion of the total variance of the test that is caused by the true score, i.e.

$$R = \frac{V_T}{V_O}$$

而信度是指测验的总变异中真实得分造成的变异所占的比例，即

$$R = \frac{V_T}{V_O}$$

For example, when the reliability coefficient is 0.80, it can be assumed that 80% of the variance in the observed scores is due to true scores and only 20% comes from measurement error.

例如，当信度系数为0.80时，可以认为观察到的得分中有80%的变异是由真实得分造成的，仅有20%来自测量误差。

1.5 Factors Affecting Reliability(影响信度的因素)

Several factors may affect the reliability coefficients as follows.

下面几个因素都可能会影响到信度系数：

(1)For observation-type scales, different observers may get different results, so uniform training can be provided to the observer.

对于观察类的量表，不同的观察者可能得到不同的结果，因此，可以对观测人员进行统一的培训。

(2)Reliability is related to the heterogeneity of the sample being measured. If there is less variation among the samples being measured, it will be difficult for the instrument to distinguish those samples with different attributes, and the reliability coefficient will be lower.

信度与被测样本的异质性有关，如果被测样本之间的差异越小，工具就很难区分那些具有不同属性的样本，信度系数就会越低。

(3) Related to the sample size, the larger the sample size is, the more accurate the estimated reliability will be, all other things being equal.

与样本容量相关，在其他条件不变的情况下，样本的容量越大估计出的信度就越准确。

(4)the content of the measurement instrument, in general, the more entries in the scale, the higher the reliability, but as the number of entries increases, the subject may become inattentive, which in turn increases the error and decreases the reliability. Therefore, it is sometimes necessary to weigh the two, and a large number of scales can be divided into multiple subscales.

测量工具的内容，在一般情况下，量表的条目越多，信度越高。但是，随着条目的增多，受测者可能出现注意力不集中，反而使误差增大，信度降低。因此，有时需要权衡两者，可以将一个大量表分为多个分量表。

2. Internal Consistency(内部一致性)

Internal consistency (internal consistency) refers to the intrinsic correlation between the items of a measurement instrument. Since a single item is not sufficient to measure a concept, a multi-item research instrument needs to be constructed, and the formation of a research instrument in which all items measure the same indicators indicates a high internal consistency and good reliability of the instrument.

内部一致性是指测量工具各条目间的内在相关性。由于单条目不足以测量一个概念，因此需要构建多条目的研究工具，而组建研究工具的各条目都是测量相同的指标，就说明工具的内在一致性较高，信度较好。

3. Measurement Error(测量误差)

Measurement error is closely linked to reliability and can only be absent if the reliability is 1.00, and measurement error statistics can be used to estimate the possible range of true scores. One of the most widely used indicators of measurement error is the standard deviation of measurement (SEM), which can be calculated in conjunction with either reliability or internal consistency. The confidence factor does not have units of measurement, while SEM has units of measurement associated with the actual measurement. For example, when measuring weight, SEM is measured in grams or kilograms, etc. SEM is not affected by sample homogeneity and is more stable than the reliability coefficient. If the subject's score is 45 and the SEM is 2.5, we can assume that there is about a 95% chance that his true score is between 40 and 50.

测量误差与信度紧密联系，只有当信度为 1.00 时，测量误差才有可能不存在，测量误差统计可以用于估计真实得分可能的范围。其中，使用最广泛的测量误差的指标是测量标准差(SEM)，它可以结合信度或者内部一致性计算出来。信度系数没有测量单位，而 SEM 有与实际测量相关的测量单位。例如测量重量时，SEM 以克或者千克等为单位。SEM 不受样本同质性的影响，比信度系数更稳定。若受试者的得分为 45，SEM 为 2.5，我们就可以认为他的真实得分为 40~50 的概率为 95%。

Section Ⅲ　Reliability
第三节　效度

1. Validity(效度)

Another attribute of a measurement instrument is validity, also known as accuracy, which refers to the degree to which a measurement instrument reflects the concept of the variable it is studying, the higher the degree to which it reflects, the better the validity. Validity can be expressed as content validity, face validity, scale validity, and structural validity. Validity is more difficult to be evaluated compared to reliability, because some of its evaluation methods lack objective statistical data.

测量工具的另一个属性为效度，也称精确度，指某一测量工具能够反映它所研究的变量概念的程度，它所反映的程度越高，效度则越好。效度可用内容效度、表面效度、效标效度和结构效度表示。相对于信度来说，效度较难被评价，因为它的一些评价方法缺少客观的统计学数据。

2. Content and Face Validity(内容效度和表面效度)

Face validity is the judgment of researchers, subjects, or other reviewers as to whether a measurement instrument reflects the characteristics of a variable concept based on their understanding of the variable concept to be measured. Face validity is a subjective method of evaluating whether an instrument "appears" to be valid, and therefore is not strong evidence of instrument validity (DeVon et al., 2007). Researchers typically use face validity in the initial stages of assessing the validity of a measurement instrument, which is a basis for other validity assessments.

表面效度指的是研究人员、受试者或其他评议员根据对需要测量的变量概念的理解，对测量工具是否能够反映变量概念的特征所做出的判断。表面效度属于一种主观评价方法，它的评价标准为是否"看起来"有效，不能体现效度的高低，因此，它不是测量工具有效性的有力证据（DeVon 等，2007）。研究者通常在评价测量工具效度的初始阶段使用表面效度，把它作为进行其他效度评价的基础。

Content validity refers to the extent to which the items in the measurement instrument （quantity, quality, and proportion of content distribution）reflect the content of the study variables. Since content validity requires a high level of reviewers, the review is usually conducted by an expert committee consisting of at least three experts with expertise in the field of the research instrument and up to 10 experts, usually five, with an odd number of experts preferred. In addition, the experts consider whether the items contained in the instrument reflect the full composition of the measured concepts and, if the instrument is a multidimensional scale, the balance of the items in each dimension.

内容效度指的是测量工具中的条目(数量、质量和内容分配比例)反映研究变量内容的程度。由于内容效度对评议者的要求较高，所以评议通常由专家委员会进行，专家委员会由至少 3 位具有研究工具涉及领域的专业知识的专家组成，最多由 10 位专家组成，一般为 5 位，专家个数最好为奇数。专家委员会对研究工具所包含的条目与要测量的变量概念的相关程度进行评议。此外，专家们还需考虑研究工具包含的条目是否能全面地反映测量概念的组成，如果研究工具为多维度量表，还需考虑每个维度里条目分配的均衡性。

Researchers develop measurement instruments with a detailed and comprehensive conceptualization of the instrument to facilitate the instrument's ability to obtain accurate and valid information about the variables, and conduct conceptualization based primarily on extensive literature review, expert consultation, and in-depth communication with the target population.

研究者在开发测量工具时要对该工具进行详细全面的概念化定义，便于工具能够获得准确有效的变量信息，进行概念化定义主要基于大量的文献查阅、专家咨询、与目标人群的深入交流。

Content validity is evaluated with a quantitative evaluation index, the content validity index (CVI). Expert members score the relevance of each item to the study content, usually using a four-point scale (Lynn, 1986), with 1, 2, 3, and 4 representing not relevant, the item must be modified or not relevant, relevant but needs minor modification, and very relevant, respectively. For each item, the item CVI (I-CVI) is obtained by dividing the total number of experts with scores of 3 and 4 by the total number of experts, and scale-level CVI (S-CVI) is obtained by calculating the average of the CVI of all individual items(S-CVI/Ave). Polit et al. (2017) concluded that the research instrument has good content validity when the CVI of individual items is 0.78 and above and the S-CVI/Ave is 0.9 and above. If the CVI is undesirable, the researcher should revise the measurement instrument based on the experts' comments and invite the experts to review it again after the revision, with an interval of preferably 10-14 days between the two reviews to avoid the experts being influenced by the results of the first review.

内容效度采用定量评价指标——内容效度指数（CVI）进行评价。专家委员对每个条目与研究内容的相关程度进行打分，通常采用四分制（Lynn, 1986），1、2、3、4 分别代表不相关、条目必须经过修改否则不相关、相关但需要稍微修改和非常相关。单个条目的内容效度指数通过评分为 3 和 4 的专家总数除以总的专家数得出，总量表的内容效度指数通过计算所有单个条目的内容效度指数的平均值得出，Polit 等（2017）认为当单个条目的内容效度指数为 0.78 及以上，总量表的内容效度指数为 0.9 及以上时，表明研究工具有良好的内容效度。如果内容效度较低，研究者要根据专家的评议修改测量工具，修改后再次邀请专家进行评议，两次间隔时间最好为 10~14 天，避免专家们受第一次的评议结果的影响。

Although the CVI is quantitative data, it is highly influenced by the subjective factors of experts and therefore are not strong evidence of measurement validity. In addition, content validity suffers from the problem of occasional chance consistency among reviewers and is therefore not applicable to measurement instruments with few evaluation items.

内容效度指数虽然是量化的数据，但受专家们的主观因素影响较大，因此也不是测量效度的有力证据，此外，内容效度存在评议者间偶然一致性的问题，因此，不适用于评价条目较少的测量工具。

3. Criterion Validity(校标效度)

Criterion validity represents the degree of correlation between a measurement instrument and other measurement standards for the same study variable; the higher the correlation between them, the better the validity. A measurement standard refers to the ideal measure of the same study concept, i. e., the gold standard, which is reliable but may sometimes be costly, inefficient, cause discomfort or harm to patients, have limited measurement conditions, and cannot predict the occurrence of future conditions, so even with the existence of a gold standard, we still need to develop new measurement tools. Sometimes there are situations where there is no gold standard to use for comparison, such as happiness, fear, patient satisfaction with hospitalization, and nurse motivation, and in such cases, construct validity is the most appropriate evaluation method.

效标效度代表测量工具与针对相同研究变量的其他测量标准之间的相关程度，两者的相关程度越高，效度越好。测量标准指理想的测量相同研究概念的指标，即金标准，金标准的测量结果是可靠的，但是有时可能存在成本高、效率低、对病人造成不适或伤害、测量条件受限和无法预测未来情况的发生等问题，所以即使有金标准的存在，我们还需要开发新的测量工具。有时会存在没有金标准可以用来比较的情况，如幸福感、恐惧感、患者的住院满意度和护士的工作积极性等，这种情况下，结构效度是最适合的评价方法。

Criteria validity is divided into concurrent validity and predictive validity based on differences in time. Concurrent validity refers to the degree of correlation between a new research instrument and an existing measurement standard, and predictive validity refers to the degree to which a measurement instrument is valid for predicting future conditions.

根据时间上的差异，标准效度分为同时效度和预测效度。同时效度指新的研究工具与现有的测量标准之间的相关程度，预测效度指的是测量工具对未来情况预测的有效程度。

Researchers can use statistical methods to test the hypothesis of criterion validity, and the choice of statistical method depends on whether the type of data measured by the focal measure and the gold standard is continuous or categorized. Three common scenarios are described below：

研究者可以使用统计学方法验证标准效度的假设，统计学方法的选择取决于焦点测量和金标准测量的数据类型是连续型还是分类型。下面介绍了常见的三种情况：

3.1 Criterion Validity with a Continuous Measure and a Continuous Criterion
（连续型测量标准及连续型测量结果）

The results of both the focal and standard measures are continuous data, and in this case, researchers usually choose Pearson's r to calculate the degree of correlation between the two scores; the higher the correlation coefficient, the higher the criterion validity.

焦点测量和标准测量的结果都是连续性数据，这种情况下，研究者通常选择皮尔逊相关系数计算两者分数之间的相关程度，相关系数越高，标准效度越高。

3.2 Criterion Validity with a Dichotomous Measure and a Dichotomous Criterion
（二分类测量标准及二分类测量结果）

The results of both focal and standard measures are dichotomous data, and in this case, researchers usually use the method of assessing diagnostic accuracy, with sensitivity and specificity, as metrics to evaluate diagnostic accuracy. Sensitivity and specificity are inversely related, and in order to consider them together, the researcher can summarize their relationship in a single number by calculating the likelihood ratio, predictive value, percent correct, and

Youden index.

焦点测量和标准测量的结果都是二分类数据，这种情况下，研究者通常使用的是评估诊断准确率的方法，灵敏度和特异度是评价诊断准确度的指标。灵敏度和特异度成反比关系，为了综合考虑两者的关系，研究者可以通过综合指标（即似然比、预测值、正确百分率和 Youden 指数）来概括他们之间的关系。

Sensitivity, also known as true-positive rate (TPR), is calculated as the number of true-positive cases divided by the sum of the number of true-positive cases and false-positive cases, with larger values indicating the better ability of the measurement tool to correctly diagnose, screen and predict a true condition. The specificity, also known as the true-negative rate (TNR), is calculated as the number of true-negative cases divided by the sum of the number of true-negative cases and the number of false-negative cases, with a larger value indicating a greater ability of the instrument to correctly rule out non-true conditions.

灵敏度又称真阳性率，计算公式为真阳性例数除以真阳性例数与假阳性例数的和，其值越大，表明测量工具正确地诊断、筛选和预测一种真实情况的能力越强。特异度又称真阴性率，计算公式为真阴性例数除以真阴性例数与假阴性例数的和，其值越大，表明测量工具正确地排除非真实情况的能力越强。

Likelihood ratio (LR) refers to the ratio of the probability of a certain result in the "diseased" group to the probability of the same result in the "non-diseased" group, and is divided into the likelihood ratio-positive (LR+) and the likelihood ratio-negative (LR−). LR+ is the ratio of the true positive rate to the false positive rate, i. e., sensitivity divided by 1 minus specificity, and the larger the value, the better the ability of the measurement method to correctly diagnose disease. LR− is the ratio of the false negative rate to the true negative rate, i. e., the difference between 1 minus sensitivity divided by specificity, and the smaller the value, the better the ability of the measurement to rule out "non-disease".

似然比指"患病组"组出现某结果的概率与"非患病组"组出现相同结果的概率之比，分为阳性似然比和阴性似然比。阳性似然比是真阳性率和假阳性率的比值，即灵敏度除以1 减去特异度，其值越大，表明测量方法正确诊断"疾病"的能力越强。阴性似然比是假阴性率与真阴性率的比值，即1 减敏感性的差除以特异性，其值越小，越能证明测量方法排除"非疾病"的能力越强。

The predictive value is divided into the positive predictive value (PPV) and the negative predictive value (NPV). PPV refers to the probability of a target positive event occurring in a person with a positive test result, the number of true positive cases divided by the sum of the number of true positive cases and false positive cases, and NPV refers to the probability of a target positive event not occurring in a person with a negative test result the number of true negative cases divided by the sum of the number of true negative cases and false negative cases. The higher the value of the likelihood ratio, the more accurate the measurement result, given the same prevalence.

预测值被分为阳性预测值和阴性预测值，阳性预测值指检测结果为阳性的人发生目标阳性事件的概率，为真阳性例数除以真阳性例数与假阳性例数的和，阴性预测值指检测结果为阴性的人未发生目标阳性事件的概率，为真阴性例数除以真阴性例数与假阴性例数的和。在患病率相同的情况下，似然比的值越大，测量结果越准确。

The correct rate refers to the ratio of the number of true positive and true negative test results to the total number of subjects; the higher the correct rate, the more reliable the measurement results. The Youden index is calculated as the sum of sensitivity and specificity minus 1. The larger the value, the more accurate the measurement method.

正确率指检测得到的真阳性和真阴性人数占受试者总人数的比例，正确率越高，测量结果越可靠。Youden 指数的计算公式为灵敏度与特异度之和减去 1，其值越大，表明测量方法越准确。

3.3　Criterion Validity with a Continuous Measure and a Dichotomous Criterion
（连续型测量标准及二分类测量结果）

The results of the focal measurement are continuous type data and the results of the standard measurement are dichotomous data, in which case researchers usually use a receiver operating characteristic curve (ROC curve) to test the hypothesis of criterion validity. The purpose of the ROC curve is to find the balance between sensitivity and specificity and to select the optimal measurement cut-off value, i. e., the optimal cut-off value, for a particular measurement method. As shown in Figure 12.3.1, the ROC curve has the true positive rate (sensitivity) as the vertical coordinate and the false positive rate (1−specificity) as the horizontal coordinate. If the ROC curve is tighter along the left line and then along the top line, the more accurate the test is. In the ROC curve space, if the curve is tighter along the chance line (45-degree diagonal), the less accurate the test is. The area under the ROC curve (AUC) is an important indicator to evaluate the accuracy of the measurement. Less than 0.7 of the AUC indicates low accuracy, 0.7-0.9 indicates moderate accuracy, and 0.9 or more indicates high accuracy. The slope of the tangent line at the truncated value is the LR+ corresponding to that test value. The LR+ is greatest in the lower left corner of the ROC curve space and decreases as the curve moves from the lower left to the upper right.

焦点测量的结果是连续型数据，标准测量的结果是二分类数据，在这种情况下，研究者通常采用接受者工作特性曲线(ROC曲线)验证标准效度的假设。ROC曲线的目的是找到灵敏度与特异度间的平衡，选择出某一测量方法最佳的测量界限值，即最佳截断值。如图12.3.1所示，ROC曲线以真阳性率(灵敏度)为纵坐标，以假阳性率(1-特异性)为横坐标，如果ROC曲线沿着左边线，然后沿着上边线越紧密，则试验准确度越高。在ROC曲线空间，如果曲线沿着机会线(45°对角线)越紧密，则试验准确度越低。ROC曲线下面积是评价测量准确度的重要指标，ROC曲线下面小于0.7表明准确度较低，0.7~0.9表明准确度中等，0.9以上表明准确度高。在截断值处的正切线的斜率就是该试验值对应的阳性似然比。在ROC曲线空间的左下角阳性似然比最大，随着曲线从左下方往右上方移动，阳性似然比逐渐减小。

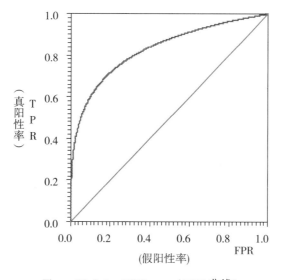

Figure 12.3.1　ROC curve(ROC曲线)

4. Construct Validity(结构效度)

Construct validity refers to the degree to which a test measures the theoretical structure or properties of a concept, and is the agreement between the test and the theory, focusing primarily on the properties measured by the research instrument rather than the outcome of the measurement. Construct validity reflects the extent to which the instrument matches the theoretical or conceptual framework on which it is based. In validating construct validity, the instrument developer needs to have a clear conceptualization not only of the construct itself but also of the relationship between the construct and other constructs. Construct validity consists of three aspects: hypothesis-testing construct validity, structural validity, and cross-cultural validity.

结构效度是指测验测量到的概念的理论结构或属性的程度，是测验与理论之间的一致性，主要关注的是研究工具测量的属性，而不是测量的结果。结构效度反映的是工具与其所依据的理论或者概念框架的相符程度，在验证结构效度时，工具开发者不仅需要对结构本身有明确的概念化，而且还需要对构造物与其他构造物之间的关系有明确的概念化。结构效度包括三个方面：假设检验结构效度、构造效度和跨文化效度。

Hypothesis-testing construct validity refers to the extent to which the hypothesis can be confirmed about how scores on one measure work in relation to scores on measures on other constructs (or the same construct), which in turn includes convergent validity and discriminant validity. Convergent validity refers to the fact that if two tests measure a unifying trait, the correlation between them should be high even if different research instruments are used, and discriminant validity refers to the fact that if two tests measure different traits or clusters, the correlation between them should be low even if the same instruments are used.

假设检验结构效度是指能够在多大程度上证实假设，即一个测量上的分数与其他结构（或同一结构）上的测量上的分数之间是如何发挥作用的，其中又包括聚合效度和辨别效度。聚合效度是指如果两个测验是测量统一特质的，即使使用不同的研究工具，他们之间的相关也应该是高的；辨别效度是指如果两个测验测量的是不同的特质或群组，即使使用相同的工具，他们之间的相关性也应该是低的。

Structural validity refers to the extent to which the structure in a multi-item scale reflects the hypothesized dimensions of the structure being tested, and structural validity is often assessed by factor analysis. Factor analysis is a method for identifying clusters of related items and includes validating factor analysis and exploratory factor analysis. Exploratory factor analysis is an important tool for developing and refining multi-item scales, and validating factor analysis is the preferred method for testing the structural validity of scale dimensions.

构造效度是指多条目量表中的结构反映被测结构的假设维度的程度，构造效度常用因子分析来评估。因子分析是一种识别相关条目群集的方法，包括验证性因子分析和探索性因子分析。探索性因子分析是编制和完善多条目量表的重要工具，验证性因子分析是测试量表维度结构效度假设的首选方法。

Cross-cultural validity is related to measures that have been translated or adapted for use with different cultural groups, and refers to the extent to which translated or culturally adapted measurement instruments work relative to how well they work on the original instrument.

跨文化效度与已翻译或改编用于不同文化群体的测量相关，是指翻译的或文化适应的测量工具相对于它们在原始工具上发挥作用的程度。

5. Critiquing Data Quality in Quantitative Studies(评判量性研究中的数据质量)

Measures should be taken in the study to ensure that the measurement, if the data are flawed, the conclusions of the study will not be convincing. Information on data quality (reliability and validity) needs to be provided in the study report, and the reliability and internal consistency coefficients in the report should be calculated from the data in the study rather than from previous studies. For observational studies, inter-rater reliability is particularly important. In addition, the value of the reliability coefficient should be high enough to make the study's findings more valid. As for validity, researchers need to cite publications that provide valid information from the developer of the study instrument and, if the study uses screening or diagnostic measures, information on sensitivity and specificity.

在研究中应该采取措施来确保测量，如果数据存在缺陷，研究的结论就不能让人们信服。关于数据质量的信息(信度和效度)需要提供在研究报告中，而且报告中的信度和内部一致性系数应该根据研究中的数据计算，而不是通过之前的研究。对于观察性的研究来说，评定者间的信度尤其重要。另外，信度系数的值应该足够高，从而使得研究的结论更有效。至于效度，研究人员需要引用研究工具开发者提供有效信息的出版物，如果研究使用筛查或诊断措施，还需要提供有关敏感性和特异性的信息。

Therefore, the following questions need to be considered when judging the quality of data in quantitative studies.

因此，在评判量性研究中的数据质量时，需要考虑以下问题：

(1)Are the study variables described consistently in the introduction and methods sections? 研究变量在引言和方法部分中描述的是否一致?

(2) Does the report state the reasons for selecting these research instruments for measurement? Are there better research instruments available? 报告中是否说明选择此研究工具进行测量的原因? 是否有更好的研究工具?

（3）Is the process of collecting data sound? Was training provided to the collectors?

收集数据的过程是否合理？是否对收集人员进行培训？

（4）Is the reliability of the research instruments provided in the study report? Does the evidence come from the study data itself or is it based on previous studies? Is the methodology for reporting the reliability appropriate? Is a reliability coefficient calculated? Is the confidence level sufficiently high?

研究报告中是否提供研究工具的信度？证据是来自研究数据本身还是基于之前的研究？报告的信度的方法合适吗？是否计算信度系数？信度是否足够高？

（5）Is the validity of the research instrument provided in the report? Is the methodology of the reported reliability appropriate?

报告中是否提供了研究工具的效度？报告的信度的方法合适吗？

（6）Are the hypotheses of the study supported? If not, was the quality of the data one of the reasons for not confirming the hypotheses?

研究的假设是否得到了支持？如果没有，数据质量是未能证实这些假设的原因之一吗？

Studies Cited in Chapter 12（第十二章参考文献）

[1] Kaplan, A. The conduct of inquiry: Methodology for behavioral science[M]. New York, NY: Harper & Row, 1963.

[2] Waltz, C. F., Strickland, O. L., Lenz, E. R. Measurement in nursing and health research [M]. 4th ed. New York: Springer Publishing Company, 2010.

[3] Bialocerkowski, A., Klupp, N., Bragge, P. Research methodology series: How to read and critically appraise a reliability article [J]. International Journal of Therapy & Rehabilitation, 2010, 17(3): 114-120.

[4] DeVon, H. A., Block, M. E., Moyle-Wright, P., et al. A psychometric toolbox for testing validity and reliability[J]. Journal of Nursing Scholarship, 2007, 39(2): 155-164.

[5] Lynn, M. R. Determination and quantification of content validity[J]. Nursing Research, 1986, 35(6): 382-385.

[6] Polit, D. F., Beck, C. T., Owen, S. V. Is the CVI an acceptable indicator of content validity? Appraisal and recommendations[J]. Research in Nursing & Health, 2007, 30: 459-467.

Chapter 13: Developing and Testing Self-Report Scales
第十三章 自我报告量表的编制和测试

Standard scales are often used in questionnaire survey. If there's no recognized scale suitable for the study, or the existing scales have certain limitations, a new scale should be developed. This chapter will discuss the steps to develop a high-quality self-report scale.

问卷调查法中常需要使用标准的量表。如果没有发现符合研究的公认量表，或是现有的量表存在某些局限性，则需要自行研制新的量表。本章将讨论高质量自我报告量表的编制步骤。

Section Ⅰ Developing Self-Designed Questionnaire
第一节 自设问卷的编制

A complete self-designed questionnaire should include three parts: instructions, form-filling explanation and questions.

一份完整的自设问卷应包括指导语、填表说明和问题三个部分。

1. Instruction(指导语)

Instruction refers to the brief description to the respondents on the first page of the questionnaire, mainly including the identity of the investigator, the purpose, significance, content and requirements of the investigation, and the guarantee of anonymity.

指导语是指在问卷的首页上给调查对象的简短说明，主要包括调查者的身份、调查目的和意义、内容和要求，以及匿名保证等内容。

2. Form-filling Explanation(填表说明)

The function of the form filling explanation is to explain the meaning of certain indicators in the questionnaire and to guide the respondent or the investigator how to fill in the questionnaire.

填表说明的作用是解释问卷中某些指标的含义，并指导被调查者或调查者如何填写。

【Example 1】 "Please read each question in the questionnaire carefully and answer it according to your actual feelings. If you don't know what the questions are saying, you don't have to answer. The answer to all questions is a subjective judgment. There is no right or wrong."

【例1】 "请您认真阅读问卷中的每一道题目，并根据自身的实际感受作答。如果您对某些题目所说的内容不了解，您可以不回答。所有问题的回答都是一种主观判断，没有对与错、是与非之分。"

3. Questions(问题)

3.1　The Construction of Questions(问题的构建)

First of all, according to the purpose of our research, on the basis of consulting a large number of relevant literature and combining our own professional knowledge and theoretical framework, list the problems in several aspects that we want to investigate. Then use a number of specific small questions to further explain the content of each aspect. Start by writing down as many questions as possible under each aspect without thinking too much about whether the words are appropriate, similar or repetitive. The more specific and comprehensive the questions, the more accurate and persuasive the results are, the easier it will be for in-depth analysis. Finally, the questions are combined, sorted and selected, compose the first draft of the questionnaire. The preliminary draft of the questionnaire was used in a small-scale pre-survey to find the problems in the questionnaire and the problems that might be encountered in the practical application, and the questionnaire is modified according to the feedback information.

首先，要根据自己的研究目的，在查阅大量相关文献并结合自己专业知识及理论框架的基础上，列出想要调查的几方面的问题。然后，运用多个具体的小问题进一步说明每个方面的内容。开始时不用过多考虑用词是否恰当是否类似或重复等，尽可能写下每道题目下可能包含的小题目。题目越具体、越周全，结果越准确和越有说服力，就越易于深入分析。最后，对问题进行组合、整理和精选，组成问卷的初稿。将问卷初稿用于小规模的预调查，以发现问卷中存在的问题和在实际应用中可能遇到的问题，并根据反馈的信息来修改问卷。

3.2　Deciding on the Type of Questions(问题的类型)

3.2.1　**Open questions**(开放式问题)

Open questions refer to only asking questions without setting alternative answers, and respondents can answer freely according to their own situation, for example, "What do you think about diabetes?". Open questions are suitable for exploratory research and can provide in-depth information. However, due to the large difference in the survey results, it is not easy to standardize, so researchers need to further sort out and summarize the data. Answering open-ended questions takes more time and is easily rejected.

开放式问题是指只提出问题，不设立备选答案，被调查者根据自己的情况进行自由回答，例如"您如何看待糖尿病问题?"开放式问题适用于探索性研究，能提供较深入的信息。但调查结果差异较大，不易标准化，需要对资料进行进一步整理和归纳。开放式问题的回答，花费时间相对较多，且易产生拒答现象。

3.2.2　Closed Questions(闭合式问题)

Closed questions refer to the alternative answers attached to each question, and the respondents can choose the answer according to their own situation. The response rate of closed questions is high, for some sensitive questions, such as income, sexual life, etc., closed questions are easier to obtain more realistic answers. However, due to the fixed answers of closed questions, the creativity of respondents is limited, so it is not conducive to discover new problems and easy to cause data bias.

闭合式问题是指在每道问题后面附备选答案，被调查对象可根据自己的情况选择答案。闭合式问题问卷应答率高，对于某些敏感性问题，如收入、性生活情况等，闭合式问题更容易获得较为真实的答案。然而由于闭合式问题的答案较为固定，限制了被调查者的创造性，故不利于发现新问题，易使资料产生偏倚。

3.3　Deciding on the Number of Questions(问题的数目)

The number of questions in the questionnaire cannot be generalized. According to psychological knowledge, it is generally considered that the respondents can answer the questions in about 30 minutes, and the longest time cannot be more than 45 minutes. Children's questionnaires usually take no more than 15 minutes.

问卷中问题的数目不能一概而论，根据心理学知识，一般以回答者在 30 分钟左右能够答完为度，最长不能超过 45 分钟。儿童问卷一般不超过 15 分钟。

3.4　Deciding on the Arrangement of Question(问题的排列)

The order of the questions in the questionnaire also has certain rules, which are designed to make it easier for the respondent to think and reduce the possibility of rejection. The principles of question ordering are as follows：

问卷中问题排列的顺序也有一定的规则，其目的是便于回答者思考，减少拒答的可能性。问题排序的原则有：

（1）The easy questions come first; the hard ones come later.

容易回答的问题在前，难回答的问题在后。

（2）The questions should be arranged in a logical order. Similar questions and related questions should be put together. If the questions are related to time, they should be listed in order from far to near or near to far.

问题按一定的逻辑顺序排列，同类问题、有关联的问题放在一起。问题若关联到时间，应按由远至近或由近至远的顺序排列。

（3）Sensitive questions（such as questions about personal privacy）come later.

敏感问题(如个人隐私问题)排在后面。

（4）Closed questions come first, open questions come later.

封闭式问题在前，开放式问题在后。

（5）The layout is neat, the font is appropriate, and the jump question filling method is clearly marked.

排版整齐，字体适宜，明确标注跳跃式问题填写方式。

3.5 Deciding on the Language used in the Questionnaire(问卷中所使用的语言)

The understanding and answer of the questionnaire questions depend on the language of the questions, so attention should be paid to the design：

对问卷问题的理解和回答取决于问题的语言，设计时应加以注意：

（1）The language is clear and clear, and should be suitable for patients with low education level to understand.

语言清楚明白，要适于文化程度较低的患者理解。

（2）Questions should be positive and objective, not tendentious or suggestive.

问题的提法应肯定和具有客观性，不应带有倾向性或暗示性。

（3）Don't ask two things or two sides of the same thing in one question.

一个问题中不要询问两件事或一件事情的两个方面。

（4）Ask questions in the third person on sensitive issues.

对于某些敏感性问题使用第三人称进行提问。

Section Ⅱ　Developing and Testing Self-Report Scales
第二节　量表的编制和测试

1. Beginning Steps：Conceptualization and Item Generation（初始步骤：概念化及生成条目）

1.1　Conceptualizing the Construct(量表概念的界定/构架概念化)

The development of the questionnaire needs to base on relevant professional theories and be guided by a clear idea. If there is no relevant theory, a clear concept needs to be available to guide what is to be measured. Therefore, the concepts associated with the scale need to be defined before it is developed. For example, the dimensions of the scale, the population to which the scale is adapted, and cultural adaptability need to be determined in advance.

调查问卷的编制需要以相关的专业理论为基础，以明确的思路为指导。如果没有相关的理论，就需要有一个清晰的概念来指导测量内容的制定。因此，需要在量表开发之前对量表相关的概念进行界定。例如，需要事先确定量表的维度、适用的人群，以及文化适应性等。

1.2　Deciding on the Type of Scale(确定量表类型)

Before items can be generated, it is necessary to decide on the type of scale to be created, as the item characteristics vary by scale type. Scales are divided into two main categories：traditional summated rating（Likert-type）scales and latent trait scales.

在生成条目之前，有必要预先确定要创建的量表类型，这也决定了条目的特征。量表主要分为两大类：传统的累加评分(李克特式)量表和潜在特质量表。

1.3　Generating an Item Pool(生成条目池)

Items that reflect the latent variables of the scale are selected to form an item pool. Item homogeneity of the scale requires that all items should reflect the same latent variable. Items can be generated from the following sources：

选择反映量表潜变量的条目，形成一个条目池。量表的条目同质性要求所有条目都应反映相同的潜变量。量表的条目可由以下来源产生：

（1）Literature review.（文献回顾）

（2）Expert consultation.（专家咨询）

（3）Concept analysis.（概念分析）

（4）Qualitative studies.（质性研究）

（5）Clinical observation.（临床观察）

【**Example 2**】Sources of Items：Choe（2014）developed a scale to measure hope in people with schizophrenia. Forty items were initially developed, based on concept clarification research, a qualitative study, and an extensive literature review.

【**例 2**】条目来源：Choe（2014）开发了一个量表来衡量精神分裂症患者的希望。根据概念澄清类的研究、质性研究和大量的文献综述，最初形成了 40 个条目。

1.4 Making Decision About Item Features（决定条目特征）

1.4.1 Numbers of Item（条目数量）

When building an item pool, a fairly exhaustive set of item possibilities should be generated, given the construct theoretical demands. Our recommendation is to generate a very large pool of items. DeVellis（2012）recommends starting with as many items as possible with 3 to 4 times as many items, but at least 50% more.

当构建一个条目池时，应该生成一个相当详尽的条目集合，以满足构建量表的理论需求。我们的建议是先生成一个非常大的条目池。随着这一进程的继续，其中的许多条目将被逐步排除。DeVellis（2012）建议可以尽量设计 3~4 倍数量的条目，至少要多 50% 的数量。

1.4.2 Response Options（回答选项）

Scale items consist of a stem（usually a declarative statement）and response options. It is important to note that variability is essential. Variability can be enhanced by including many items, by providing a large number of response options, or both.

量表的条目通常由一个题干（通常是一个陈述性语句）和回答选项组成。需要注意的是，可变性是必不可少的。可以通过设计多个条目、提供大量的回答选项或两者兼有来提高可变性。

1.4.3　Positive and Negative Stems(正向和负向措辞)

Psychometricians recommend that scale developers consciously include both positive and negative wording and reverse the calculation of negative item scores. Some research suggests that acquiescence can be minimized by placing the most positive response option (e. g., "strongly agree") at the end of the list, rather than at the beginning.

心理测量学家建议量表开发者有意识地同时使用正向和负向的措辞，并反向计算负向条目的分数。一些研究表明，可以通过把最积极的回答选项(例如"非常同意")放在最后，而不是放在开头，来尽量减少默许。

1.4.4　Item Intensity(条目措辞强度)

In a traditional composite rating scale, the strength of the statements should be similar and fairly strongly worded. If the wording of the item is agreed by almost everyone, then the scale will not be able to distinguish between people with different underlying traits.

在传统的综合评分表中，条目陈述的强度应该相似，并且措辞较为强烈。如果条目的措辞使得某些选项几乎被所有人认同，那么该量表将无法区分具有不同潜在特征的人。

1.4.5　Item Time Frames(条目的时间框架)

Sometimes the scale instructions can specify a time frame of reference (e. g., indicate how you felt in the past week when answering the following question).

有时，量表指导语可能会指定一个参考的时间范围(例如，"在回答以下问题时，表明你在过去一周的感受")。

1.4.6　Wording the Items(条目的措辞)

Items should be worded in such a way that each respondent answers the same question. There are some basic requirements for the wording of items:

条目应合理措辞，以使每个受访者回答相同的问题。对条目的措辞有以下几点基本要求：

(1) Clarity. (清晰)

Words should be carefully chosen according to the education and reading level of the target population.

要根据目标人群的教育程度和阅读水平，精心挑选词语。

(2) Terminology. (术语)

The use of jargon should be avoided.

应该尽量避免使用术语。

（3）Length.（长度）

Avoid long sentences or phrases. In particular, delete unnecessary words.

应当避免使用长句子或短语。特别是要删除不必要的词语。

（4）Double negatives.（双重否定）

It is better to say affirmatively（I am usually happy）than to say negatively（I am usually not sad）, but double negatives should always be avoided.

肯定的陈述(我通常很快乐)比否定的陈述(我通常不悲伤)要好，特别是要避免使用双重否定句式。

【Example 3】Examples of wording the items(条目措辞示例)

Target: Income

Question 1: How much do you earn per month?

Question 2: What was the total income earned by you and your family last year?

Clarify the research questions and goals, that is, answer the questions of what to test and why. The above two questions are about income, but the survey results are quite different. It is necessary to decide which question is more appropriate according to the research purpose.

【例3】目标：收入

问题1：你每个月的收入是多少?

问题2：去年一年，你和家人的总收入是多少?

明确研究问题和目标，即回答测什么和为什么测。上述两个问题都是询问经济收入，但调查结果却大不相同。需要根据研究目的决定哪种问法比较恰当。

2. Preliminary Evaluation of Items(条目的初步评估)

2.1　Internal Review(内部审查)

A preliminary evaluation is performed after a large item pool is generated. Attention should be paid to whether a single item fits the overall structure, whether it is grammatically correct, and whether it is worded appropriately. The internal review should also consider whether the items taken together adequately embrace the full nuances of the construct. At the same time, we should consider whether the scale language expression is applicable to all target populations, and whether the length of time required to complete the scale is appropriate.

产生条目池后要进行内部审查。内部审查应该注意的问题有：单个条目是否能满足整体结构，合乎是否语法，用词是否恰当。内部审查还应该考虑将条目组合在一起是否充分地包含了该概念的所有方面。同时，应该考虑该量表语言表述是否对所有目标人群均适用，完成该量表所需的时间长短是否适宜。

2.2 External Review by Experts（专家外部评审）

After an internal review, an external review of the revised items should be conducted by a panel of experts in order to assess the content validity of the scale. It is advisable to undertake two rounds of review, if feasible the first to refine or weed out faulty items or to add new items to cover the domain adequately and the second to formally assess the content validity of the items and scale. Expert external review steps are as follows：

在进行内部审查后，为了评估量表的内容效度，应该由专家小组对修订条目进行外部审查。建议进行两轮审查，第一轮对有缺陷的项目进行改进或剔除，或增加新的项目以充分覆盖该领域，第二轮对条目和量表的内容有效性进行正式评估。专家外部评审步骤如下：

2.2.1 Selecting and Recruiting the Experts（挑选和招募专家）

In the initial phase of a two-part review, we advise having an expert panel of 8-12 members, with a good mix in terms of roles and disciplines. If the scale is intended for broad use, it might also be advantageous to recruit experts from various countries or areas of a country, because of possible regional variations in language. The second panel for formally assessing the content validity of a more refined set of items should consist of 3-5 experts in the content area.

第一轮评估的专家小组成员应为 8~12 名，在角色和学科方面能进行良好的组合。如果该量表打算在世界各地广泛使用，专家小组成员应从不同国家及地区招募。第二轮正式评估小组由于其评估改进后的条目的内容有效性，其组成应为 3~5 名该内容领域的专家。

2.2.2　Preliminary Expert Review: Content Validation of Items

（初步专家评审：条目的内容检验）

The expert's job is to evaluate individual items and the overall scale (as well as any subscales) using the guidelines established by the scale developer. The evaluation content includes: whether the wording of each item of the scale is appropriate, whether the expression of the item is clear, and whether all items of the scale can be comprehensively evaluated.

专家的工作是利用量表开发人员建立的指导方针，评估单个条目和整体量表(以及任何子量表)。评估内容包括：量表每个条目措辞是否恰当，条目表述是否清晰，量表所有条目是否能够全面地评估需要评估的内容。

The formula for evaluating agreement among experts on individual items is the number agreeing, divided by the number of experts. When the aspect being rated is relevance, the standard method for computing an item-level content validity index (I-CVI) is the number giving a rating of 3 or 4 on the 4-point relevance scale, divided by the number of experts. Items with lower than desired I-CVIs need careful scrutiny. It may be necessary to recontact the experts to better understand genuine differences of opinion or to strive for greater consensus. If there are legitimate disagreements among the experts on individual items (or if there is agreement about lack of relevance), the items should be revised or dropped.

评估专家对单个条目的意见一致程度的评价公式是同意人数除以专家人数。当被评级的方面是相关性时，用条目内容效度指数 (I-CVI) 表示。计算 I-CVI 的标准方法为在 4 分的相关性量表上给出 3 或 4 的评级的专家除以专家总数。I-CVIs 值低于期望的条目需要仔细审查。可能有必要重新与专家接触，以便更好地了解真正的意见分歧或争取达成更大的共识。如果专家对个别条目存在合理的分歧(或一致认为缺乏相关性)，则应修订或删除这些条目。

2.2.3　Content Validation of the Scale（量表内容检验）

In the second round of content validation, a smaller group of experts (3-5) can be used to evaluate the relevance of the revised set of items and to compute the scale content validity (S-CVI). The experts in the second round may be newly recruited experts in the field or a subset of the members of the first round.

在第二轮的内容验证中，可以使用较小的专家小组(3~5 人)来评估修订后的条目集的相关性，并计算量表水平的内容效度(S-CVI)。第二轮的专家可以是本领域新聘请的专家，也可以是第一轮成员的一部分。

There is more than one way to compute an S-CVI. We recommend the approach that averages across I-CVIs.

计算 S-CVI 的方法不止一种。我们推荐在 I-CVIs 中取平均值的方法。

Section Ⅲ   Field Testing the Instrument
第三节   测量工具的现场测试

The steps of the measurement tool mainly include sampling plan, data collection plan and data collection.

测量工具的步骤主要包括制订抽样计划、制订数据收集计划和进行数据收集。

1. Developing a Sampling Plan(制订抽样计划)

First of all, not only sample size but also sample composition should be considered in sample selection. The properties of the predicted objects are the same as those to be measured by formal questionnaires in the future. In addition, the process of sample collection should follow the principle of randomness, which is conducive to improving sample representativeness. If randomness is not possible in the sampling process, it can be used to sample people of different genders, ages and nationalities from different regions to evaluate the application differences of the scale in different regions and different populations, so as to improve sample representativeness.

首先，选择样本时不仅要考虑样本的大小，还要考虑样本的构成。预测对象的性质与将来正式问卷要测量的对象性质相同。另外，样本收集的过程要遵循随机原则，有利于提高样本代表性。如果抽样过程中不能做到随机，则可以对不同地区的不同性别、年龄及民族等人群进行抽样，评估量表在不同地域和不同人群的应用差异，以提高样本代表性。

Second, there is hard and fast rule on sample size among experts. It is generally considered from the scale items and the proportion of respondents. The empirical method can also provide some reference for determining the sample size. For example, the sample size of the investigation study should be at least 100 cases. The sample size of descriptive studies should be 10%~20% of the total. A large sample size is crucial to improve the stability of inter-item relationships. If a retest is required to evaluate the reliability and validity of the scale, fewer samples are usually selected to participate in the retest.

其次，专家们对样本的大小有严格的规定。一般从量表条目与调查人数比例进行考虑。经验法也可以在确定样本量时提供一些参考，例如，调查性研究样本量至少需要 100 例以上；描述性研究一般样本量应为总体的 10%~20%。样本量足够大对于提高条目间关系的稳定性至关重要。如果要进行复测来评估量表信度和效度，通常会选取较少的样本参与复测工作。

Finally, in the collection process, efforts should be made to collect samples that have heterogeneity with the target attributes of the scale. If the results are not diversified enough, the stability and internal consistency of the scale will be affected to some extent.

最后，在收集过程中，应努力收集与量表目标属性有异质性的样本。如果结果不够多样化，对量表的稳定性和内在一致性会产生一定影响。

2. Developing a Data Collection Plan(制订数据收集计划)

The formulation of data collection plan mainly includes determining data types, selecting data collection methods, pretesting data software collection packages, and developing data collection forms and procedures. There are many methods for data collection, including on-site questionnaire, telephone questionnaire, network questionnaire and mail/email questionnaire. Therefore, it is necessary to choose a method that is most suitable for subjects to fill in and has a high recovery rate. In addition, it will be critical to consider incorporating other measures into the scale if a separate study is not conducted to assess the scale's reliability and validity.

制订数据收集计划主要包括确定数据类型、选择数据收集方法、对数据软件收集包进行预测试、开发数据收集表格和程序。数据的收集方式有很多，包括现场问卷法、电话问卷法、网络问卷法和邮寄/电子邮件问卷法，因此，应该选择一种最适宜研究对象填写和回收率高的方法。另外，如果不进行单独的研究来评估量表的信度和效度，还应考虑将其他测量方法纳入量表中，这将是至关重要的。

3. Data Collection(数据收集)

In the process of data collection, the filling form of the scale should be clear and clear, and it is necessary to evaluate the readability of the words. How to rank the items in the scale also needs to be considered. The "proximity effect" is the idea that when people respond to something, they are often influenced by the response to the previous thing. This effect tends to artificially exaggerate estimates of the scale's internal consistency. There are two ways to deal with this problem. For a scale designed to measure several related dimensions, items can be randomly sorted, or items that are expected to be scored can be systematically alternated into different subscales.

在数据收集过程中，量表的填写形式应该清楚明了，对其文字进行可读性评估是有必要的。如何对量表中的条目进行排序也是需要考虑的问题。"邻近效应"，即人们在回应某一事物时，往往会受到对前一事物回应的影响。这种效应往往会人为地夸大对量表内在一致性的估计。处理这种问题有两种方法，对于旨在测量几个相关维度的量表来说，可以对条目进行随机排序，另一种方法是系统地将预计会被打分的条目交替放入不同的子量表。

Section Ⅳ   Analysis of Scale Development Data
第四节   分析量表编制数据

1. Basic Item Analysis(基本项目分析)

According to the principle of item analysis, each item of the questionnaire was analyzed one by one to enhance the effectiveness of the questionnaire in distinguishing and identifying the psychological trait level of the subjects. The commonly used evaluation index is critical specific decision value (CR), which is suitable for multi-level or continuous variables, the questionnaire compiled is 5-level scoring data. Each item of the questionnaire was analyzed, the critical ratio value (decision value, CR value) of each item of the scale was calculated, and the items that did not reach the level of significance test were deleted. The main operation steps of item analysis are as follows:

依据项目分析的原则，对问卷每个条目逐一进行鉴别分析，增强问卷对被试者心理特质水平的区分、鉴别效力。常用的评价指标是临界比决断值（CR），CR 适用于多级或连续变量，编制的问卷为 5 级计分的资料。对问卷各条目进行分析，计算量表各条目的临界比值比(决策值、CR 值)，删除未达到显著性检验水平的条目。

2. Exploratory Factor Analysis(探索性因子分析)

After item analysis, factor analysis was used to test the scale's structural validity. The purpose of exploratory factor analysis is to find out the potential structure of the scale, determine the dimension of the factors, and make them into a group of small variables that are relatively correlated with each other. Basic steps of exploratory factor analysis as follows:

项目分析后，通过因子分析检验量表的结构效度。探索性因子分析的目的是找出量表潜在的结构，确定因子的维度，使其成为一组相互之间相对相关的小变量。

In exploratory factor analysis, the commonly used principles for determining the number of factors are as follows: (1) According to Kaiser's view, factors with a value greater than 1 should be retained; (2) It is determined by the decreasing variation of screen plot factors. In a steep slope plot, if the factor variation graph changes from slope to flatness, the factors after flatness can be removed.

探索性因子分析中，常用的确定因子个数的原则有：(1)根据 Kaiser 的观点，保留特征值大于 1 的因素；(2)根据碎石图上的因子变异递减情形来决定。在碎石图中，如果因子变化图呈现由斜坡转为平坦，平坦以后的因子可以去掉。

After determining the number of factors, the factors are named according to the connotation of the items in each factor. In the actual research, the construction of scale validity sometimes requires 2-3 factor analyses.

确定因子数后，根据各因子中条目的内涵进行因子命名。在实际研究中，量表效度的构建有时需要进行 2~3 次因子分析。

3. Internal Consistency Analysis(内部一致性分析)

After factor analysis, to further understand the reliability of the questionnaire, internal consistency test should be performed. Cronbach'α coefficient and semicircular reliability are commonly used to test the reliability of internal consistency in the Likert scale. The internal consistency of the scale includes the total scale and the measurement of the internal consistency of each subscale.

因子分析之后，为进一步了解问卷的可靠性，要做内在一致性检验。在李克特型量表中常用的内部一致性信度检验方法为 Cronbach'α 系数和折半信度。量表的内在一致性包括总量表以及各分量表的内在一致性测定。

4. Test-Retest Reliability Analysis(重测信度分析)

Test-retest reliability refers to the repeated testing of the same group of subjects with the same scale at an interval of time, and then calculate the correlation coefficient of the scores obtained twice.

重测信度指间隔一段时间，以同一量表重复对同一组研究对象施测，然后计算两次所得分数的关系系数。

Section V　Scale Refinement and Validation
第五节　量表的完善及验证

1. Revising the Scale(量表的修订)

Items often need to be modified or added in the process of scale formulation. For example, if the Cronbach'α coefficient of the subscale is below 0.80, additional items should be considered for subsequent testing.

在量表制订的过程中常常需要修改或增加条目。例如，如果子量表的Cronbach'α 系数低于 0.80，就应该考虑增加条目进行后续测试。

Before the final scale is finalized, the contents of items in the scale should be carefully checked and improved. Sometimes, the Cronbach'α value of the scale will be inflated because the contents or words between items are similar. To avoid such problems, not only their contribution to Cronbach'α values but also their content validity should be considered when deciding to keep or delete items. Finally, it is necessary to re-examine the item-level content validity index (I-CVI) of each item. I-CVI can not only be used for the evaluation of content validity, but also provide information for the modification or deletion of items in the early stage of scale compilation.

在最终的量表定型之前，需要认真检查和完善量表中条目的内容。因为有时条目之间内容或文字相似，会导致量表Cronbach'α 值虚高。为避免出现此类问题，在决定保留或删除条目时，不仅要考虑它们对 Cronbach'α 值的贡献，还要考虑其内容效度。最后，重新审查每个条目的内容效度指数是有必要的。I-CVI 不仅可以用于内容效度的评价，在量表编制的初期还可以为条目的修改或删除提供信息。

2. Conducting a Validation Study(进行验证研究)

The final finalization and market use of the scale need to be verified and studied. Scale developers can use data from original development samples to conduct multiple validation activities if they are unable to conduct a separate validation study. Design validation studies require many of the same questions and recommendations as design development studies in terms of sample composition, sample size, and data collection strategies. Our main concern here is with analyses performed in confirmatory studies, where internal consistency should be recalculated in confirmatory samples. CFA is preferred to Exploratory Factor Analysis (EFA) because CFA is a hypothesis testing method that tests the assumptions that items belong to a particular factor, rather than allowing a set of project dimensions to emerge empirically, as Exploratory Factor Analysis does.

量表最终的定型和投入市场使用需要经过验证研究。量表开发者如果不能进行单独的验证研究，可以利用原始开发样本的数据进行多种验证活动。在样本构成、样本大小和数据收集策略方面，设计验证研究需要很多设计开发研究相同的问题和建议。我们在此主要关注验证性研究中进行的分析，应在验证样本中重新计算内部一致性。验证性因子分析比探索性因子分析更可取，因为验证性因子分析是一种假设检验方法，检验条目属于特定因素的假设，而不是像探索性因子分析那样让一组项目的维度通过经验出现。

Section Ⅵ Cross-cultural Validation of the Scale
第六节 国外量表的跨文化调适

In the field of nursing research, many researchers use measurement tools developed by foreign researchers because of the late development of scales in China. Different cultural backgrounds have a certain degree of influence on people's health care behaviors and their knowledge and understanding of things. Therefore, the purpose of cross-cultural adaptation is to achieve equivalence between the original scale and the target scale. Cross-cultural adaptation includes both translation and psychological testing. According to Brislin's (Brislin, 1970) questionnaire translation-back translation principle, the cross-cultural adaptation process of the scale(see Figure 13.6.1) mainly includes translation, back translation, cultural adaptation, and pre-survey. The elements of the psychometric assessment of the scale are: number of translations, reliability, validity, and responsiveness, respectively. The following are guidelines for the cross-cultural accommodation process as recommended by the American Academy of Orthopedic Surgeons Committee on Evidence-Based Medicine (Beaton D., 2000).

在护理研究领域，由于国内的量表发展起步较晚，很多研究人员运用国外研究者编制的测量工具。不同的文化背景对人们的健康保健行为、对事物的认识与理解都有一定程度的影响。因此，量表跨文化调适的目的是达到原量表和目标量表之间的对等性。跨文化调适包括翻译和心理学测试两项内容。根据 Brislin（Brislin，1970）问卷翻译-回译原则，量表的跨文化调适过程（见图 13.6.1）主要包括翻译、回译、文化调适、预调查。量表心理测评的要素分别有：翻译次数、信度、效度和反应度。以下是美国矫形外科医师学会循证医学委员会推荐的跨文化调适过程的指南（Beaton D，2000）。

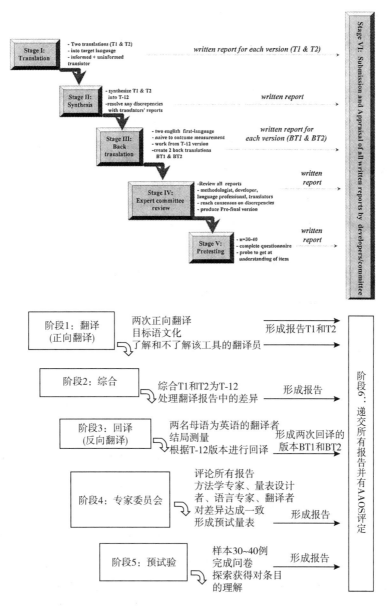

Figure 13.6.1　The Cross-Cultural Adaptation Process of the Scale（量表的跨文化调适过程）

Section Ⅶ Critiquing Scale Development Studies
第七节 评判量表编制的研究

There are many articles on scale formulation and development in nursing related journals. If scales are to be used in a substantive study, not only should methods be found for constructing scales and measuring psychological characteristics, but the evidence on scale psychometric measures should be carefully examined to warrant their use. In addition, if a scale with low reliability and validity is used in the research, the validity and reliability of the research results may be affected.

在护理相关杂志上有许多关于量表制定和开发的文章。如果要在一项实质性研究中使用量表，不仅要找到用于构建量表和测量心理特性的方法，还应仔细检查关于量表心理测量的证据是否足够充分，以保证其使用。另外，如果在研究过程中使用了信度和效度低的量表，有可能会影响研究结果的有效性和可靠性。

📖 Studies Cited in Chapter 13（第十三章参考文献）

[1] Choe, K. Development and preliminary testing of the Schizophrenia Hope Scale, a brief scale to measure hope in people with schizophrenia[J]. International journal of nursing studies, 2014, 51(6): 927-933.

[2] DeVellis, R. F., Thorpe, C. T. Scale development: Theory and applications[M]. London: Sage Publications, 2021.

[3] 李峥，邹海欧，王凌云，等. 社区老年人认知功能和抑郁情绪的纵向研究[J]. 中华护理杂志，2020.

[4] Brislin, R. W. Back-translation for cross-cultural research[J]. Journal of Cross-Cultural Psychology, 1970, 1(3): 185-216.

[5] Leplège, A. The adaptation of health status measures: a discussion of certain methodological aspects of the translation procedure[J]. The international assessment of health-related quality of life: theory, translation, measurement and analysis, 1995.

[6] Guillemin, F., Bombardier, C., Beaton, D. Cross-cultural adaptation of health-related quality of life measures: literature review and proposed guidelines[J]. Journal of clinical

epidemiology, 1993, 46(12): 1417-1432.

[7] Beaton, D. E., Bombardier, C., Guillemin, F., et al. Guidelines for the process of cross-cultural adaptation of self-report measures[J]. Spine, 2000, 25(24): 3186-3191.

Chapter 14：Descriptive Statistics
第十四章　统计描述

According to research purpose, researchers might need to measure a certain attribute of the research sample. This attribute of the research sample is named variable, the value of the variable is named data.

根据研究目的，对研究对象的某个或某些特征(亦称研究指标或项目)实施测量，这些特征称为变量，变量的观测值(即变量值)构成数据或资料。

For a practical problem that needs to be studied, after the data collection according to the research design, it is necessary to analyze the data to obtain the required information and achieve the research purpose. Data analysis is known as statistical analysis, its purpose is to express the characteristics of the data, clarify the internal relationship and regularity of things. Statistics can be descriptive or inferential.

对于一个需要研究的实际问题，依据设计方案收集到数据后，需要对数据进行分析以获取所需信息，达到研究目的。数据分析又称为统计分析，其目的是表达数据特征，阐明事物的内在联系和规律性。统计分析的方法包括统计描述和统计推断。

Descriptive statistics use proper descriptive index, tables and graphs to measure and describe the quantitative characteristics and distribution of the data. A descriptive index from a sample is a statistic, while a descriptive index calculated from population data is called a parameter. For statistical analysis, the first step is using descriptive statistics to understand the range, centrality and shape of the data distribution. Descriptive statistics provide a basis for the subsequent inferential statistics. The main content of this chapter includes: the basic concepts of descriptive statistics, descriptive statistics for quantitative data and qualitative data (Polit & Beck, 2017).

统计描述是指用恰当的统计指标、统计表与统计图等，对数据的数量特征及其分布规律进行测定和描述。用于描述样本的统计指标称为统计量，而通过总体计算出的统计指标称为参数。进行数据分析的首要步骤即为通过统计描述了解数据的分布范围、集中位置以及分布形态等特征。统计描述可为选择统计推断的方法提供基础。本章的主要内容包括：统计描述的基本概念，计量资料的统计描述和计数资料的统计描述(Polit 和 Beck, 2017)。

Section Ⅰ　Levels of Measurement and Frequency Distributions
第一节　测量水平和频数分布

1. Levels of Measurement(测量水平)

The object of statistical analysis is data. Different statistical methods should be used for different forms of data. Many ways of classifying data are available according to different rules and rationales. This chapter classifies data depending on how variables are measured. There are four levels of measurement: nominal measurement, ordinal measurement, interval measurement, and ratio measurement.

统计描述的对象为数据。不同数据需采用不同的统计分析方法。根据不同的原则和理解，统计数据有不同的分类方法。本书按照数据的测量方式对数据进行分类。测量水平可分为：名义测量，次序测量，间距测量(定距测量)和比率测量(定比测量/等比测量/比例测量)。

Nominal measurement refers to qualitative measurement that counts the research objects in categories according to certain attributes. It is the lowest level of measurement and its data is named qualitative data (or count data) or categorical data. Examples of variables amenable to nominal measurement include gender, blood type, and marital status.

名义测量是指将观察单位按某种属性进行分组计数的定性测量，所获取的资料为计数资料或分类资料，是测量水平最低的测量。例如：性别、血型和婚姻状况的测量。

Ordinal measurement involves sorting people based on their relative ranking on an attribute. Its data is named ordinal data or qualitative data (or count data). Examples of variables amenable to ordinal measurement is measuring ability to perform activities of daily living, which can be ranked as (1) completely dependent, (2) needs another person's assistance, (3) needs mechanical assistance, (4) completely independent. This measurement level is semi-quantitative.

次序测量是指将观察单位按某种属性的不同程度或次序分成等级后分组计数的定性测量，所获取的资料为等级资料或计数资料。例如：日常生活活动能力可分为完全依赖、需要他人协助、需要器械协助和完全独立。

Interval measurement occurs when researchers can assume equivalent distance between rank ordering on an attribute. Its data is quantitative data (or measurement data) and often given a unit. Interval measurement has all the characteristics of ordinal measurement. Moreover, it requires the distance between two value is numeric and quantitative with a unit. However, "0" as the value of an interval measurement is meaningless. Value of an interval measurement can be calculated by addition and subtraction but cannot be calculated by multiplication and division. For example, the data of temperature measurement indicate that the distance between 30 Celsius and 40 Celsius is 10 Celsius. However, 30 Celsius cannot be understood as 30 times more than 1 Celsius, as 0 Celsius is meaningless.

当研究人员可以假设一个属性的排序之间的距离相等时，就会发生定距测量。它所获取的资料为计量资料，一般有计量单位。定距测量不仅具有次序测量的所有特征，还要求任何两个测量值之间的距离是已知的、有单位的，但没有绝对零点，测量值之间可以做加减运算，不能做乘除运算。例如：体温的测量中，30℃和40℃有10℃的差别，但不能认为30℃是1℃的30倍，因为0℃并不代表没有温度。

Ratio measurement is the highest measurement level. In addition to having all the characteristics of distance measurements, its 0 value has absolute meaning. For example, the measurement of age, weight and pulse.

定比测量是最高级的测量，它除了具有间距测量的所有特征外，其0值具有物理上的绝对意义。例如：年龄，体重，脉率的测量。

In general, nominal measurement and ordinal measurement result in qualitative data (including categorial data and ordinal data). Interval measurement and ratio measurement result in quantitative data (or measurement data). The statistical methods and indicators for describing these two kinds of data are different (Polit & Beck, 2006).

综上所述，名义测量和定序测量所获取的资料均为计数资料（包括分类资料和等级资料）。定距测量和定比测量所获取的资料均为计量资料。计量资料与计数资料的统计描述方法不同，采用的描述指标不同（Polit 和 Beck, 2006）。

2. Frequency Distribution(频数分布)

When describing large sample or data, frequency distribution can be used for both of qualitative data and quantitative data to understand the general distribution of the data. A frequency distribution is a systematic arrangement of values from lowest to highest and the number of times of each value is summarized. Table 14. 1. 1 presents the age of the 160 participants which are quantitative data. This set of data is used to illustrate the method of calculating frequency distribution. When presenting frequency distribution, both of tables and graphs can be used with different purposes.

无论是计数资料还是计量资料，在描述大样本数据时，可通过编制频数分布表了解数据的基本分布情况。频数分布是系统地将数据值由小到大排列并列出每个数值或每段数值出现的次数。表格 14.1.1 中是 160 名研究对象的年龄，是计量资料。以这组数据说明计算频数分布的方法。呈现频数分布的方法包括频数分布表和频数分布图，两者目的不同。

Table 14.1.1   **Age of the 160 participants**（160 名研究对象的年龄）

86	25	81	28	99	29	27	65	34	38
35	31	81	46	97	96	31	93	39	68
20	42	85	83	56	53	52	93	26	50
85	93	96	63	54	61	97	81	37	44
59	37	38	79	32	77	25	88	65	94
47	99	66	24	81	71	81	61	31	44
62	87	83	44	20	72	50	44	79	62
97	47	44	76	30	32	66	40	70	27
47	83	29	26	95	89	51	80	54	91
74	22	97	24	65	83	43	65	75	90
39	78	26	71	50	36	83	90	41	62
22	97	79	87	54	47	36	88	41	50
52	71	58	32	65	28	97	26	40	49
69	30	67	36	67	49	68	48	57	44
51	29	43	60	84	95	36	37	34	66
26	39	33	78	52	67	51	99	67	75

2.1 Frequency distribution for quantitative data（计量资料的频数分布）

For quantitative data, constructing a frequency distribution is actually dividing the range of the score values into several groups that are mutually exclusive and collectively exhaustive, and then counting the frequency of cases at each value group. Scores are listed in order in one column, and corresponding frequencies are listed in another. The sum of numbers in the frequency column must equal the sample size, as shown in Table 14.1.2.

对于计量资料，编制频数分布表本质上就是把资料的取值范围分割成若干个互不相交的组段，统计每个组段内的观察值个数作为应对的频数。分数在一列中按顺序列出，相应的频率在另一列中列出。频率列中的数字之和必须等于样本容量，如表 14.1.2 所示。

Table 14.1.2   **Frequency distribution for the age of the 160 participants**

（160 名研究对象的年龄频数分布表）

Age group 年龄组	Frequency 频数	Percent(%) 频率	Cumulative frequency 累计频数	Cumulative percent(%) 累计频率
20~29	20	12.50	20	12.50
30~39	24	15.00	44	27.50
40~49	21	13.12	65	40.62
50~59	18	11.25	83	51.87
60~69	22	13.75	105	65.62
70~79	15	9.38	120	75.00
80~89	20	12.50	140	87.50
90~99	20	12.50	160	100.00
Total 合计	160	100	—	—

Frequency data can also be displayed graphically. Figure 14.1.1 is the graph for the frequency distribution in Table 14.1.2, and this kind of graph is histogram. In histograms, score values are arrayed on a horizontal dimension, with the lowest value on the left, ascending to the highest value on the right. Frequencies or percentages are displayed vertically. A histogram is constructed by drawing bars above the score classes to the height corresponding to the frequency for that score.

还可用频数分布图直观地描述计量资料的频数分布。图 14.1.1 是表 14.1.2 对应的频数分布图，称为直方图。在直方图中，分数值按水平维度排列，最低值在左边，最高值在右边。频率或百分比垂直显示。直方图是通过在得分类的上方绘制与该得分频率对应的高度的条形图来构造的。

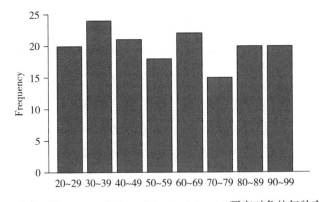

Figure 14.1.1   Histogram of Age of the Participants(研究对象的年龄直方图)

2.2 Frequency Distribution for Qualitative Data(计数资料的频数分布)

For qualitative data, a frequency distribution can be constructed by directly calculating the frequency and percentage for each value. A table for frequency distribution can be made by listing the frequency, percentage, cumulative frequency and cumulative frequency.

对于计数资料，编制频数分布表的方法是直接计算出每一个观察值的频数和频率，以及累计频数和累计频率，然后将它们列在一个表中。

For Example, age in Table 14.1.1 can be transformed into qualitative data or count data by classifying the participants as youth (19-35 years old), middle-aged adults (36-59 years old) and older adults (60 years and older). Then the frequency distribution of the age as qualitative data could be obtained as Table 14.1.3.

例如，可将表14.1.1中的年龄处理为计数资料，划分为青年(19~35岁)，中年(36~59岁)和老年(60岁及以上)三个等级进行计数统计，则可得到计数资料的频数分布表14.1.3。

Table 14.1.3　**Frequency distribution for the age of the 160 participants**

(160 名研究对象的年龄频数分布表)

Age group 年龄组	Frequency 频数	Percent(%) 频率	Cumulative frequency 累计频数	Cumulative percent(%) 累计频率
Youth 青年	32	20.00	32	20.00
Middle-aged adults 中年	51	31.88	83	51.88
Older adults 老年	77	48.12	160	100.00
Total 合计	160	100	—	—

2.3 Table and Graph for Frequency Distribution(频数分布表和频数分布图)

Histograms can reveal the type of data distribution more directly. The type of data distribution can be divided into symmetric distribution and skewed distribution. For skewed distribution, the peak is off center and one tail is longer than the other. There are two types of skewed distribution, positively skewed distribution and negative skewed distribution. When the longer tail points to the right, the distribution is positively skewed. If the tail points to the left, the distribution is negatively skewed.

频数分布图可比频数分布表更直观地揭示数据分布类型。数据的分布类型可分为对称分布和偏态分布两种。偏态分布的顶点不位于中间，顶点两侧分布长短不一。包含右偏态和左偏态两种。右偏态分布也称为正偏态分布，即频数集中位置偏向数值小的一侧，长尾向右侧延伸。左偏态分布，也称为负偏态分布，即频数集中位置偏向数值大的一侧，长尾向左侧延伸。

Section Ⅱ　Descriptive Statistics for quantitative data
第二节　计量资料的统计描述

Basic characteristics of the data can be seen from the frequency distribution. For drawing more specific and accurate information from the data, calculating a certain series of statistical index is crucial. For quantitative data, detailed descriptive statistics include statistics for central tendency (average level) and variability (degree of variation).

从数据的频数分布表和频数分布图可以看出样本观察值的分布情况，但要从中得到数据特征的准确信息需计算相应的统计指标。对计量资料进行统计描述，常从集中趋势(平均水平)和离散趋势(变异程度)两个方面进行描述。

1. Describing Central Tendency(集中趋势的描述)

An index of typicalness is come from the center of a distribution, such indexes are called measures of central tendency. There are several main indexes of central tendency: the mode, the median, and the mean.

集中趋势指的是一组计量资料的大多数观察值所在的中心位置。描述集中趋势的主要统计指标包括：众数、中位数和算数均数，也称为位置度量指标。

1.1　The Mean(均数)

The mean, or arithmetic mean, is the sum of all scores divided by the number of scores. The mean reflects the average level of all the score values and it is the most stable index of central tendency.

算术均数，简称为均数，等于一个指标变量所有观察值的和除以观察值的个数。算术均数描述了一个变量所有观察值的平均水平，是描述集中趋势最稳定的指标。

1.2　The Mode(众数)

The mode is the most frequently occurring score value in a distribution. In multimodal distributions, there is more than one score value that has high frequencies. Modes are a quick way to determine a "popular" score but are rather unstable.

众数是指一组数据中出现次数最多的数值。有时，在一组多峰数据中有多个众数。众数是常用的快速描述一组数据平均水平的一个集中趋势指标，但是它不稳定。

1.3　The Median(中位数)

The median is the point in a distribution above which and below which 50% of cases fall. It is often symbolized as M. As median is not sensitive to abnormal values, it's proper to use median to describe the central tendency of a group of data when the data has abnormal or unknown value, as well as when the data presents a skewed shape or an unknown shape. For symmetric distribution, the median is close to the mean; for positive distribution, the mean is larger than median; for negative distribution, the mean is smaller than median. Therefore, the shape of the data can be roughly estimated by comparing the median and the mean.

中位数指的是在按"从小到大顺序"排列后，位置居于中间的数值，记为 M。因为中位数对极端值不敏感，所以当数据中有极端值或含不确定值的资料，数据呈偏态分布或分布类型未知时，均宜采用中位数来描述集中趋势。当数据呈对称分布时，均数和中位数接近；当数据呈右偏态分布时，均数大于中位数；当数据呈左偏态分布时，均数小于中位数。因此，也可根据中位数和均数的差别大小，粗略判断数据的分布类型。

2. Describing Variability(离散趋势的描述)

Variability reflects how spread out or dispersed the data are from the center. There are several main indexes of variability: the range, the quantile, the variance, the standard deviation and the coefficient of variance.

离散趋势是指计量数据的所有观察值与中心位置的偏离程度。描述离散趋势的主要统计指标包括：极差、分位数、方差、标准差和变异系数，也称为变异性度量指标。

2.1　Range(极差/全距)

The range is simply the highest score minus the lowest score in a distribution. For variables with the same unit, the larger the range is, the data has a higher degree of variance and is more disperse. As the larger the sample size is, the larger the range, it is not often used to describe the variability of a data.

极差(或全距)等于一个变量的所有观察值中的最大值与最小值之间的差值。对于计量单位相同的变量，极差越大，变量的观察值越发散，表明变异度越大。由于样本量越大，极差往往越大，所以一般不太直接用极差描述离散趋势。

2.2 Quantile(分位数)

Quantile is a value between the maximum and minimum values of a variable. It makes some observed values of a variable less than or equal to it and others greater than or equal to it. The distance between two quantiles can be used to describe the degree of dispersion of the data. The commonly used quantile in statistics is the percentile. The percentile is a position indicator, expressed by p%, and p is expressed by percentage, $0 \leqslant p \leqslant 100$. In statistics, 25%, 50% and 75% are referred as quartiles. The difference between Q3 and Q1 is called quartile range.

分位数是介于变量的最大值和最小值之间的一个数值，它使得变量的一部分观察值小于或等于它，另一部分观察值大于或等于它。两个分位数之间的距离可以用来描述数据的离散程度。统计学中常用的分位数是百分位数。百分位数是一个位置指标，用 p 表示，p 用百分数表述，$0 \leqslant p \leqslant 100$。统计学将特殊的三个分位数 25%、50%、75%统称为四分位数，且称 Q3 与 Q1 的差值为四分位间距。

2.3 Variance(方差)

Variance indicates the average amount of deviation of values from the mean and is calculated using every score. Usually, X stands for the variance of the population while S^2 stands for the variance of the sample. It is calculated by the following formula:

方差是描述一个变量的所有观察值与均数的平均离散程度的指标(指一组数据百中的各个数减这组数据的平均数的平方和的平均数)。通常，X 表示总体的方差，S^2 表示样本的方差。计算公式如下：

$$S^2 = \frac{1}{n} \sum_{i=1}^{n} (X_i - \overline{X})^2$$

2.4 Standard Deviation(标准差)

Standard deviation (SD) is the arithmetic square root of variance. X represents the standard deviation of the population and S represents the standard deviation of the sample. The unit of standard deviation is consistent with that of the variable. For variables with the same unit of measurement, the greater the standard deviation, the greater the dispersion of the data.

标准差是方差的算术平方根。一般用 X 表示总体标准差，用 S 表示样本标准差。标准差的单位与原变量的单位一致。对于计量单位相同的变量，标准差越大，数据的离散程度就越大。

2.5 Coefficient of Variance(变异系数)

Coefficient of variation（CV）is an index to measure the degree of relative dispersion, and its calculation formula is:

变异系数是一个度量相对离散程度的指标，其计算公式为:

$$CV = \frac{S}{\bar{X}} \times 100\%$$

The formula decides that CV is a dimensionless index. It can be used to compare the dispersion degree among several variables with different dimensions or unites. It can also be used to compare the degree of dispersion among variables varying largely in mean although their dimensions or unites are the same. The greater the degree of dispersion, the greater the CV value.

从公式可以看出，变异系数是无量纲的指标，可用于比较几个量纲不同的指标变量之间的离散程度的差异，也可以用来比较维度或量纲相同但均数相差悬殊的变量之间的离散程度的差异。变异系数值越大，表示离散程度越大。

Section Ⅲ Descriptive Statistics for qualitative data
第三节 计数资料的统计描述

Similar with descriptive statistic for the quantitative data, specific indexes are needed to be calculated to obtain the detailed and accurate information of the variables, although basic distribution of the variable can be known from the frequency distribution. When describing quantitative data, absolute numbers are used to reflect the total scale and level of objective phenomenon at a certain time and place. Relative numbers are used to describe qualitative data and are calculated by comparing two related indicators. Commonly used indexes to describe qualitative data are ratio, proportion, rate, relative risk, odds ratio, etc.

与计量资料类似，要获取数据特征的准确信息，需要计算相应的用于描述计数资料的统计指标。描述计量资料时通常使用的是绝对数，旨在反映客观现象总体在一定时间、地点条件下的总规模、总水平。描述计数资料时通常使用的是相对数，是由两个有联系的指标对比产生的，包括：比、比例、率、相对危险度、比数比等。

1. Commonly Used Indexes for Relative Number(常用的相对数指标)

1.1　Ratio(比)

The ratio represents the quotient of the values of two related indicators. It describes how many times or percent an indicator is of the value of another indicator. Its calculation formula is：

$$Ratio = \frac{\text{Value of Indicator A}}{\text{Value of Indicator B}}$$

比表示两个相关指标的值之商，它描述了一个指标是另一个指标值的几倍或百分之几，其计算公式为：

$$Ratio = \frac{\text{指标 A 的值}}{\text{指标 B 的值}}$$

1.2　Proportion(比例)

Proportion refers to the ratio of the number of the component to the number of the whole. It describes the proportion of the internal components of the observations. The calculation formula is as follows：

比例指的是某事物内部各组成部分的观察单位数与所有组成部分的总观察单位数之比。它描述事物内部各组成部分所占的比例。其计算公式如下：

（1）Proportion indicating distribution structure 表示分布结构的比例：

$$\text{Constituent Ratio} = \frac{\text{number of one component}}{\text{number of the whole observations}} \times 100\%$$

$$\text{构成比} = \frac{\text{该事物内部某组成部分的观察单位数}}{\text{某事物内部各个组成部分的总观察单位数}} \times 100\%$$

（2）Proportion indicating the frequency of a phenomenon 表示某现象发生的频率：

$$\text{Frequency} = \frac{\text{the number of the observations}}{\text{the number of all of the potential observations}} \times K$$

$$频率 = \frac{某现象实际发生的观察单位数}{可能发生该现象的观察单位总数} \times K$$

K could be 100%, 1000% and etc. to make the final number having 1 to 2 bits of integers.

K 是比例基数，它可以取值 100%、1000%等。比例基数的选择主要根据习惯用法，使得计算结果能保留 1~2 位整数。

1.3 Rate(率)

The rate is an index with time notion. It is also called the absolute risk which is the proportion of people or observations who experienced an undesirable outcome in each group during a certain period of time. Commonly used rates include incidence rate and mortality.

率是一个具有时期概念的指标，也称为绝对危险度，是指某一段时间内发生某事件的人或观察单位数占该时期开始时暴露的人数或观察单位数之比。通常为发病率、死亡率。

1.4 Relative Risk (相对危险度)

Relative risk, or the risk ratio, represents the ratio of two rates of the same event in two different circumstances.

相对危险度指的是同一事件在两种不同情况下发生率之比。其计算公式是：

$$RR = \frac{P1}{P2}$$

In epidemiology study, P1 represents the rate of an event exposed to risk factors, and P2 represents the rate of an event not exposed to risk factors.

在流行病学中，用 P1 表示暴露于危险因素下某事件的率，用 P2 表示未暴露在危险因素下某事件的率。

In the experimental study, P1 represents the rate of exposure to an event in the intervention group and P2 represents the rate of an event in the control group which is not exposed to the intervention.

在干预性研究里，P1 表示暴露于干预组中某事件的率，P2 表示未暴露于干预的对照组中某事件的率。

The events generally refer to death, recurrence of diseases, morbidity, etc.

这里所说的事件一般为死亡、复发、发病等。

1.5 Odds Ratio(比数比)

For odds, if P is the incidence rate or probability of an event, then odds$=P/(1-P)$. That is，the odds is the proportion of people with the adverse outcome relative to those without it. The calculation formula is：

比数比设 P 是某事件的发生率或发生概率，则比数 odds＝P/(1－P)。也可以理解为，发生某事件的观察单位数与未发生某事件的观察单位数之比。其计算公式是：

$$OR = odds1 / odds2$$

The OR is a widely reported index. It is varied useful when the incidence of an event (such as incidence rate) is very small, then $1-p$ is approximately equal to 1, so OR is approximately equal to RR. That is, when the probability of an event is small, the ratio is approximately equal to the relative risk. In addition, when OR equals to 1, then RR would definitely equal to 1. On the contrary, when RR equals to 1, there must be OR equals to 1.

OR 被广泛使用，其重要意义在于：当某事件的发生率(如发病率)很小的情况下，1－P 约等于 1，从而，OR 约等于 RR。即，在某事件发生概率较小的情况下，比数比近似地等于相对危险度。另外，当 OR＝1 时，一定有 RR＝1；反之，当 RR＝1 时，一定有 OR＝1。

2. Notes for Using Indexes for Relative Number(应用相对数指标的注意事项)

(1)When using the relative number, the total number of observations should be sufficient. If the number of observations is too small and inadequate of representativeness, the relative number will be unstable and cannot accurately reflect the overall population parameter. (Zhenqiu Sun & Yongyong Xu, 2014).

计算相对数时总观察单位数应足够多。观察单位数过小，缺乏代表性，会造成相对数不稳定，不能准确反映总体的客观规律(孙振球、徐勇勇，2014)。

(2) Distinguish the difference between proportion and rate. Proportion is an indicator independent of time or is only an indicator of a time point, and rate is an indicator of a period. While the rate is an indicator of a period. Due to historical reasons, some indicators are nominally rate, but actually not rate. For example, the prevalence rate is a frequency index at a time point, but not rate.

要区分比例与率的差异。比例是与时间无关的指标或者仅是一个时点的指标，率是一个时期的指标。

(3)Distinguish the role of constituent ratio and frequency in proportion. The constituent ratio indicates the proportion of the internal parts of a thing. It cannot be used to explain the frequency or intensity of a phenomenon.

区别比例中的构成比和频率的作用。构成比表示事物内部各部分所占比例，不能用构成比来说明某现象发生的频率或强度。

（4）Correctly calculate the total sample rate. To calculate the rate for total sample, the correct numerator and denominator should be defined first according to the definition of rate.

正确计算总样本率。应当严格按照患病率的定义找出正确的分子和分母，然后计算合计率。

（5）Pay attention to the correction for the total sample rate. When estimating the rate of the population based on the rate of the sample, we often need to pay attention to the correction of the sample rate.

注意总样本率的校正计算。如果要根据样本来推断总的样本率，往往需要注意样本率的校正计算问题。

（6）Pay attention to the comparability of relative numbers. As many confounding factors could affect relative numbers, if the homogeneity requirements cannot be met, they cannot be directly compared with each other. If the internal composition affects the total sample rate, the relative number shall be standardized.

注意相对数的可比性。由于影响相对数的混杂因素很多，如果不能满足同质性要求，通常不能直接相互比较。若由于内部构成影响总样本率时，应当对相对数进行标准化。

（7）The purpose of rate standardization is to eliminate the influence of different internal components (e. g. age, sex, duration of disease, etc.) that cannot be directly compared when comparing the prevalence, incidence rate, mortality and other data of two different populations.

率的标准化是为了在比较两个不同人群的患病率、发病率、死亡率等资料时，消除其内部构成（如年龄、性别、病程长短等）不同而不能直接比较所产生的影响。

📖 Studies Cited in Chapter 14（第十四章参考文献）

[1] Polit, D. F., Beck. C. T. Nursing Research: Generating and Assessing Evidence for Nursing Practice[M]. 10th ed. Philadelphia: Lippincott Williams & Wilkins, 2017.

[2] Polit, D. F., Beck. C. T. Essentials of Nursing Research-Methods, Appraisal, Utilization [M]. 6th ed. Philadelphia: Lippincott Williams & Wilkins, 2006.

[3] 孙振球，徐勇勇. 医学统计学：第 4 版[M]. 北京：人民卫生出版社，2014.

Chapter 15: Inferential Statistical Analyses
第十五章 推断性统计分析

Inferential statistics is a statistical method that uses probability numbers to determine the possibility of a certain relationship between a certain group (or groups) of numbers, and inferring overall characteristics by sample characteristics. Inferential statistics provide a framework for making objective judgments about the reliability of sample estimates. Statistical inference consists of two techniques: (1) estimation of parameters and (2) hypothesis testing.

统计推断是用概率数字决定某两组(或多组)数字之间存在某种关系的可能性，并由样本特征来推断总体特征的统计方法。统计推断为对样本估计的可靠性做出客观判断提供了框架。包括两种重要方法：(1)参数估计；(2)假设检验。

Section I Estimation of Parameters
第一节 参数估计

Parameter estimation can make inferences about unknown population parameters from sample information obtained from a survey or experiment. In this section, we present general concepts relating to parameter estimation.

参数估计，可通过一次调查或试验获得的样本信息，对未知的总体参数做出推断。在这一部分中，我们给出了参数估计的一般概念。

1. Sampling Distributions(抽样分布)

Sampling distribution refers to the distribution of sample estimators.

抽样分布也称为统计量分布，是指样本估计量的分布。

Taking the sample mean as an example, it is an estimator of the population mean. If the samples are drawn repeatedly according to the same sample size and the same sampling method, an average can be calculated each time, and the average of all possible samples is formed. This distribution is a sampling distribution of the mean.

以样本平均数为例，它是总体平均数的一个估计量。如果按照相同的样本量，相同的抽样方式，反复地抽取样本，每次可以计算一个平均数，所有可能样本的平均数所形成的分布，就是样本平均数的抽样分布。

Sampling distributions of means are normally distributed, and the mean of a sampling distribution with an infinite number of sample means always equals the population mean.

均值的抽样分布是正态分布的，具有无穷多个样本均值的抽样分布的均值总是等于总体均值。

The standard deviation of a sampling distribution of the mean is called the standard error of the mean (SEM). It reflects the degree of dispersion between the sample means and the difference between the sample means and the population mean. The smaller the SEM—that is, the less variable the sample means—the more accurate are the means as estimates of the population value. The equation for the SEM is:

$$SEM = SD/\sqrt{N}$$

均值抽样分布的标准差称为标准误（SEM）。它反应样本均数之间的离散程度，也反应样本均数与相应总体均数之间的差异。SEM 越小——即样本均值的变量越小——作为总体估计的均值越准确。均值标准差的公式为：

$$SEM = SD/\sqrt{N}$$

2. Confidence Intervals(置信区间)

Parameter estimation is used to estimate a parameter. Estimation can take two forms: point estimation or interval estimation. The point estimation involves calculating a single descriptive statistic to estimate the population parameter. Point estimates convey no information about margin of error, so we could not make inferences about the accuracy of the parameter estimate. Interval estimation is useful because it indicates a range of values within which the parameter has a specified probability of lying. With interval estimation, we construct a confidence interval (CI) around the estimate; Confidence intervals are generally made up of two values, the upper and lower limits are confidence limits. Constructing a confidence interval around a sample mean establishes a range of values for the population value as well as the probability of being right—the estimate is made with a certain degree of confidence. By convention, researchers usually use either a 95% or a 99% confidence interval.

　　参数估计用来估计一个参数。可以采取两种方式进行估计：点估计和区间估计。点估计是计算一个单一的描述性统计来估计总体参数。但是，点估计没有考虑抽样误差范围，因此我们不能对参数估计的准确性做出推断。应采用区间估计，因为它给出了一个取值范围内的参数，这些参数具有一定的错误概率。我们围绕参数估计构建的区间称为置信区间，置信区间一般由两个数值构成，其中较小的值为可信下限，较高的值为可信上限。围绕样本均值构造一个置信区间，以一定的置信度建立总体的取值范围，以及被正确估计的概率。按照惯例，研究者通常使用95%或99%的置信区间。

3. Confidence Intervals around a Mean(总体均数的区间估计)

Confidence intervals reflect the researchers' risk of being wrong. With a 95% CI, researchers accept the probability that they will be wrong 5 times out of 100. Calculating confidence limits around a mean involves using the SEM. In a normal distribution, 95% of the scores lie within about 1.96 SDs from the mean. We can build a 95% confidence interval with the following formula:

$$CI\ 95\% = (X \pm 1.96 \times SEM)$$

　　置信区间反映了研究者出错的风险。在95% CI的情况下，研究者接受100次中5次出错的概率。我们利用SEM计算均值周围的置信限。在正态分布中，95%的分数距离平均值约1.96个SEM。我们可以用下列公式建立95%的置信区间：

$$CI\ 95\% = (X \pm 1.96 \times SEM)$$

4. Confidence Intervals around Proportions and Risk Indexes
(总体率和危险度指标的区间估计)

For proportions based on dichotomous variables, the applicable theoretical distribution is not a normal distribution but rather a binomial distribution. Certain features of confidence intervals around proportions are worth noting. First, the CI is rarely symmetric around a sample proportion. Second, the width of the CI depends on both the value of the proportion and the sample size. The larger the sample, the smaller the CI. Also, the closer the sample proportion is to 0.50, the wider the CI. Finally, the CI for a proportion never extends below 0 or above 1.0, but a CI can be constructed around an obtained proportion of 0 or 1.0.

对于基于二分变量的比例，适用的分布理论不是正态分布而是二项分布。关于比例的置信区间的某些特征值得注意。首先，CI 围绕一个样本比例很少是完全对称的。其次，CI 的宽度取决于比例的大小和样本量的大小。样本越大，CI 越小。而且，样本比例越接近 0.5，CI 越宽。最后，一个比例的 CI 不会小于 0 或大于 1，但 CI 可以围绕得到的 0 或 1 来构造。

<h1 style="text-align:center">Section Ⅱ　Hypothesis Testing
第二节　假设检验</h1>

1. Hypothesis Testing(假设检验)

Hypothesis testing is another method of statistical inference, also known as significance testing. Hypothesis testing is based on negative inference. There are two explanations for the between-group differences：（1）the effect of the intervention（2）the difference caused by chance factors such as sampling error. The first hypothesis is our research hypothesis, called the alternative hypothesis, denoted as H_1, and the other is the null hypothesis, denoted as H_0, that is, the null hypothesis indicates that there is no relationship between the variables.

假设检验是另一种统计推断方法，也称作为显著性检验。假设检验是基于否定推理的。对组间差异，有两种解释：(1)是干预措施的作用；(2)是抽样误差等偶然因素引起的差异。第一个假设是我们的研究假设，称为备择假设，记作 H_1，另一种就是零假设，记作 H_0，也就是说，零假设表明变量之间没有关系。

2. Two Type of Errors(假设检验的两类错误)

We decide whether to accept or reject a null hypothesis by determining how probable it is that observed results are due to chance. We can only conclude that hypotheses are probably true or probably false based on data from a sample, and there is always a risk of error. There are two types of statistical errors that we can make：reject the true null hypothesis or accept the false null hypothesis.

我们决定是否接受或拒绝一个零假设，是通过确定观察到的结果偶然发生的可能性。根据样本数据，我们只能得出结论，假设很可能是真的或可能是假的，并且总是存在错误的风险。我们可能会犯两种类型的统计错误：拒绝真零假设或接受假零假设。

Errors in which the null hypothesis H_0 is true and are rejected are called Type I errors, also known as false positive errors. The probability of making a Type I error is denoted as α, which is the maximum allowable probability of making a Type I error pre-specified in the study design.

零假设 H_0 为真且被拒绝的错误被称为第一类错误，也称 I 型错误、假阳性错误。犯 I 类错误的概率记作 α，是在研究设计时预先规定的允许犯 I 类错误概率的最大值。

Conversely, when the null hypothesis H_0 is not true and H_1 is true, the hypothesis test conclusion accepts H_0 and rejects H_1, which is called Type II error, false negative error, and denoted as β.

相反，当零假设 H_0 不真而 H_1 为真时，假设检验结论接受了 H_0 而拒绝了 H_1，称 II 型错误、假阴性错误，记作 β。

3. Level of Significance(显著性水平)

In practice we never know when we have made an error in statistical decision making. The validity of a null hypothesis could be known only by collecting data from the population. We usually control the risk of a Type I error by selecting a level of significance (referred to as α), which signifies the probability of incorrectly rejecting a true null hypothesis.

实际工作中我们从来不知道自己在统计决策中什么时候出错。只有从总体中收集数据，才能知道零假设的有效性。我们可以通过选择显著性水平(记作 α)来控制 I 型错误的风险，这意味着错误地拒绝一个正确的零假设的概率。

The two most frequently used significance levels are 0.05 and 0.01. With a 0.05 significance level, we accept the risk that out of 100 samples drawn from a population, a true null hypothesis would be rejected 5 times. The minimum acceptable level for α usually is 0.05.

最常用的两个显著性水平是 0.05 和 0.01。在 0.05 的显著性水平下，我们接受的风险是，在从一个总体中抽取的 100 个样本中，一个真实的零假设将被拒绝 5 次。α 的最低可接受水平通常为 0.05。

4. Critical Regions(临界区域)

There is a decision criterion in hypothesis testing based on the distribution of the test statistic. The rule is to reject the null hypothesis if the test statistic falls at or beyond the limits that establish acritical region on an applicable theoretical distribution and don't refuse the null hypothesis otherwise.

假设检验中根据检验统计量的分布，有一个决策规则。该规则是，如果检验统计量落在或超过在适用的理论分布上建立临界区域的界限，则拒绝零假设，反之则不拒绝零假设。

5. One-Tailed and Two-Tailed Tests(单尾检验与双尾检验)

In most hypothesis-testing situations, we use two-tailed tests. This means that both tails of the sampling distribution are used to determine improbable values.

在大多数假设检验中，我们都采用双尾检验，也就是说抽样分布的两个尾部都用来确定不可能的值。

When we have a strong basis for a directional hypothesis, we can use a one-tailed test. In one-tailed tests, the critical region of improbable values is in only one tail of the distribution——the tail corresponding to the direction of the hypothesis. It is easier to reject the null hypothesis with a one-tailed test than with a two-tailed test.

当我们有很强的方向性假设基础时，可以使用单尾检验。在单尾检验中，小概率值的临界域只在分布的一个尾部——对应于假设方向的尾部。单尾检验比双尾检验更容易拒绝零假设。

6. Parametric and Nonparametric Tests(参数检验与非参数检验)

If based on experience or α theory, some assumptions about the population can be made before inference, these assumptions are conducive to improving the efficiency of statistical inference. The statistical inference method is called parametric testing.

若根据经验或者某种理论能在推断之前就对总体作一些假设，这些假设有利于提高统计推断的效率，这种情况下的统计推断方法叫作参数检验。

If you know so little about the characteristics of the population that you cannot make assumptions about the population or only make general assumptions before inference, such as continuous distribution, symmetric distribution, etc. In statistics, statistical inference methods that make no assumptions about the overall distribution or only make general assumptions become nonparametric tests.

若对总体特征知之甚少，以至于在推断前不能对总体做出假设或仅能作一般性假设，如连续分布、对称分布等。在统计学上，对总体分布不做假设或仅作一般性的假设统计推断方法成为非参数检验。

7. Overview of Hypothesis-Testing Procedure(假设检验步骤概述)

（1）Select an appropriate test statistic. We must consider such factors as which measurement levels were used, whether a parametric test is justified, whether a dependent groups test is needed, and whether the focus is correlations or group comparisons—and how many groups are being compared.

选择适当的测试统计量。我们必须考虑使用哪种测量水平、参数检验是否合理、是否需要进行独立性检验、关注的焦点是相关性还是组间比较，以及有多少组数据在进行比较。

（2）Establish the level of significance. An α of 0.05 is usually acceptable.

建立检验水准。一般选择 $\alpha = 0.05$ 水平。

（3）Select a one-tailed or two-tailed test. In most cases, a two-tailed test should be used.

选择单尾或双尾检验。在大多数情况下，应该使用双尾检验。

（4）Compute a test statistic. Using collected data, we can calculate a test statistic using appropriate computational formulas or instruct a computer to calculate the statistic.

计算测试统计量。利用收集到的数据，我们可以使用适当的计算公式计算测试统计量，或者通过计算机计算统计量。

（5）Determine the degrees of freedom (symbolized as df). The degree of freedom refers to the number of independent or freely changing data in the sample when the parameters of the population are estimated by the statistic of the sample, it is easy to compute, the formula for df is as follows：

$$df = n-k$$

确定自由度(符号为 df)。自由度是指当以样本的统计量来估计总体的参数时，样本中独立或能自由变化的数据的个数，易于计算。计算公式如下：

$$df = n-k$$

where n is the number of samples, k is the number of restricted conditions or variables, or the number of other independent statistics used in computing a statistic.

其中 n 为样本数量，k 为被限制的条件数或变量个数，或计算某一统计量时用到其他独立统计量的个数。

(6) Compare the test statistic with a tabled value. Theoretical distributions for test statistics enable researchers to determine whether obtained values of the test statistic are beyond the range of what is probable if the null hypothesis were true. If the absolute value of the test statistic is larger than the tabled value, the results are statistically significant. If the computed value is smaller, the results are nonsignificant.

将计算的测试统计量与表值进行比较。检验统计量的理论分布可以帮助我们确定，检验统计量的测得值是否超出了零假设成立的可能范围。如果检验统计量的绝对值大于表中值，则结果具有统计学意义。如果计算值较小，则结果不显著。

Section Ⅲ   Testing Differences Between Two Group Means
第三节   两样本均数比较的假设检验

In the hypothesis testing of the comparison between means of two samples in measurement data, the commonly used methods are the t-test and the Z test. This section focuses on the t test. The parametric procedure for testing differences in group means is the t-test.

在计量资料两个样本均数比较的假设检验中，常用的方法有 t 检验和 Z 检验。本节着重讲解 t 检验。组间均数差异检验的参数化过程为 t 检验。

1. t-Tests for Independent Groups(两独立样本均数的 t 检验)

The two independent sample t test, also known as the group t-test, is suitable for the comparison of the means of two independent samples in a completely random design, and its purpose is to test whether the unknown population means represented by the two independent sample means are different. Its application conditions are: the two groups of data obey the normal distribution and the two populations corresponding to the two samples have equal variance, that is, the homogeneity of variance.

两独立样本 t 检验又称为成组 t 检验，适用于完全随机设计两独立样本均数的比较，其目的是检验两个独立样本均数所代表的未知总体均数是否有差别。其应用条件是：两组数据均服从正态分布且两样本对应的两总体方差相等，即方差齐性。

【Example 1】To compare the effects of regular-discharge and early-discharge nursing on maternal perception of mothers. The scale scores are as follows:

【例1】比较常规出院和早期出院护理对产妇母性感知能力的影响。量表得分如表 15.3.1 所示：

Table 15.3.1　**Scores on a Perceived Maternal Competence Scale for Regular-Discharge and Early-Discharge Mothers(常规出院和早期出院的母亲母性感知能力量表得分)**

Regular-Discharge Mothers 常规出院组	Early-Discharge Mothers 早期出院组
30	23
27	17
25	22
20	18
24	20
32	26
17	16
18	13
28	21
29	14
Mean(均值)= 25.0	Mean(均值)= 19.0

Notes(注): t=2.86; df=18; p=0.011

As shown in example 1, there are differences in the maternal perception data between the two groups in the table. This difference may indeed be due to the factors we studied, or it may be due to measurement errors. The question we face is: Can a portion of the variability reliably be attributed to the independent variable—time of discharge from the hospital? The hypotheses are: H_0: $\mu_1 = \mu_2$; H_1: $\mu_1 \neq \mu_2$

如例1所示，表中两组的母性感知能力数据是存在差异的。这种差异有可能确实是由于我们的研究因素导致的，也有可能是测量误差导致的。我们面临的问题是：能否将数据间的差异可靠地归因于出院时间这一自变量？我们建立假设：H_0: $\mu_1 = \mu_2$; H_1: $\mu_1 \neq \mu_2$。

To test these hypotheses, we would compute a t-statistic. We can do this through computer software. Then we get the value of t is 2.86. Next, degrees of freedom are calculated, df=20−2=18. We can get the values for α=0.05 for a two-tailed test by appendix 15.3.1, we find in this column that for df=18, the tabled value of t is 2.10. Thus, the calculated t of 2.86, which is larger than the tabled value of the statistic, is improbable. We can now say that the primiparas discharged early had significantly lower perceptions of maternal competence than those who were not discharged early. The group difference in perceived maternal competence is sufficiently large that it is unlikely to reflect merely chance fluctuations.

为了检验这些假设，我们将计算 t 统计量。我们可以通过计算机软件来实现这一过程。得到 t 值为 2.86。其次，计算出自由度。在这种情况下，df＝20－2＝18。查附录表 15.3.1 可见，对于 df＝18，α 取值 0.05 时双尾检验 t 的表值为 2.10。因此，计算出的 t 为 2.86，大于 2.10，有统计学意义。也就是说，早出院的初产妇对母亲能力的感知低于未早出院的初产妇。两组之间差异足够大，不太可能仅仅反映抽样误差。

2. Confidence Intervals for Mean Differences(均差的置信区间)

Confidence intervals can be constructed around the difference between two means, and the results provide information about both statistical significance and precision of the estimated difference. Because CI information is richer and more useful in clinical applications than p values, it is sometimes preferred.

围绕两组均数的差异构建置信区间，其结果能提供关于差异估计的统计意义和精度信息。由于 CI 信息比 p 值更丰富，在临床应用中更有用。

In the example in Table 15.3.1, the mean maternal competence scores were 25.0 in the regular discharge group and 19.0 in the early discharge group. Using a formula to compute the standard error of the difference, CIs can be constructed around the mean difference of 6.0. For a 95% CI, the confidence limits in our example are 1.6 and 10.4. This means that we can be 95% confident that the true difference in population means for early-and regular-discharge mothers lies somewhere between these limits.

在表 15.3.1 中的例子中，常规出院组平均得分 25.0 分，早期出院组得分 19.0 分。利用公式计算差值的标准误差，可以在均值差值 6.0 附近构造 CI。对于 95% 的 CI，我们的例子的置信限是 1.6 和 10.4。这意味着我们可以 95% 地确信，早期出院与常规出院的总体均值确实在此区间存在差异。

3. Paired t-Tests(配对样本均数的检验)

We sometimes obtain two measurements from the same people or from paired sets of participants. When means for two sets of scores are not independent，we should use a paired t-test—a t-test for dependent groups. A t-statistic then would be computed from pretest and posttest data，using a different formula than for the independent group t-test. The obtained t would be compared with tabled t values.

我们有时从同一个人或成对的参与者中获得两个测量值。当两组分数的均值不独立时，应该使用配对 t 检验。然后从测试前和测试后的数据计算 t 统计量，使用与独立样本 t 检验不同的公式，将得到的 t 与查表所得 t 值进行比较。

For this type of t-test，the formula for df is as follows：

$$df = N-1$$

此时的自由度公式如下：

$$df = N-1$$

Confidence intervals can be constructed around mean differences for paired as well as independent means.

置信区间可以围绕配对和独立的均值差异构造。

4. Nonparametric Two-group Tests(两样本的非参数检验)

If the application conditions of the t-test are not met，the nonparametric two-group tests should be used.

若不符合 t 检验的应用条件，则应使用两独立样本的非参数检验。

For instance，the Mann-Whitney U test，the nonparametric analog of an independent group's t-test，involves assigning ranks to the two groups of scores. The sum of the ranks for the two groups can be compared by calculating the U statistic. When ordinal-level data are paired，the Wilcoxon signed-rank test can be used.

例如，Mann-Whitney U 检验是独立组 t 检验的非参数方法，是对两组分数进行等级赋值，通过计算 U 统计量可以比较两组秩和。当有序等级数据成对时，可以使用 Wilcoxon 符号秩检验。

Section Ⅳ　Testing Mean Differences with Three or More Groups
第四节　三组及以上样本均数比较的假设检验

Analysis of variance（ANOVA）is the parametric procedure for testing differences between means when there are three or more groups. In practical work, we usually encounter the situation of comparing multiple sample means. At this time, using t-test may increase the possibility of making Type I errors, so ANOVA is more suitable than t-tests. This section describes the ANOVA method applicable to the comparison of multiple sample means.

方差分析是检验三组或三组以上组间均数差异的参数检验方法。实际工作中我们常常会遇到多个样本均数进行比较的情况，此时使用 t 检验可能会增加 I 型错误的可能性，所以方差分析比 t 检验更适合。本节将介绍适用于多个样本均数进行比较的方差分析方法。

ANOVA decomposes total variability in a dependent variable into two parts：（1）variability attributable to the independent variable and （2）all other variability, such as individual differences, measurement error, and so on. Variation between groups is contrasted to variation within groups to get an F-ratio. When differences between groups are large relative to variation within groups, the probability is high that the independent variable is related to, or has caused, group differences.

方差分析将因变量中的总变异性分解为两部分：（1）归因于自变量的变异性；（2）其他所有变异性，如个体差异、测量误差等。组间差异与组内差异进行对比，以获得 F 值。当组间差异相对于组内差异较大时，自变量与组间差异相关或引起组间差异的概率较大。

1. One-Way ANOVA(单因素方差分析)

One-way analysis of variance is to randomly group according to one treatment factor, and statistically analyze whether the mean difference between groups at each level of the treatment factor is statistically significant.

单因素方差分析是按一个处理因素随机分组，统计分析处理因素各个水平组间均数差别有无统计学意义。

In calculating an F-statistic, total variability in the data is broken down into two sources. The portion of the variance due to group status is reflected in the sum of squares between groups, or SS_B.

在计算 F 统计量时，数据的总变异性被分解为两个部分。处理组引起的方差部分反映在组间平方和即 SS_B 中。

The second component is the sum of squares within groups, or SS_W.

第二部分是组内平方和，即 SS_W。

In an ANOVA context, the variance is conventionally referred to as the mean square （MS）. The formulas for the mean square between groups and the mean square within groups are

$$MS_B = SS_B / df_B \qquad MS_W = SS_W / df_W$$

在方差分析中，通常要计算均方（MS）。组间均方和组内均方的计算公式为

$$MS_B = SS_B / df_B \qquad MS_W = SS_W / df_W$$

The F-ratio statistic is the ratio of these mean squares.

F 值就是这两者之比，即

$$F = MS_B / MS_W$$

At present, the calculation process can usually be done by computer software.

目前，计算过程通常可以由计算机软件完成。

【Example 2】 To compare the effectiveness of alternative interventions for smoking cessation. Thirty smokers were randomly divided into 3 groups, one group of smokers received intensive nurse consultation, the second group received nicotine patch therapy, and the third group as control group received no special treatment. The 1-day cigarette consumption measured 1 month after the intervention is shown in the table below, and one-way ANOVA tests the following hypotheses. Try to analyze whether the intervention is working. (see Table 15.4.1)

【例2】 比较戒烟替代干预措施的有效性。将30名吸烟者随机分为3组，第一组吸烟者接受密集的护士咨询，第二组接受尼古丁贴剂治疗，第三组对照组不接受特殊治疗。干预后1个月测量的1天香烟消费量如下表，试着分析干预措施是否有效。（见表15.4.1）

Table15.4.1　**Number of Cigarette Smoked in One day After One-month Intervention**

（干预一月后一天内吸食香烟的数量）

Group 1 Nurse Counseling （一组 护士咨询组）	Group 2 Nicotine Patch （二组 尼古丁贴组）	Group 3 Control Group （三组 对照组）
28	0	33
0	31	54
17	26	19
20	30	40
35	24	41
19	27	35
24	0	0
0	3	43

续表

Group 1 Nurse Counseling （一组 护士咨询组）	Group 2 Nicotine Patch （二组 尼古丁贴组）	Group 3 Control Group （三组 对照组）
21	24	39
2	27	36

First，establish the hypothesis，the hypothesis of one-way ANOVA is：

$$H_0： \mu_1 = \mu_2 = \mu_3； H_1： \mu_1 \neq \mu_2 \neq \mu_3$$

首先建立假设，单因素方差分析的假设为：

$$H_0： \mu_1 = \mu_2 = \mu_3； H_1： \mu_1 \neq \mu_2 \neq \mu_3$$

The Table 15.4.2 shows that the calculated F-statistic in our example is 4.98. For df = 2 and 27 and $\alpha = 0.05$，the tabled F-value is 3.35 (see Appendix 15.4.1). Because our obtained F-value of 4.98 exceeds 3.35，we reject the null hypothesis that the population means are equal.

表 15.4.2 显示我们的例子中计算的 F 统计量是 4.98。对于 df = 2 和 27 以及 $\alpha = 0.05$，查附录表 15.4.1 可知 F 值为 3.35。由于我们得到的 4.98 的 F 值超过了 3.35，我们拒绝零假设。

Table 15.4.2　**ANOVA Summary Table for Posttreatment Smoking Example**

干预后吸烟实例的方差分析汇总表

Source of Variance （变异来源）	SS	df	MS	F	P
Between Groups（组间）	1761.9	2	880.9	4.98	0.014
Within Groups（组内）	4772.0	27	176.7		
Total（总差异）	6533.9	29			

Notably，the data support the research hypothesis that different treatments were associated with different cigarette smoking，but we cannot tell from the test whether the first treatment was significantly more effective than the second treatment.

值得注意的是，这些数据支持了研究假设，即不同的治疗与吸烟数量不同有关，但我们无法从测试中判断第一组治疗方法是否比第二组更有效。

2. Two-Way ANOVA(双因素方差分析)

Two-way ANOVA is to group the data in two directions and perform ANOVA on the two grouping variables.

双因素方差分析就是将数据按照两个方向进行分组，并对两个分组变量进行方差分析。

Suppose we wanted to test whether the two smoking cessation treatments (nurse counseling and a nicotine patch) were equally effective for men and women. We need to randomly assign women and men, separately, to the two treatment conditions. The resulting data can be processed by the two-way ANOVA method.

假设我们尝试检验两种吸烟代替治疗(戒烟)方法(护士咨询和尼古丁贴片)对男女是否同样有效，这需要我们将男、女受试者随机分配至两组。得到的数据可以采用双因素方差分析法来处理。

With two independent variables, three hypotheses are tested. Firstly, we are testing the effectiveness, for both men and women, of nurse counseling versus the nicotine patch. Secondly, we are testing whether postintervention smoking differs for men and women, regardless of treatment approach. These are tests for main effects. Thirdly, we are testing for interaction effects (i. e., differential treatment effects on men and women). Interaction concerns whether the effect of one independent variable is consistent for all levels of a second independent variable.

在两个自变量的情况下，对三个假设进行检验。首先，我们测试护士咨询与尼古丁贴剂对男性和女性的有效性。其次，我们测试干预后男性和女性吸烟是否有差异，不管治疗方法如何。这些都是对主效应的检验。第三，我们测试交互效应(即对男性和女性的差别对待效应)。交互作用涉及一个自变量的效应对第二个自变量的所有水平是否一致。

By performing a two-way ANOVA on the differences in the data, we can learn whether these differences are statistically significant.

通过对数据的差异进行双因素方差分析，我们可以了解这些差异是否具有统计学意义。

3. Repeated-measures ANOVA(重复测量方差分析)

ANOVA on repeated measures data needs to consider two factors. One is to deal with grouping, by applying intervention and randomization; the other is to measure time. Therefore, the variance for repeated measures data can be decomposed into five components, namely treatment group, measurement time, interaction between treatment group and time, subject random error, and repeated measures error.

对重复测量数据的方差分析需要考虑两个因素。一个是处理分组，通过施加干预和随机分组来实现；另一个是测量时间。因此，对于重复测量数据的变异可分解为5个部分，分别是处理组、测量时间、处理组与时间的交互作用、受试对象的随机误差，以及重复测量误差。

4. Nonparametric "Analysis of Variance"（方差分析的非参数方法）

When comparing multiple groups of measurement data, if the data does not meet the conditions of variance analysis, the Kruskal-Wallis test, also known as the H-test or the K-W test, can be used. Infer whether there are differences in the multiple population distributions from which multiple independent samples of measurement data or grade data are derived.

多组计量资料比较时，若数据不满足方差分析的条件时，可以用 Kruskal-Wallis 检验，又称为 H 检验或 K-W 检验。可以推断计量资料或等级资料的多个独立样本来自的多个总体分布是否有差别。

Section V Testing Differences in Proportions
第五节　检验率的差异

1. The Chi-square Test(卡方检验)

The chi-square (χ^2) test is applied to count data to determine whether there is a difference between two or more rates or constituent ratios, and whether there is a correlation between two categorical variables. The chi-square statistic is computed by comparing observed frequencies and expected frequencies. Expected frequencies are the cell frequencies that would be found if there were no relationship between the two variables.

卡方(χ^2)检验是适用于计数资料的检验方法，其目的是推断两个或多个总体率或构成比之间有无区别，以及两个分类变量之间有无关联性。卡方统计量通过比较观测频率和期望频率来计算。期望频率是指如果两个变量之间没有关系，那么期望频率是期望在单元格中出现的个案数。

If null hypothesis is established, the difference between the actual observation frequency of each cell and the theoretical frequency will not be too large, that is, the value of χ^2 will not be too large, so null hypothesis will not be rejected; if the value of χ^2 obtained by the formula is large, which is greater than the pre-determined level α the corresponding χ^2 critical value, then reject the null hypothesis H_0, accept H_1, the difference is statistically significant.

如果原假设成立，则各格子实际观察频数与理论频数相差不会太大，即 χ^2 值不会太大，因此不拒绝原假设；如果公式计算获得 χ^2 值较大，大于事先确定的水准 α 所对应的 χ^2 临界值，则拒绝原假设 H_0，接受 H_1，差异具有统计学意义。

【Example 3】 Try to compare the efficacy of two drugs in the treatment of lung cancer, the experimental results are shown in Table 15.5.1:

【例3】尝试比较两种药物治疗肺癌的效果，实验结果见表 15.5.1:

Table15.5.1　**The experimental results of the two drugs in the treatment of lung cancer**

（两种药物治疗肺癌疗效的实验结果）

Drugs（药物）	Efficacy（疗效）		Total（合计）	Efficient Ratio （有效率(%)）
	Efficient（有效）	Invalid（无效）		
A	28(15)	2(15)	30	93.33
B	12(8)	4(8)	16	75.00
Total 合计	40	6	46	86.96

Notes（注）: $\chi^2=1.69$, $df=1$, $P=0.194$

Formulas and computations are not shown here, but in our example, $\chi=1.69$. For chi-square tests, df equals the number of rows minus1 times number of columns minus 1. In the current case, $df=1\times1=1$. According appendix 15.5.1, at the level of $df=1$ and $\alpha=0.05$, the theoretical chi-square value is 3.84. In this case $\chi^2=1.69<3.84$, the null hypothesis is not rejected, so it cannot be considered that there is a difference in the efficacy of the two drugs in the treatment of lung cancer.

公式和计算在这里没有显示，但在我们的例子中，$\chi^2=1.69$。对于卡方检验，df 等于行数减 1 乘以列数减 1。在当前情况下，$df=1\times1=1$。查阅附录表 15.5.1 可知，在 $df=1$，$\alpha=0.05$ 的水平下，卡方的理论值为 3.84。本例 $\chi^2=1.69<3.84$，不拒绝原假设，因此尚

不能认为两种药物在治疗肺癌的疗效上有差异。

2. Confidence Intervals for Differences in Proportion(率差及其置信区间)

Using the difference $p_1 - p_2$ of the two population rates as the point estimation of the difference $\pi_1 - \pi_2$ of the two population rates cannot take into account the size of the sampling error, so it is necessary to estimate the confidence interval of the population rates of the two samples. As with means, it is possible to construct confidence intervals around the difference between two proportions.

用两样本率之差 $p_1 - p_2$ 作为两个总体率之差 $\pi_1 - \pi_2$ 的点估计无法考虑抽样误差的大小，所以要估计两样本总体率的置信区间。与均值一样，可以围绕两个比例之间的差异构造置信区间。

3. Other Tests of Proportions(其他率的差异检验)

Sometimes a chi-square test is not appropriate. When the total sample size is small (total N of 30 or less) or when there are cells with small frequencies (five or fewer), Fisher's exact test should be used to test the significance of differences in proportions. Because chi-square test results may be biased, this method is to directly calculate the probability, so it is also called the Fisher's exact probability test method.

有时使用卡方检验并不合适。当样本含量较小时(小于 30 例)或者是有小格频率小于 5 时，需要采用 Fisher 确切检验法进行分析，因为卡方检验结果可能会有偏性。此方法是直接计算概率，因此也叫 Fisher 确切概率检验法。

Section Ⅵ　Testing Correlations
第六节　相关性检验

The statistical tests discussed thus far are used to test differences between groups—they involve situations in which the independent variable is a nominal-level variable. In this section, we consider statistical tests used when both the independent and the dependent variables are ordinal, interval, or ratio.

迄今为止讨论的统计检验用于检验组间差异，即自变量是名义水平变量的情形。在本节中，我们考虑当自变量和因变量都是序数、间隔或比率时使用的统计检验。

1. Pearson's r(皮尔逊相关系数)

Pearson's r, the correlation coefficient calculated when two variables are measured on at least the interval scale, is both descriptive and inferential. Descriptively, the correlation coefficient summarizes the magnitude and direction of a relationship between two variables. As an inferential statistic, r tests hypotheses about population correlations, which are symbolized as ρ.

Pearson's r, 是当两个变量至少在区间尺度上测量时计算的相关系数，既是描述性的，也是推断性的。从描述性来看，相关系数概括了两个变量之间关系的大小和方向。作为一个推断统计量，r 检验关于总体相关性的假设，其符号为 ρ。

The null hypothesis is that there is no relationship between two variables:

$$H_0: \rho = 0; \quad H_1: \rho \neq 0$$

它的原假设是，两个变量之间不存在相关性，即：

$$H_0: \rho = 0; \quad H_1: \rho \neq 0$$

The values of this statistics range from −1.00 to +1.00. A positive r value indicates a positive correlation, a negative r value indicates a negative correlation, $|r| = 1$ indicates a complete correlation, and $r = 0$ is zero correlation.

皮尔逊相关系数取值为 $-1 \leqslant r \leqslant 1$。r 值为正表示正相关，r 值为负表示负相关，$|r| = 1$ 表示完全相关，r=0 为零相关。

2. Other Test of Bivariate Relationships(双变量相关性的其他检验方法)

Pearson's r is a parametric statistic. When the assumptions for a parametric test are violated, then the appropriate coefficient of correlation is either Spearman's rho. Another correlation statistic that is used to correlate a dichotomous variable with a continuous one is called a point-biserial correlation coefficient.

皮尔逊相关系数是参数统计量。当数据不符合参数检验的条件时，那就应该用 Spearman 值相关。另一个用来将一个二分变量与一个连续变量相关联的统计量称为点二列相关系数。

Section Ⅶ　Power Analysis and Effect Size
第七节　检验效能和效应量

Power analysis is used to reduce the risk of Type Ⅱ errors and strengthen statistical conclusion validity by estimating in advance how big a sample is needed. There are four components in a power analysis, three of which must be known or estimated:

检验效能用于预先估计需要多少样本来降低第二类错误的风险并加强统计结论的有效性。检验效能由 4 个组成，其中 3 个必须已知或估计:

(1)The significance criterion α. Other things being equal, the more stringent this criterion, the lower the power.

显著性水平 α。在其他条件相同的情况下，这一标准越严格，检验效能越低。

(2)Power 1−β. This is the probability of rejecting a false null hypothesis.

检验效能 1−β。这是拒绝错误原假设的概率。

(3)The effect size ES. ES is an estimate of how wrong the null hypothesis is, that is, how strong the relationship between the independent variable and the dependent variable is in the population.

效应大小 ES。ES 是对原假设的错误程度的估计，即自变量和因变量之间的关系在总体中的强度。

(4)The sample size N. As sample size increases, power increases.

样本量 N。随着样本量的增加，效能增加。

We usually establish the risk of a Type I error (α) as 0.05. The conventional standard for 1−β is 0.80. With power equal to 0.80, there is a 20% risk of committing a Type Ⅱ error. The effect size is the magnitude of the relationship between the research variables. When relationships are strong, they can be detected at significant levels even with small samples. With modest relationships, large sample sizes are needed to avoid Type Ⅱ errors. In using power analysis to estimate sample size needs, the population effect size is not known; if it were known, there would be no need for the new study. So the effect size must be estimated using available evidence and theory.

我们通常将犯第一类错误的风险 α 设定为 0.05。1−β 的常规标准为 0.80。检验效能为 0.80 时，犯第二类错误的风险为 20%。效应量是研究变量之间联系的大小。当联系很强时，即使在小样本情况下也能在显著水平上检测到它们。对于适中的关系，需要较大的样本容量以避免类型 Ⅱ 错误。在使用检验效能估计样本量时，总体效应量的大小是不可知的；如果已知，就没有必要进行新的研究。因此效应量必须利用现有的证据和理论进行估计。

【Example 4】 We were testing the hypothesis that cranberry juice reduces the urinary pH of diet-controlled patients. We plan to assign some patients randomly to a control condition（no cranberry juice）and others to an experimental condition in which they will be given cranberry juice for 7 days. How large a sample is needed for this study, given a desired α of 0. 05 and power of 0. 80?

【例4】 在蔓越莓汁降低饮食控制患者尿液 pH 值的研究中，将受试者随机分配到 2 个组，对照组和计划给予 7 天蔓越莓汁的干预组。考虑到所需的 α 为 0. 05 和检验效率为 0. 80，这项研究需要多大的样本?

To answer this, we must first estimate ES. In a two-group situation in which mean differences are of interest, ES is usually designated as d, the formula for which is:

$$d = \frac{\mu_1 - \mu_2}{\sigma}$$

为了回答这个问题，我们必须首先估计 ES。在关注两组均值差异的情形中，ES 通常被指定为 d，计算公式为:

$$d = \frac{\mu_1 - \mu_2}{\sigma}$$

These population values are never known, they can be estimated by earlier study. Suppose the results of prior research were as follows: $X_1 = 5. 70$, $X_2 = 5. 50$, SD $= 0. 50$, Then, the estimated value of d would be:

$$d = \frac{5. 70 - 5. 50}{0. 50} = 0. 4$$

这些总体数值从来不是已知的，我们可以通过预实验进行估计。假设在我们的例子中得到的预实验结果，$\overline{X}_1 = 5. 70$，$\overline{X}_2 = 5. 50$，SD $= 0. 50$，则我们例子中:

$$d = \frac{5. 70 - 5. 50}{0. 50} = 0. 4$$

The Table 15. 7. 1 presents approximate sample size requirements for various effect size and powers, in a two-group mean-difference situation. We find in this table that the estimated n (number per group) to detect an effect size of 0. 40 with power equal to 0. 80 is 99 people.

表 15. 7. 1 给出了在两组均差情形下，各种效应量和检验效能的样本量要求。我们在这个表中发现，在检验效率等于 0. 80，效应大小为 0. 40 的情况下每组的样本量为 99 人。

Table 15. 7. 1 **Approximate sample size per Group for various effect size and powers, for α= 0. 05**

（α= 0. 05 下不同检验效能与效应量每组需要的大致样本量）

Power	Estimated effect size(d)估计效应量										
效能	0. 10	0. 15	0. 20	0. 25	0. 30	0. 35	0. 40	0. 50	0. 60	0. 70	0. 80
0. 60	979	435	245	157	109	80	62	40	28	20	16
0. 70	1233	548	309	198	137	101	78	50	35	26	20
0. 80	1576	701	394	253	176	129	99	64	44	33	25
0. 90	2103	935	526	337	234	172	132	85	59	43	33
0. 95	2594	1154	649	416	289	213	163	105	73	53	41

Assuming that the earlier study provided a good estimate of the population effect size, the total number of people needed in the new study would be about 200, with half assigned to the control group (no cranberry juice) and the other half assigned to the experimental group. With a sample size smaller than 200, there would be a greater than 20% chance of a false negative conclusion, that is, a Type II error. For example, a sample size of 128 (64 per group) would result in an estimated 40% chance of incorrect nonsignificant results.

假设我们的预实验能够提供合适的总体效应量，新的研究需要的总样本量约为 200，其中一半分配给对照组(无蔓越橘汁)，另一半分配给实验组。当样本量小于 200 时，会有大于 20 ％的概率出现假阴性结论，即 II 型错误。例如，样本容量为 128 (64 只/组)会导致估计 40 ％的不正确的非显著性结果。

If there is no prior research, researchers can, as a last resort, estimate whether the expected effect is small, medium, or large. By convention, the value of ES in a two-group test of mean differences is estimated at 0. 20 for small effects, 0. 50 for medium effects, and 0. 80 for large effects.

如果没有事先的研究，研究人员可以估计预期效果大小作为最后手段。根据惯例，两组均值差异检验中的 ES 值估计为：小效应为 0. 20，中等效应为 0. 50，大效应为 0. 80。

We'd better avoid using the conventions in favor of more precise estimates based on existing evidence. If the conventions cannot be avoided, conservative estimates should be used to minimize the risk of obtaining nonsignificant results.

我们最好避免使用惯例，而是根据现有证据进行更精确的估计。如果不能避免，应使用保守的估计，以尽量减少获得不显著结果的风险。

Section Ⅷ   Critiquing Inferential Statistical Analyses
第八节   评判推断性统计分析

Different inspection methods have their own application conditions, we must learn to choose the correct inspection method. Statistical analyses and design issues are sometimes intertwined, and both can affect statistical conclusion validity. It is also very important whether the appropriate statistical method is used according to the research design, and even affects whether the conclusion is correct.

不同的检验方法有各自的应用条件，我们要学习选择正确的检验方法。统计分析和研究设计往往是交织在一起的，它们都会对统计结论的有效性产生影响。是否根据研究设计选用合适的统计学方法也是非常重要的，甚至会影响结论是否正确。

In addition, we need to clarify whether the report presents the results of statistical tests for all study hypotheses and whether the researchers undertook analyses to address questions about the study's internal validity.

另外，我们要明确研究报告中是否提供了所有研究假设的统计检验结果，以及研究人员是否进行了分析以解决关于研究内部效度的问题。

📖 Studies Cited in Chapter 15（第十五章参考文献）

[1]Beck, Cheryl Tatano. Polit, Denise, F. Nursing research-generating and assessing evidence for nursing practice[J]. Wolters Kluwer Health, 2017.

[2]颜虹. 医学统计学[M]. 北京：人民卫生出版社，2015.

[3]李峥，刘宇. 护理学研究方法. [M]. 北京：人民卫生出版社，2018.

[4]胡雁. 护理学研究[M]. 北京：人民卫生出版社，2017.

Chapter 16: Multivariate Statistics
第十六章　多元统计分析

In nursing research, the observable indicator of interest to researchers is often influenced by multiple factors, such as the pain score of hospitalized patients not only related to disease type, but also gender, age, and the hospital environment. For this type of research, bivariate research is no longer suitable, and multivariate statistical analysis methods can be used to analyze the relationship between observed indicators and these factors.

在护理学研究中，研究人员感兴趣的某个观察指标往往受多种因素的影响，如住院患者的疼痛评分不仅与疾病类型有关，还与性别、年龄、医院环境有关。对于这类研究，已不再适合双变量研究，可以采用多元统计分析方法来分析观察指标和这些因素之间的关系。

As the focus of this chapter, multiple regression analysis is the most widely used multivariate statistical analysis method, which is used to analyze the influence of two or more independent variables on continuous dependent variables. In order to better understand the multiple regression analysis methods, this chapter first introduces the related content of simple linear regression (bivariate).

多元回归分析是应用最为广泛的多元统计分析方法，用于分析两个或两个以上的自变量对连续因变量的影响，是本章学习的重点。为了更好地理解多元回归分析方法，本章节首先讲述了简单线性回归(双变量)的相关内容。

Section I　Simple Linear Regression
第一节　简单线性回归

In data containing only two variables, if one variable Y changes linearly with the other variable X, which is called simple linear regression. In regression analysis, the variable Y is called the response variable, also known as the dependent variable; the variable X is called the explanatory variable, also known as the independent variable. For example, when studying the change of children's height with age, age is the independent variable, and children's height is the dependent variable. The variable X (such as age) can be used to predict the variable Y (height), and the stronger the correlation between the two variables, the higher the accuracy of the variable X in predicting the variable Y. If the correlation coefficient of the two variables is equal to 1, we can consider that the variable Y can be completely predicted by the variable X. However, few variables can be completely correlated in real life, so the regression analysis we usually do cannot be completely predicted.

在只包含两个变量的资料中，如果一个变量 Y 随另一个变量 X 呈线性变化趋势，称之为简单线性回归。回归分析中，将变量 Y 称为反应变量，又称因变量；将变量 X 称为解释变量，又称自变量。如研究儿童身高随年龄的变化时，年龄为自变量，儿童身高为因变量。变量 X(如年龄)可以用来预测变量 Y(身高)，当两个变量间的相关性越强，变量 X 预测变量 Y 的准确性越高。如果两个变量的相关系数等于 1 时，我们可以认为变量 Y 能够由变量 X 完全预测。然而实际生活中很少有变量能够做到完全相关，因此我们通常做的回归分析都无法做到完全的预测。

The simple linear regression equation is(简单线性回归方程的一般表达式为)

$$\hat{Y}=a+bX$$

$\hat{Y}$ is the point estimate of the mean of Y; a is the intercept of the Y-axis in the regression line; b is the regression coefficient, also the slope of the regression line, whose statistical significance is that when X increases (or decreases) by one unit, $\hat{Y}$ changes b units. If $b>0$, indicating that Y increases with the increase of X; $b<0$, indicating that Y decreases with the increase of X; $b=0$, indicating that there is no linear relationship between Y and X. For a fixed value of X, the relationship between the actual observed value Y of the individual and $\hat{Y}$ is as follows: $Y=\hat{Y}+\varepsilon$ (ε is the residual, also the difference between Y and $\hat{Y}$).

$\hat{Y}$ 为 Y 的均数的点估计值；a 为回归直线在 Y 轴上的截距；b 为回归系数，即回归直线的斜率，其统计学意义是 X 每增加(或减少)一个单位，$\hat{Y}$ 改变 b 个单位。$b>0$，表示 Y 随 X 的增大而增大；$b<0$，表示 Y 随 X 的增大而减小；$b=0$，表示 Y 与 X 不存在线性关系。对于固定的 X 值，个体实际观测值 Y 与 $\hat{Y}$ 的关系如下：$Y=\hat{Y}+\varepsilon$(ε 为残差，即 Y 与 $\hat{Y}$ 的差值)。

The construction of a linear regression model must meet the following four conditions: (1) Linear: when the independent variable X is quantitative data or rank data without dummy variables, X has a linear relationship with the dependent variable Y; (2) Independence: the observed value of an individual is not affected by other individuals; (3) Normal: when given the value of X, the value of Y is required in a normal distribution, and the residuals are also required in a normal distribution; (4) Equal variance: when given different explanatory variables X, the variances of the response variable Y are equal.

线性回归模型成立必须满足以下四个条件：(1)线性：当自变量 X 为定量资料或不设哑变量的等级资料时，X 与因变量 Y 呈直线关系；(2)独立性：个体的观测值不受其他个体的影响；(3)正态性：给定 X 值，Y 的取值服从正态分布，同时要求残差也服从正态分布；(4)方差齐性：给出不同解释变量 X 时，反应变量 Y 的方差相等。

For example, Table 16.1.1 lists the math scores (Y) and study time (X) of 5 students in a class. If these data are drawn into a scatter plot, as shown in Figure 16.1.1, it is not difficult to find that there is a certain linear relationship between X and Y, and X is strongly correlated with Y ($r=0.996$). We can solve a and b through these five sets of data, and get the regression equation $\hat{Y}=8.1+15.6X$. If any X value is given, the predicted value $\hat{Y}$ corresponding to the X value can be obtained. Comparing the actual value Y corresponding to the X value with the estimated value $\hat{Y}$ in Figure 16.1.1, it is found that Y is not equal to $\hat{Y}$, which indicates that there will be a certain prediction error in predicting Y entirely by X. The prediction error occurs because X and Y are not fully correlated, which is $r \neq 1$. Therefore, if we minimize the prediction error, we can get an approximately standardized regression equation, which is called the least-squares method. Specifically, in simple linear regression, we minimize the sum of the squares of the prediction errors (called residuals ε) to obtain the standard regression equation, such as ε^2 in Table 16.1.1, so standard regression is also called the least-squares regression.

例如在表 16.1.1 中，列出了一个班级中的 5 名同学数学成绩(Y)与学习时间(X)的数据。若将这组数据绘制成散点图，如图 16.1.1 所示，不难发现，X 与 Y 存在一定的线性关系，且呈强相关($r=0.996$)。我们可以通过这五组数据求解出 a 和 b，得到回归方程 $\hat{Y}=8.1+15.6X$，若给出任意 X 值，就能够得到与 X 相对应的预测值 $\hat{Y}$。将图 16.1.1 中 X 所对应的实际值 Y 与估计值 $\hat{Y}$ 比较发现，Y 并不等于 $\hat{Y}$，这表明完全由 X 来预测 Y 会存在一定的预测误差。预测误差的产生是因为 X 与 Y 并没有达到完全相关，即 $r \neq 1$。因此，我们如果将预测误差最小化，便可以得到近似标准化的回归方程，这种方法称作最小二乘法。具体来说，在简单线性回归中，我们是将预测误差(称为残差 ε)的平方和最小化，如表 16.1.1 中的 ε^2，进而得到标准回归方程，因此标准回归也被称为最小二乘回归。

To describe the effect size of the independent variable on the dependent variable, the square of the correlation coefficient (r^2) is used to reflect the percentage that X can explain in the total variance of Y. In the above example, $r=0.996$ and $r^2=0.992$, indicating that 99.2% of the total variance in math scores is related to study time.

为了描述自变量对因变量影响的大小，相关系数的平方(r^2)用来反映 Y 的总变异中 X 所能解释的百分比。在上述的例子中，$r = 0.996$，$r^2 = 0.992$，表明数学成绩总变异的 99.2%与学习时间有关。

Table 16.1.1 　　**Example of Simple Linear Regression**(简单线性回归的例子)

X	Y	$\hat{Y}$	ε	ε^2
1.75	33	35.4	−2.44	5.96
2.5	48	47.2	0.83	0.68
3.25	62	58.9	3.09	9.57
4.75	82	82.4	−0.37	0.14
5.5	93	94.1	−1.10	1.22
$\overline{X}=3.55$	$\overline{Y}=63.6$		0.00	$\overline{\sum \varepsilon} = 17.57$
$r=0.996$				
$\hat{Y}=a+bX=8.1+15.6X$				

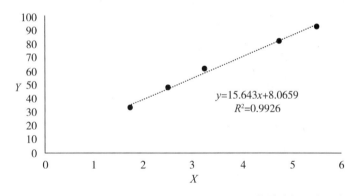

Figure 16.1.1　Example of Simple Linear Regression(简单线性回归的例子)

Section Ⅱ　Multiple Linear Regression
第二节　多元线性回归

In nursing research, research indicators are often affected by multiple factors, so researchers often try to improve the accuracy of the prediction for the variable Y through multiple independent variables X. In this process, X is also called the predictor variable.

在护理学研究中，研究指标往往受多种因素影响，因此研究人员往往尝试通过多个自变量 X 来提高对变量 Y 预测的准确性，在这个过程中，X 也被称作预测变量。

1. Basic Concepts for Multiple Regression(多元线性回归的基本概念)

Multiple linear regression refers to a statistical method to explore the linear relationship between a dependent variable Y and multiple independent variables X, also referred to as multiple regression, which is an extension of simple linear regression. The multiple regression equation is:

多元线性回归是指探讨一个因变量 Y 与多个自变量 X 之间线性关系的一种统计学方法，简称多元回归，是简单线性回归的延伸。多元回归方程的表达式为：

$$\hat{Y} = a + b_1X_1 + b_2X_2 + \cdots + b_kX_k$$

As with simple linear regression, $\hat{Y}$ is the point estimate of the mean of Y; a is the constant term, the intercept of the regression line. k is the number of independent variables, bk ($k=1$, 2...) is the partial regression coefficient, which means that when the independent variables other than X_k are fixed and unchanged, each time X_k changes by one unit, the average value of the corresponding Y changes, the positive or negative of b_k determines the direction of Y change. In addition to the four items listed in the simple linear regression above, the prerequisites for the construction of the multiple linear regression model also need to consider the relationship between multiple independent variables. If the two independent variables are highly correlated, it is considered that there is multicollinearity between the independent variables, which can easily lead to unstable regression results. Correlation processing should be performed before regression analysis.

与简单线性回归相同，$\hat{Y}$ 为 Y 的均数的点估计值；a 为常数项，即回归直线的截距。k 为自变量的个数，$b_k(k=1，2，\cdots)$ 为偏回归系数，表示在除 X_k 以外的自变量固定不变的情况下，X_k 每改变一个单位，相应的 Y 平均变化的值，b_k 的正负决定 Y 变化的方向。多元线性回归模型成立的前提条件除上述简单线性回归列出的四条之外，还需要考虑多个自变量之间的关系。若两个自变量间高度相关，则称自变量间存在多重共线性，这很容易导致回归结果不稳定，应进行相关处理后再进行回归分析。

For example, Wang Huali (2014) collected data on the height of parents and sons in 20 families to analyze the effect of parental height on the height of sons, as shown in Table 16.2.1.

例如，王华丽(2014)为研究父母身高对儿子身高的影响，调查收集了 20 个家庭的父母身高和儿子身高的数据，见表 16.2.1。

Table 16.2.1 **The data on the height of parents and sons in 20 families**
(20 个家庭父母身高和儿子身高资料)

Number （编号）	Father's Height（X_1） （父亲身高（X_1））	Mother's Height（X_2） （母亲身高（X_2））	Son's Height（Y） （儿子身高（Y））
1	172	163	176
2	171	159	172
3	169	158	170
4	171	161	174
5	167	159	169
6	172	163	177
7	172	160	171
8	170	162	173
9	175	166	182
10	179	166	183
11	176	164	180
12	171	159	174
13	167	158	172
14	176	163	177
15	172	162	175
16	181	169	186
17	174	167	182
18	170	161	174
19	183	169	187
20	176	165	182

Taking the son's height as the dependent variable Y, the father's height and the mother's height as the independent variables X_1 and X_2, respectively, the linear regression analysis was performed in SPSS software, and the regression equation $Y = -63.5 + 0.381X_1 + 1.072X_2$ was obtained. The partial regression coefficient $b_2 = 1.072$, which means that when the father's height remains unchanged, each time the mother's height increases 1cm, the son's height average changes 1.072cm.

以儿子身高为因变量 Y，父亲身高和母亲身高分别为自变量 X_1 和 X_2，在 SPSS 软件中进行线性回归分析，得到回归方程 $Y = -63.5 + 0.381X_1 + 1.072X_2$。偏回归系数 $b_2 = 1.072$，表示在父亲身高不变的情况下，母亲身高每增加1cm，儿子的身高平均变化1.072cm。

The multiple linear regression involved multiple independent variables, and corresponding to the multiple linear regression is multiple correlation coefficient, which is called R and used to represent the degree of correlation between multiple independent variables and a dependent variable. Different from the correlation coefficient r, the value range of the multiple correlation coefficient R is between 0 and 1, and does not determine the direction in which Y changes with X. The square of the multiple correlation coefficient R (R^2, called as the coefficient of determination) reflects the percentage of the total variance of Y explained by all the multiple independent variables X, and also reflects the quality of the regression equation model.

在多元线性回归中，涉及多个自变量，与之相对应的是复相关系数，称为 R，用来表示多个自变量和一个因变量的相关程度。与相关系数 r 不同的是，复相关系数 R 的取值范围在 0 和 1 之间，且不决定 Y 随 X 变化的方向。复相关系数 R 的平方（R^2，也称为决定系数）反映了在 Y 的总变异中多个自变量 X 所共同解释的百分比，也反映了回归方程模型效果的好坏。

Multiple linear regression analysis requires that the dependent variable Y is the random continuous variable, such as blood pressure and weight, while the independent variable X can be the continuous variable or the categorical variable. However, only after quantifying and coding, binary variables can be included in the regression model. For multi-category variables, it is necessary to perform "dummy". Assuming that the variable has m categories, it is transformed into (m−1) binary variables, and these (m−1) binary variables are called "dummy variable".

多元线性回归分析要求因变量 Y 是连续性随机变量，如血压、体重，而自变量 X 可以是连续性变量，也可以是分类变量。对于二分类变量，需要对其进行数量化编码后纳入回归模型，而对于多分类变量，则需要进行"哑元化"，假设变量有 m 个分类，将其变换为(m-1)个二分类变量，这(m-1)个二分类变量称为"哑变量"。

2. Tests of Significance(显著性检验)

In statistical analysis, most of the data and information we use come from samples, so can the results of the final regression equation reflect the characteristics of the population? Therefore, the following significance tests are required.

在统计分析中，我们所用的资料信息大多来自样本，那么最终回归方程的结果能否反映总体的特征呢？因此，需要进行以下几个显著性检验。

2.1　Tests of the Overall Equation and R(回归方程和 R 的检验)

Analysis of variance was used to test whether the entire regression equation was statistically significant, as follows:

采用方差分析的方法来检验整个回归方程是否有统计学意义。

In the example of Table 16.2.1, the results of variance analysis (Table 16.2.2) obtained by SPSS show that $F = 148.4$, $P < 0.001$, so reject H_0 and accept H_1, it can be considered that b_1 and b_2 are not all 0, and the entire regression equation was statistically significant.

在表 16.2.1 的例子中，由 SPSS 得出的方差分析的结果(表 16.2.2)可知，$F = 148.4$，$P < 0.001$，因此拒绝 H_0，接受 H_1，可以认为 b_1 和 b_2 不全为 0，整个回归方程有统计学意义。

Table 16.2.2

Results of ANOVA

(方差分析结果)

Model 模型	Sum of square 平方和	df 自由度	Mean square 均方	F	P
Regression 回归	517.561	2	258.780	148.427	0.000[b]
Residual 残差	29.639	17	1.743		
Total 总计	547.200	19			

Notes(注): a. Dependent variable: the son's height(因变量：儿子身高); b. Predictors: the constant, the mother's height, the father's height. (预测变量：常量，母亲身高，父亲身高)

【Example 1】Multiple regression: Yiqiu Shi et al. (2020) used multiple regression to analyze the influencing factors of the nurse's psychological resilience during the prevalence of COVID-19. The results showed that education level, self-reported health status, knowledge of prevention and control of COVID-19 infection, mood when told to go to the frontline, time spent working at the frontline of the epidemic so far, and daily time spent on information about COVID-19 through the Internet or other ways were the main predictors of psychological resilience among nurses, with all predictors explaining 41.7% of the total variance in psychological resilience ($R^2=0.417$, $P<0.001$).

【例1】多元回归：史逸秋等(2020)使用多元回归分析了新冠疫情期间护理人员心理弹性的影响因素，结果显示文化程度、自评健康状况、新型冠状病毒感染防控知识掌握程度、被告知赴一线时心情、到目前为止在疫情一线工作时间、每天通过网络或者其他途径了解新型冠状病毒的信息花费时间等是护理人员心理弹性的主要预测因素，所有的预测因子解释了心理弹性总变异的41.7%($R^2=0.417$，$P<0.001$)。

2.2　Tests of the Regression Coefficients(回归系数的检验)

Due to sampling error, when the population partial regression coefficient is 0, the sample partial regression coefficient is not necessarily 0, so it is necessary to perform hypothesis testing on the partial regression coefficient. Generally, t-test is used to infer whether the population partial regression coefficient is 0. If the population partial regression coefficient is 0, which means that the corresponding independent variables have no effect on the dependent variable, the specific methods are as follows：

由于抽样误差，当总体偏回归系数为0时，样本偏回归系数也不一定为0，因此需要对偏回归系数进行假设检验。一般采用t检验推断总体偏回归系数是否为0，若总体偏回归系数为0，则表明相对应的自变量对因变量没有影响，具体方法如下：

For the data in Table 16.2.1, SPSS obtained the result of regression coefficient b_2(Table 16.2.3), $t=2.408$, $P=0.028<0.05$, so according to the test level of $\alpha=0.05$, H_0 is rejected, and it can be considered that there is a linear relationship between the father's height and son's height.

对于表16.2.1中的数据，SPSS得出回归系数 b_2 的结果(见表16.2.3)，$t=2.408$，$P=0.028<0.05$，因此按 $\alpha=0.05$ 的检验水准，拒绝 H_0，可以认为父亲的身高与儿子的身高存在线性关系。

Table 16. 2. 3   **Regression coefficient(回归系数)**

Model(模型)	b (非标准化系数)	S_b (标准误差)	B (标准系数)	t	P
Constant(常量)	−63. 495	14. 357		−4. 423	0. 000
Father's height(父亲身高)	0. 381	0. 158	0. 306	2. 408	0. 028
Mother's height(母亲身高)	1. 072	0. 198	0. 689	5. 426	0. 000

Notes(注): Dependent variable: the son's height(因变量: 儿子身高)

3. Strategies for Handling Predictors in Multiple Regression (在多元回归中处理预测变量的方法)

Multiple regression analysis methods can be divided into simultaneous multiple regression, hierarchical multiple regression and stepwise multiple regression according to the different input regression model methods of predictors.

多元回归分析方法按预测变量输入回归模型方法的不同可分为同步多元回归、分层多元回归和逐步多元回归。

3. 1 Simultaneous Multiple Regression(同步多元回归)

Simultaneous multiple regression is the most basic method in multiple regression analysis, which is a statistical method that inputs all the predictors into the regression equation and then performs regression analysis. This method is suitable for regression analysis in which all predictors have equal importance, and there is no one independent variable that has priority over any other independent variable to affect the dependent variable.

同步多元回归是多元回归分析中最基本的一种方法，就是将所有的预测变量都输入回归方程中再进行回归分析的一种统计方法。这种方法适用于所有预测变量都具有同等的重要性，不存在某一个自变量优先于其他任何自变量去影响因变量的回归分析中。

3. 2 Hierarchical Multiple Regression(分层多元回归)

Different from simultaneous multiple regression, hierarchical multiple regression divides all predictors into several steps in order of priority and then inputs them into the regression equation step by step based on the theory. Hierarchical multiple regression can not only solve the problem of sequential causality in predictors but also control related confounding variables.

与同步多元回归不同的是，分层多元回归是基于理论将所有的预测变量按优先顺序分为几个步骤再逐步输入回归方程。分层多元回归不仅可以解决预测变量中先后因果关系的问题，还可以控制相关的混杂变量。

【**Example 2**】Hierarchical multiple regression：Ban et al.（2021）explored the effect of fear progression on the quality of life of breast cancer patients and the mediating role of social support. Hierarchical multiple regression was used to divide the independent variables into four steps into the regression model. The first step was to input age and potential control variables，the second step to input fear progression，the third step to input social support，and the fourth step to input simultaneously fear progression and social support.

【**例 2**】分层多元回归：Ban 等（2021）研究了恐惧进展对乳腺癌患者生活质量的影响以及社会支持的中介作用。采用分层多元回归，将自变量分为四步输入回归模型，第一步输入年龄和潜在的控制变量，第二步输入恐惧进展，第三步输入社会支持，第四步将恐惧进展和社会支持同时输入。

3.3 Stepwise Multiple Regression（逐步多元回归）

Stepwise multiple regression is a method of constructing the optimal regression equation by screening the optimal variables one by one in multiple regression. The most commonly used method is the forward method，and the specific method is as follows：firstly，select the optimal predictor of the dependent variable，which is also the independent variable with the highest correlation with the dependent variable，and enter it into the regression equation as the first step of regression analysis；the second step selects the variable with the largest contribution to the dependent variable to enter the equation on the basis of the independent variables included in the first step；repeat the second step until all the independent variables with statistically significant contribution increments to the dependent variable are included in the model.

逐步多元回归是多元回归中通过逐个筛选最优变量，建立最优回归方程的一种方法。最常用的方法是前进法，具体方法如下：首先选择因变量的最佳预测因子，即与因变量相关性最高的自变量，作为回归分析的第一步输入回归方程中；第二步在第一步纳入的自变量的基础上选择对因变量贡献增量最大的变量进入方程；重复第二步，直至对因变量贡献增量有统计学差异的自变量全部纳入模型为止。

【**Example 3**】 Stepwise multiple regression: Hsu et al. (2021) analyzed the predictors of sleep quality through stepwise multiple regression when exploring the association between sleep quality and heart rate variability in female nurses. The variable most correlated with sleep quality (Total power of heart rate variability, TP) was entered first; heart rate was entered second. The results showed that TP and heart rate explained 23.1% of the variance in sleep quality.

【例3】 逐步多元回归：Hsu 等(2021)在探讨女护士睡眠质量与心率变异性之间的关联时，通过逐步多元回归分析睡眠质量的预测因素。首先输入与睡眠质量相关性最强的变量(心率变异的总功率，TP)；其次输入心率。结果显示，TP 和心率解释了睡眠质量方差的 23.1%。

4. Relative Contribution of Predictors(预测变量的相对贡献)

In practical research, we may not only want to predict a phenomenon but also understand the relative contribution of the predictors to the prediction of the dependent variable. In the case of Table 16.2.1, if we want to know which of X_1(the father's height) and X_2(the mother's height) has more impact on the son's height (Y), we can directly compare the partial regression coefficients b_1 and b_2 to get that the mother's height has more impact on the son's height. If the exercise time is added to the regression equation as the independent variable X_3, then the contribution of father's height and exercise time to son's height is compared. At this time, we cannot directly compare the partial regression coefficients b_k, because the independent variables X_1 and X_3 have their own measurement units and different degrees of variation. The unit of X_1 is centimeters (cm), and the unit of X_3 is hours (h).

在实际研究中，我们可能不仅仅想要预测某种现象，更想了解预测因子对因变量预测的相对贡献。在表 16.2.1 的案例中，如果我们想要知道 X_1(父亲身高)和 X_2(母亲身高)中谁对儿子身高(Y)的影响更大，我们可以直接比较偏回归系数 b_1 和 b_2 的大小，得出母亲的身高对儿子身高的影响更大。若将锻炼时间作为自变量 X_3 加入回归方程中，比较父亲身高和锻炼时间对儿子身高的贡献大小。此时我们不能直接比较偏回归系数 b_k，因为自变量 X_1 和 X_3 都具有各自的计量单位及不同的变异程度，X_1 的单位是厘米(cm)，而 X_3 的单位是小时(h)。

If you want to compare the contribution of X_1 and X_3 to the dependent variable Y, you must standardize the original observation data of the independent variable, as follows:

如果要比较 X_1 和 X_3 对因变量 Y 的贡献大小，必须对自变量的原始观测数据进行标准化，方法如下：

$$X'_k = \frac{X_k - \overline{X}_k}{SD_k}$$

Then use the standardized data for regression analysis, and the obtained partial regression coefficient b'_k is called the standard partial regression coefficient, b'_k has no unit of measurement, and can be compared to reflect the contribution of the independent variable to the dependent variable. The original data can be standardized directly in SPSS software to obtain standard partial regression coefficients, such as 0. 306 and 0. 689 in Table 16. 2. 3, which is simpler than the above formula method.

再用标准化的数据进行回归分析，得到的偏回归系数 b'_k 称为标准偏回归系数，b'_k 没有度量单位，可以进行比较来反映自变量对反映变量的贡献大小。在 SPSS 软件中可以直接对原始数据进行标准化，得到标准偏回归系数，如表 16. 2. 3 中的 0. 306 和 0. 689，相比上述公式法更为简单。

5. Regression Results(回归结果)

The results of multiple regression are generally presented in the form of a three-line table. There is no uniform standard for the table format, and there will be slight differences according to the type of regression. The parameters that are often reported are β, R^2 and P value. Below, we illustrate using the regression analysis results of a cross-sectional study on predictors of depression in Spanish children (Garaigordobil et al., 2017). The main purpose of this study was to examine the association of self-reported and adaptation (social skills, self-concept, self-esteem, resilience, personal adaptation) in children with depression and clinical variables (clinical impairment, school maladaptation, emotional symptoms, internalizing/externalizing problems, problem behaviors, childhood stress), and identify predictors of childhood depression. Table 16. 2. 4 shows the results of multiple regression analysis of overall dimension variables predicting childhood depression.

多元回归的结果一般以三线表的形式呈现，表格格式没有统一的标准，根据回归类型的不同会稍有差异，常报告的参数有 β，R^2 和 P 值。下面我们使用一项关于西班牙儿童抑郁预测因素的横断面研究(Garaigordobil 等，2017)的回归分析结果为例进行阐述。这个研究的主要目的是研究儿童抑郁自评与适应(社会技能、自我概念、自尊、韧性、个人适应)

和临床变量(临床障碍、学校适应不良、情绪症状、内化/外化问题、问题行为、童年压力)之间的关系，并确定儿童抑郁的预测因素。表16.2.4为整体维度变量预测儿童抑郁的多元回归分析结果。

Table 16.2.4 **Multiple regression analysis for global dimensions predictive of childhood depression.**

（全球维度预测儿童抑郁的多元回归分析）

Items	R	R^2	B	SE(B)	Constant（常量）	β	t
BASC. Clinical Maladjustment（临床适应不良）	0.566	0.321	0.410	0.049	36.83	0.328	7.19***
CAG. Global self-concept（整体的自我概念）	0.682	0.466	−0.412	0.076	170.65	−0.263	−5.42***
IECI. Childhood stress（儿童压力）	0.707	0.499	2.418	0.463	171.30	0.243	5.27***
SSIS. Social skills（社会技能）	0.715	0.512	−0.297	0.098	178.24	−0.142	−3.03**

Notes(注)：BASC-S2(Behavior Assessment System for Children and Adolescents 儿童和青少年行为评估系统)；CAG(Self-concept Questionnaire 自我概念问卷)；IECI(Inventory of Daily Stress in Children 儿童日常压力清单)；SSIS(Social Skills Improvement System 社会技能提升系统)；"**"表示 $P<0.01$；"***"表示 $P<0.001$.

The first column of Table 16.2.4 shows the predictors for the four overall dimensions, and each subsequent column shows the multiple correlation coefficient (R), the coefficient of determination (R^2), the partial regression coefficient (B), the standard deviation of partial regression coefficient (SE), constant, standard partial regression coefficient (β), and t-value results. The size of the P value can be judged by the * in the last column, "**" represents $P<0.01$, and "***" represents $P<0.001$. The results indicated that high clinical maladjustment, low overall self-concept, higher levels of stress, and lower social skills were predictors of depression in children, and these four variables together explained 51.2% of the variation in depression in children.

表16.2.4的第一列显示了四个整体维度的预测变量，接下来的每一列分别显示了复相关系数(R)、决定系数(R^2)、偏回归系数(B)、偏回归系数的标准差(SE)、常量、标准

偏回归系数(β)，以及 t 值的结果。p 值的大小可以通过最后一列的"*"来判断，"**"代表 $p<0.01$，"***"代表 $p<0.001$。结果表明高度的临床适应不良，整体的自我概念低，较高水平的压力以及较少的社交技能是儿童抑郁的预测因素，这 4 个变量共同解释了儿童抑郁变异的 51.2%。

Section Ⅲ Analysis of Covariance
第三节 协方差分析

Analysis of covariance can be used to compare the difference of the overall mean of two or more groups, which is similar to ANOVA, but its greatest characteristics is that it can use the idea of regression analysis to control confounding variables.

协方差分析可以用来比较两组或两组以上的总体均数的差异，这点类似方差分析，但其最大的特点是可以使用回归分析的思想来控制混杂变量。

1. Uses of Analysis of Covariance(协方差分析的应用)

In practical research, whether using one-way ANOVA or multi-variate ANOVA, there are inevitably some random variables that are difficult to control, and these variables will significantly affect our research results. So how to get the correct research results under the premise of controlling these variables?

在实际研究中，无论是采用单因素方差分析还是多因素方差分析，都难免存在一些人为难以控制的随机变量，而这些变量又会显著影响我们的研究结果。那么如何在控制这些变量的前提下，得出正确的研究结果呢?

For confounding variables that cannot be controlled by randomization in the experiment, we can control it through post hoc statistical analysis, and the analysis of covariance can achieve this purpose. For example, the Analysis of Covariance was performed on the above cases, taking the fear of childbirth before the intervention as a covariate, and adjusting the statistical model to make the effect of the fear of childbirth before the intervention on the three groups of women equal, and then analyze the effect of different intervention methods on the fear of childbirth to obtain more accurate research results.

对于在实验中无法通过随机化控制的混杂变量，我们可以事后通过统计分析进行控制，协方差分析就可以达到这个目的。如对上述的案例进行协方差分析，将干预前的分娩恐惧作为协变量，通过校正统计模型使干预前的分娩恐惧对三组产妇的影响相等，再分析不同干预方法对产妇分娩恐惧的影响，从而得到更准确的研究结果。

2. Selection of Covariates（协变量的选择）

The choice of covariates is particularly important when performing Analysis of Covariance, which is related to the accuracy of the research results. A good covariate must not only be related to the dependent variable, but must also have a certain degree of effect on the dependent variable. For most studies, demographic characteristics such as age and sex are often the best choices for covariates. In addition, the literature is also one of the sources of information for selecting appropriate covariates. In general, for experimental studies with pre-test and post-test design, the pre-test data are usually selected as covariates. However, for such studies, we can also choose ANOVA with repeated design instead of ANOVA.

在进行协方差分析时，协变量的选择尤为重要，这关系到研究结果的准确性。一个好的协变量不仅要与因变量相关，而且必须能对因变量产生一定程度的影响。对于大多数研究而言，年龄、性别这种人口学特征往往是协变量的最佳选择。除此之外，文献也是选择合适的协变量的信息来源之一。一般对于前-后测设计的实验性研究，通常选择前测数据作为协变量，不过对于这类研究，我们也可以选择重复设计的方差分析替代协方差分析。

3. Adjusted Means（校正均数）

After the Analysis of Covariance, the predicted mean of each group of dependent variables will be obtained. This mean is different from the original mean of the dependent variable, which is the mean of each group of dependent variables obtained after adjusting the covariates, which we call the adjusted mean. By comparing the adjusted means, we can directly observe the differences between groups.

在进行协方差分析之后，会得到各组因变量的预示平均值，这个平均值与因变量原始平均值不同，是在调整协变量后得到的各组因变量均值，我们称之为校正均数。通过比较校正均数，我们可以直接观察到各组的差异。

【**Example 4**】Analysis of Covariance：To explore the intervention effect of physical activity music therapy（MTPA）on the frail elderly in the community, Sun et al.（2021）

divided the elderly over 65 years old into the MTPA group and the control group for intervention. Differences in frailty scores between the two groups were compared using Analysis of Covariance with gender as a covariate.

【例4】协方差分析：Sun 等（2021）为探讨体力活动音乐疗法（MTPA）对社区虚弱老年人的干预效果，将65岁以上的老人分为 MTPA 组和对照组进行干预。将性别作为协变量，使用协方差分析比较两组虚弱评分的差异。

Section Ⅳ　Logistic Regression
第四节　Logistic 回归

Logistic regression is a widely used analysis method in multivariate statistics, which analyzes the relationship between multiple independent variables and a dependent variable (categorical variable) to obtain the predictive model. Logistic regression can be divided into conditional logistic regression (paired design) and unconditional logistic regression (group design) according to different research designs; according to the classification level of dependent variables, it can be divided into binary logistic regression and multi-category logistic regression. When we conduct data analysis, we can choose the corresponding logistic regression model according to these two classification methods.

Logistic 回归是多元统计中应用较为广泛的分析方法，通过分析多个自变量和一个因变量(分类变量)的关系得出预测模型。Logistic 回归依据研究设计的不同，可分为条件 Logistic 回归(配对设计)和非条件 Logistic 回归(成组设计)；依据因变量的分类水平，可分为二分类 Logistic 回归和多分类 Logistic 回归。我们在进行数据分析时，可以根据这两种分类方法选择相应的 Logistic 回归模型。

1. Basic Concepts for Logistic Regression Logistic(回归的基本概念)

Logistic regression uses the maximum likelihood method to estimate the regression coefficient. By establishing the likelihood function, the maximum probability value of obtaining the existing sample in one sampling is obtained.

$$\text{logit}(P) = \ln(P/1-P) = a + b_1 X_1 + b_2 X_2 + \cdots + b_k X_k$$

According to the above equation, the relationship between the independent variable and the dependent variable can be described, and the probability of a positive result under specific conditions can be calculated. It should be noted that the meaning of the logistic regression coefficient b is different from that introduced in the multiple regression. It can be understood as the change of the logit value of the relevant dependent variable when the independent variable changes each unit (on the condition that other independent variables remain unchanged).

Logistic 回归使用最大似然法对回归系数进行估计，通过建立似然函数，求解在一次抽样中获得现有样本概率最大的值。

$$\text{logit}(P) = \ln(P/1-P) = a + b_1X_1 + b_2X_2 + \cdots + b_kX_k$$

根据上述公式可描述自变量和因变量的关系，并且可以计算出特定条件下阳性结果发生的概率。需要注意的是，Logistic 回归系数 b 的意义与多元回归中介绍的不同，可以理解为自变量每变化一个单位相关因变量对数的变化值（其他自变量不变的条件下）。

2. The Odds Ratio（OR 值）

In Logistic regression, another most important indicator is the odds ratio (OR), which can be used to evaluate the effect size of exposure factors. we can according to the following equation, and finally obtained the OR value：

$$\ln(\text{OR}) = \ln(P/1-P) = a + b_1X_1 + b_2X_2 + \cdots + b_kX_k$$

Compared with the regression coefficient b, the OR value is more meaningful in explaining the influence of independent variables on the outcome, and it can explain the degree of increased risk of the outcome, so logistic regression is more widely used in the medical field.

Logistic 回归中，还有一个最重要的指标是优势比（OR），用于评价暴露因素的影响程度。我们可以通过下列等式，最终求出 OR 值。

$$\ln(\text{OR}) = \ln(P/1-P) = a + b_1X_1 + b_2X_2 + \cdots + b_kX_k$$

相比回归系数 b，OR 值在解释自变量对结局的影响更有意义，它能够说明结局风险增加的程度，因此 Logistic 回归在医学领域应用更为广泛。

3. Variables in Logistic Regression Logistic（回归中的变量）

For binary variables, positive events are generally coded as 1 and negative events as 0; if it is a multi-category variable, it needs to be coded as a series of dummy variables, with one group as the reference to analyze and compare. Generally, the variable with strong predictive ability is selected as the predictor variable. When the predictor variable is a continuous variable, the interpretation of the OR value is slightly different. For example, one of the predictors of the incidence of hypertension in the male population is body mass index (BMI), and the OR value associated with BMI is 1.42, which indicates that after controlling for other factors, for every 1 kg/m^2 increase in BMI, the risk of hypertension in the male population increased by 42%. Like multiple regression, logistic regression can also use the methods of simultaneous, stratified, and stepwise to input predictor variable into the regression equation.

通常我们需要对因变量进行虚拟编码，对于二分类变量，一般将阳性事件编码为1，阴性事件编码为0；如果是多分类变量，则需要编码为一系列虚拟变量，以其中一组为参照进行分析比较。一般选择预测能力较强的变量作为预测变量。当预测变量是连续变量时，对OR值的解释会稍有差别。例如男性人群中高血压发病率的其中一个预测因素是体重指数(BMI)，与体重指数相关的OR值是1.42，这表明在控制其他因素的情况下，BMI每增加$1kg/m^2$，男性人群中高血压的风险就增加42%。与多元回归一样，Logistic回归中的预测变量输入回归方程也可以使用同步法、分层法和逐步法。

4. Significance Tests in Logistic Regression Logistic(回归中的显著性检验)

4.1 Significance Test of the Overall Model(整体模型的显著性检验)

There are two ways to judge the quality of the overall logistic regression model：(1) likelihood ratio test；(2) goodness of fit evaluation. The likelihood ratio test determines whether the overall model is statistically significant by testing the null hypothesis that all regression coefficients are equal to 0. If $P<0.05$, it indicates that the OR value of at least one variable is statistically significant among the variables included in the fitted model, which is that the total model makes sense. The goodness of fit evaluates the degree of conformity between the effect of model construction and the real situation. Common goodness of fit indicators include −2log likelihood (−2LL) and Hosmer-Lemesho test (H-L test). -2LL is an important indicator for model evaluation, and the smaller the value, the better the model fits. The H-L test can be used to evaluate whether the model makes full use of the existing data to maximize the fitting of the model. If the result is $P<0.05$, it indicates that the effect of model fitting is good, otherwise the fitting is poor.

判断Logistic回归整体模型的好坏有两种方式：(1)似然比检验；(2)拟合优度评价。

似然比检验通过检验所有回归系数都等于 0 的零假设来确定总模型是否有统计学意义，若
$P<0.05$，则表明拟合模型纳入的变量中，至少有一个变量的 OR 值有统计学意义，即总模
型有意义。拟合优度评价的是模型构建的效果与真实情况的符合程度，常用的拟合优度指
标包括-2 对似然值(-2 log likelihood，-2LL)和 Hosmer-Lemesho 检验(H-L 检验)。-2LL
是模型评价的重要指标，该值越小表示模型拟合得越好。H-L 检验可以用于评价模型是否
充分利用现有的数据最大化拟合了模型，若结果 $P<0.05$，则表明模型拟合效果较好，反
之表示拟合欠佳。

4.2 Significance Tests for Individual Predictors(单个预测因子的显著性检验)

The significance test of each predictor in the model can use Wald's chi-square test to
calculate the statistic, so as to identify whether each predictor has a significant effect on the
outcome variable. In addition, researchers sometimes assess the significance of predictors based
on the confidence interval of the OR value. If the 95% confidence interval for the OR value
contains 1, it indicates that the OR value for that predictor is not statistically significant at the
0.05 significant level.

模型中各个预测因子的显著性检验可以采用 Wald 卡方检验计算出统计量，从而判断
各个预测因子是否对结局变量有显著影响。另外，研究者有时也根据 OR 值的置信区间来
评估预测因子的显著性。如果 OR 值 95%的置信区间内包含 1，则表明该预测因子的 OR
值在 0.05 的检验水准上没有统计学意义。

【**Example 5**】 Logistic regression: Ali et al. (2021) studied overweight and obesity in
525 women of reproductive age with iron deficiency anemia, and the multivariate logistic
regression model was used to identify the risk factors of overweight and obesity. The results
showed that women who were married (OR = 4.4), aged 30-49 years (OR = 7.6),
unemployed (OR = 1.5) and in wealthier households (OR = 3.9) had a higher risk of
overweight and obesity.

【例5】 Logistic 回归：Ali 等(2021)对 525 名缺铁性贫血的育龄女性的超重和肥胖
进行了研究，多元 Logistic 回归模型用于确定超重和肥胖的危险因素。结果显示已婚
(OR=4.4)、年龄为 30~49 岁(OR=7.6)、失业(OR=1.5)和家庭较富裕的女性(OR
=3.9) 超重和肥胖的风险更高。

Section V　Survival and Event History Analysis
第五节　生存及事件史分析

In medical follow-up studies, we usually analyze the outcome variables not only to see if the outcome occurs but also consider the length of time it has taken for the outcome to occur. For such studies of time-related outcome variables, we often use survival analysis for statistical analysis. For the univariate analysis of survival time, we can use the log-rank test for analysis; and for the multivariate analysis of survival data, the multiple regression and logistic regression introduced above are no longer applicable, and the Cox hazard proportional model (Cox regression) can be used to obtain the influencing factors of survival situation.

在医学随访研究中，通常我们对结局变量进行分析时，不仅要看是否出现了某种结局，还要考虑结局出现所经历的时间长短。关于这类与时间有关的结局变量的研究，我们常采用生存分析进行统计分析。对于生存时间的单因素分析，我们可以采用 log-rank 检验进行分析；而对于生存资料的多因素分析，前面介绍的多元回归和 logistic 回归已不再适用，可以采用 Cox 风险比例模型(Cox 回归)得出生存情况的影响因素。

【Example 6】Cox regression：Tomasdottir et al. (2021) followed up 13, 153 CHD patients to study the risk factors for atrial fibrillation in patients with coronary heart disease (CHD). The Cox regression models was used for analysis, after adjusting for clinical risk factors and biomarkers, the results showed that age, NT-proBNP and BMI were independent risk factors for developing atrial fibrillation.

【例 6】Cox 回归：Tomasdottir 等(2021)为研究冠心病(CHD)患者发生房颤的危险因素，对 13153 例 CHD 患者进行了随访。使用 Cox 回归模型进行分析，在调整临床风险因素和生物标记物之后，结果显示年龄、NT-proBNP 和身体质量指数是发生房颤的独立危险因素。

Section VI　Causal Modeling
第六节　因果模型

Nursing research often involves the study of the relationship between several variables, including correlation, mediation and causality. Causal modeling (also called as path analysis) provide a clearer approach to this research, using real data to test the hypothesis that there is a causal relationship between the studied variables.

护理研究常涉及几个变量间的关系研究，包括相关关系、中介关系和因果关系等。因果模型(也称路径分析)为这类研究提供了一种更为清晰的研究方法，通过真实数据来检验研究变量间存在因果关系的假设是否成立。

Figure 16. 6. 1 uses nurse turnover intention (V3) as the dependent variable, job-esteem (V1) as the independent variable, and job burnout (V2) as the mediator variable to establish a hypothetical model and verify the model effect. The overall fit of the model and the research data in the structural equation can be judged by the goodness-of-fit index. Commonly used fit indicators include the ratio of Chi-square value to degrees of freedom (χ^2/df), Approximate Root Mean Square Error (RMSEA)), Goodness of Fit Index (GFI), Comparative Fit Index (CFI), etc. A structural equation model is established for the hypothetical model in Figure 16. 6. 1, and the fitting indicators results obtained show that the overall model fits well. The standardized regression coefficients in the path diagram in Figure 16. 6. 2 ($b = -0.7/-0.26/0.51$, all $P<0.001$) shows that V1 has a direct negative predictive effect on V3, and can also have an indirect negative predictive effect on V3 through V2; V2 has a direct positive predictive effect on V3.

图 16. 6. 1 是以护士离职意愿(V3)为因变量，职业尊重感(V1)为自变量，职业倦怠(V2)为中介变量建立假设模型，并验证模型效应。结构方程中模型和研究数据的总体拟合程度可以通过拟合优度指标来判断，常用的拟合指标包括卡方值和自由度的比值(χ^2/df)、近似均方根误差(RMSEA)、拟合优度指数(GFI)、比较拟合指数(CFI)，等等。对图 16. 6. 1 的假设模型建立结构方程模型，得到的拟合指标结果表明总体模型拟合较好，图 16. 6. 2 路径图中的标准化回归系数($b=-0.7/-0.26/0.51$，且三者 $P<0.001$)显示，V1 对 V3 有直接的负性预测作用，也可以通过 V2 对 V3 有间接的负性预测作用；V2 对 V3 有直接的正性预测作用。

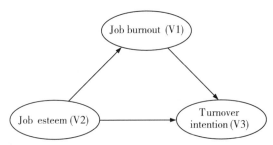

Figure 16. 6. 1　Hypothetical model of the relationship between nurses' job-esteem, job burnout and turnover intention
(护士职业尊重感、职业倦怠与离职意愿关系的假设模型)

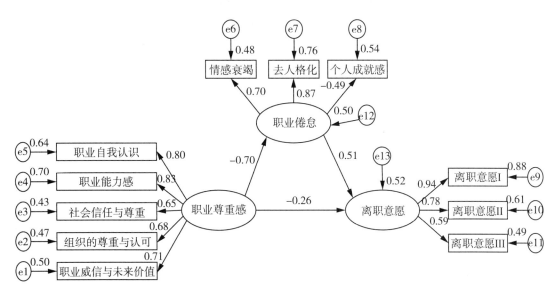

Figure 16.6.2　The path diagram of the relationship between nurses' job-esteem, job burnout and turnover intention（Shi Xiaopu et al., 2021）

护士职业尊重感、职业倦怠与离职意愿关系的路径图（史晓普等，2021）

Section Ⅶ　Critiquing Multivariate Statistics
第七节　评判多元统计分析

Multivariate statistical analysis is still widely used in the field of nursing research, and it can help researchers to conduct research more effectively. However, for most nursing researchers without statistical background, it is still difficult to choose the correct multivariate statistical analysis method and to evaluate the statistical analysis of other researchers. Therefore, at the end of this chapter, the applicable conditions of commonly used multivariate statistical methods are summarized, which can help researchers to choose the correct statistical methods to apply in nursing research, see Table 16.7.1 for details.

多元统计分析在护理研究领域应用还是比较广泛的，它能够有助于研究人员更有效地进行研究。而对于大多数无统计专业背景的护理研究者，选择正确的多元统计分析方法并对其他研究者的统计分析进行评判还是存在一定的难度。因此，本章最后对常用的多元统计方法的适用条件进行了总结，可有助于研究者选择正确的统计方法运用到护理科研中，具体见表16.7.1。

Table 16.7.1   **Selection of Multivariate Statistical Analysis Methods**

（多元统计分析方法的选择）

Statistical Methods（统计方法）	Measurement Level of Variables（变量的测量水平）			Number of Variables（变量个数）		
	IV	DV	CV	IV	DV	CV
Multiple Regression（多元回归）	Continuous, categorical（连续变量，分类变量）	Continuous（连续变量）	—	2+	1	—
ANCOVA（协方差分析）	Categorical（分类变量）	Continuous	Continuous, categorical	1+	1	1+
MANCOVA（多元协方差分析）	Categorical	Continuous	Continuous, categorical	1+	2+	1+
Logistic Regression（Logistic 回归）	Continuous, categorical	Categorical	—	2+	1	—
Cox Regression（Cox 回归）	Continuous, categorical	Binary variables, survival time（二分类变量，生存时间）	—	2+	2	—

Notes（注）：IV=Independent Variable（自变量）；DV=Dependent Variable（因变量）；CV=Covariate（协变量）；Categorical（分类变量）；Continues（连续性变量）

📖 Studies Cited in Chapter 16（第十六章参考文献）

[1]王华丽. 多元线性回归分析实例分析[J]. 科技资讯，2014，12(29)：22，24.

[2]史逸秋，戴晓婧，童为燕，李露寒，等. 新型冠状病毒肺炎疫情期间护理人员心理弹性及影响因素分析[J]. 中华护理杂志，2020，55(S1)：108-112.

[3]Ban, Y., Li, M., Yu, M., et al. The effect of fear of progression on quality of life among breast cancer patients: the mediating role of social support[J]. Health and Quality of Life Outcomes, 2021, 19(1): 1-9.

[4]Hsu, H. C., Lee, H. F., Lin, M. H. Exploring the association between sleep quality and

heart rate variability among female nurses[J]. International Journal of Environmental Research and Public Health, 2021, 18(11): 5551.

[5] Garaigordobil, M., Bernarás, E., Jaureguizar, J., et al. Childhood depression: relation to adaptive, clinical and predictor variables[J]. Frontiers in Psychology, 2017, 8: 821.

[6] Sun, F. C., Li, H. C., Wang, H. H. The effect of group music therapy with physical activities to prevent frailty in older people living in the community[J]. International Journal of Environmental Research and Public Health, 2021, 18(16): 8791.

[7] Ho, M. H., Yu, L. F., Lin, P. H., et al. Effects of a simulation-based education programme on delirium care for critical care nurses: A randomized controlled trial[J]. Journal of Advanced Nursing, 2021, 77(8): 3483-3493.

[8] Grégoire, C., Faymonville, M. E., Vanhaudenhuyse, A., et al. Randomized controlled trial of a group intervention combining self-hypnosis and self-care: secondary results on self-esteem, emotional distress and regulation, and mindfulness in post-treatment cancer patients [J]. Quality of Life Research, 2021, 30(2): 425-436.

[9] Ali, N. B., Dibley, M. J., Islam, S., et al. Overweight and obesity among urban women with iron deficiency anaemia in Bangladesh[J]. Maternal & Child Nutrition, 2021, 17(2): e13102.

[10] Tomasdottir, M., Claes Held, M. D., Hadziosmanovic, N., et al. Risk markers of incident atrial fibrillation in patients with coronary heart disease[J]. American Heart Journal, 2021, 233: 92-101.

[11] 史晓普, 李莹, 张丛丛. 护士职业尊重感、职业倦怠及离职意愿的相关性[J]. 护理研究, 2021, 35(15): 2654-2660.

PART 4：Designing and Conducting Qualitative Studies
to Generate Evidence for Nursing

第四部分　设计及开展质性研究，
为护理实践提供证据

Chapter 17: Qualitative Research Design and Approaches
第十七章 质性研究设计与方法

Simple numbers sometimes cannot very effectively answer the research questions, when we looking into an individual object at the micro level in detailed and dynamic description and analysis. At the moment, qualitative research needs to be chosen. Qualitative research is a very broad term that it is to explanatory, descriptive, and inductive in nature and to formulate the understanding of a phenomenon. This chapter now will mainly introduce the theoretical basis, characteristics and common design types of qualitative research.

当需要在微观层面对个别对象进行细致、动态的描述和分析时，简单的数字并不能有效回答研究问题。此时，可以选择质性研究。质性研究是一个广义的术语，本质上是解释、描述和归纳，来帮助我们构建出对现象的理解。因此，本章主要介绍质性研究的理论基础、特点和常见的设计类型。

Section Ⅰ The Design of Qualitative Studies
第一节 质性研究设计

1. Concept of Qualitative Study(质性研究的概念)

Qualitative research is a broad term uses a variety of data collection methods to conduct a holistic inquiry of a phenomenon and to help people formulate an understanding of the phenomenon, aiming to illuminate the underlying meaning and dimensionality of phenomena endowed by the research object.

质性研究是一个广义的术语，是在自然情境中使用各种数据收集方法，对某一现象进行整体探究，帮助人们形成对该现象的理解，旨在揭示研究对象赋予这些现象的深层含义和维度。

【Example 1】Sources of Items: Martsolf (2012) explored patterns of dating violence in 88 young adults who had experienced violent dating relationships as teenagers. Results showed four patterns of adolescent dating violence by analysis of interviews.

【例1】条目来源：Martsolf（2012）对 88 名在少年时代经历过约会暴力关系的青少年进行探讨，了解其约会暴力模式。通过分析访谈结果，得出青少年约会暴力有四种模式。

2. Characteristics of Qualitative Research Design(质性研究设计的特点)

Qualitative research is widely used in a variety of disciplines, such as anthropology, psychology, and sociology, and each has developed own methods for solving types of questions. In a general way, qualitative research design has characteristics as follows：

质性研究被广泛用于各种学科，如人类学、心理学和社会学，并且每个学科都发展了自己解决各类问题的方法。一般来说，质性研究设计具有以下特点：

High flexibility, holistic approach, multiple data collection strategies, ongoing analysis of the data, researchers are deeply involved and attention to the individual experience of the subject.

高灵活性、整体研究、多种数据收集策略、持续分析数据、研究人员高度参与和重视研究对象的个别经验。

Qualitative research can adjust to new information when data collection is conducted. During the research, the researchers are highly engaged, often combining the use of multiple data collection strategies designed to provide a holistic understanding of the content of the interviews. Meanwhile, analysis of the data is ongoing, which determines when data collection is completed.

质性研究在进行数据收集时可以根据新的信息进行调整。在研究过程中，研究人员高度参与，经常结合使用多种数据收集策略，旨在对访谈内容有一个整体的了解。同时，不断对数据进行分析，这决定何时完成数据收集。

3. Differences Between Qualitative Research and Quantitative Research (质性研究与量性研究的区别)

There are fundamental differences between qualitative research and quantitative research due to different philosophical views and methods of understanding things. Based on existing research, quantitative researchers establish hypotheses according to their own research purposes, design research schemes, obtain quantitative data through measurement indicators, and present research results in data analysis reports after a series of scientific verification. It advocates positivism, a more objective experience, and researchers are mostly not involved in the activities being studied

质性研究和量性研究由于不同的哲学观和认识事物的方法，两者存在根本的区别。量性研究者在现有研究的基础上，根据自己的研究目的建立假设，设计研究方案，通过测量指标获得量性数据，经过一系列科学验证后用数据分析报告呈现研究结果。它主张实证主义，更注重客观性体验，而研究人员多数不会参与在被研究的活动中。

4. Types of Qualitative Research(质性研究类型)

Qualitative research methods include ethnographic, phenomenological, grounded theory and other methods. These methodologies explore the substance and meaning of things similarly, but they focus on different problems and have different approaches to solve them.

质性研究方法包括民族志、现象学、扎根理论等方法。这些方法学都探索事物的实质和意义，然而他们聚焦的问题和解决问题的方法不相同。

Section Ⅱ　Ethnography
第二节　民族志研究

1. Features of Ethnographic Research(民族志研究的特点)

Generally speaking, ethnographers are required to learn the local language and look below the surface through everyday actions and rituals to identify the shared meaning and values expressed. Meanings and values may reveal power differences, gender issues, optimism, or views of diversity. It has characteristics as follows:

一般来说，民族志研究者需要学习当地的语言，通过日常的行动和仪式来观察表面之下的东西，以确定所表达的共同意义和价值。意义和价值观可能揭示出权力差异、性别问题、乐观主义或对多样性的看法。民族志的特征如下：

- Uniqueness, culture and integrity

具有特殊性、文化性、整体性

- The researcher is the tool of research

研究者是研究的工具

- Participatory observation

参与式观察

- The cycle of data collection and analysis

资料收集和分析的循环

Generally, research is terminated not because all research questions have been answered or the culture has been fully described, but because of time and resource constraints.

一般来说，研究的终止不是因为已经回答了所有的研究问题或者已经全面地描述了文化，而是受到时间和资源的限制而结束。

2. The Application of Ethnographic Research(民族志研究的适用范围)

Ethnographic research describes and interprets patterns of cultural groups of people, past and present, within a culture. Ethnography approaches are applicable to:

民族志研究描述和解释文化群体的模式，研究对象为在某一文化下的过去和现在的人，民族志学的研究方法适用于:

- Recording existing facts for research
- 记录现存事实用于研究
- Establishing and developing grounded theory
- 建立和发展扎根理论
- Understanding cultural phenomena and human behaviors
- 理解文化现象和人类行为

Ethnographic research methods can be used to describe certain social phenomena, behaviors, cultural events, etc. of an existing society or a specific cultural group in order to record the existing facts. In the face of complex social phenomena and cultural activities, ethnographic research is used to conduct in-depth analysis to understand the meaning of human behavior. In addition, grounded theory can be derived from the cultural analysis of some ethnographic studies. And grounded theory can be developed through ethnographic research.

民族志学的研究方法可以用于描述现存的某个社会或某个特定文化群体的某些社会现象、行为、文化事件等，以记录现存的事实。面对复杂的社会现象和文化活动时，通过民族志研究进行深入分析，去理解人类行为的含义。此外，扎根理论可以源于一些民族志研究的文化分析。通过民族志研究可以发展扎根理论。

3. Basic Process of Ethnographic Research(民族志研究的基本步骤)

3.1　Identifying the Research Questions(确定研究问题)

The research question of ethnographic research is determined through identifying the phenomenon.

民族志的研究问题通过对现象的识别来确定。

The research question can be a certain type of existing population or cultural issue that is not ethnographically recorded, or a theoretical or practical issue to be researched, or a study of a social phenomenon of unknown change in a transitional period. The researcher makes the final decision on the research question by combining personal abilities, interests and realities.

研究的问题可以是没有民族志记录的某类现存的人群或文化议题，或者有待研究的理论问题或实践问题，再者是对过渡时期的变化不明的社会现象的研究。研究者结合个人能力、兴趣爱好和现实情况等来最终决定研究问题。

3.2　Structuring the Study(构建研究)

By reviewing relevant literature, we can obtain the cultural background and relevant materials related to the research, have an overall grasp of the previous research, and understand the current gaps and limitations. When developing a systematic research plan, the ethnographer gathers information from general informants and from key informants. Also, field visits to the research site in advance can avoid and minimize the factors which may hinder the research.

通过回顾相关文献，获得与研究有关的文化背景和相关资料，对之前的研究有整体把握，了解当前的空白和局限。在制定系统的研究计划时，民族志学者从一般的线人和重要的线人那里收集信息。另外，考虑到实际工作中可能遇到的问题，可以提前实地考察研究现场。

3.3　Gathering and Analyzing Data(收集和分析资料)

Ethnographic data gathering involves immersion in the study setting and observation of participant, interviews of informants, and interpretation by the researcher of cultural patterns by interviewing methods, and analysis taking place in the natural setting.

民族志数据收集包括沉浸在研究设置、观察参与者、参与者访谈和研究者对文化模式的解读，通过访谈的方法收集，并在自然环境中进行分析。

3.4 Describing the Findings(描述结果)

Ethnographic studies will yield large quantities of data reflected many of evidence. Creating a cultural inventory, which provides an opportunity to collate and organize information. Then write the ethnography. Pay attention to reflect the three elements of ethnography writing in the report, namely description, analysis and interpretation. Researchers report an item-level analysis, then pattern & structure level of analysis, while providing examples from data.

民族志研究产生了大量的数据，反映了许多证据。列出文化清单，这提供了整理、组织资料的机会。然后撰写民族志，注意写作时要在报告中体现民族志写作的三要素，即描述、分析和阐释。研究人员报告项目级分析，然后是模式和结构级分析，同时提供来自数据的例子。

Section Ⅲ Phenomenological Approach
第三节 现象学研究

Phenomenology has several variants and methodological interpretations. Descriptive phenomenology and interpretive phenomenology are two main schools of thought.

现象学有几种变体和方法论的解释。描述现象学和解释现象学是两个主要的思想流派。

1. Descriptive Phenomenology(描述现象学)

Descriptive phenomenology, based on epistemology, is represented by Husserl. This philosophy is reflected in knowledge, which is to explore the source of all knowledge and construct a complete system of knowledge from it, and this source exists in "facts", that is, back to the thing itself. Descriptive phenomenology believes that the ultimate basis of knowledge is the most basic knowledge of experience, so the research focuses on phenomena (a certain experience that a person goes through), and considers that all indirect knowledge such as culture, background, history, direct knowledge of the external world and personal preconceptions related to the researcher affect the objectivity of the research. The research is conducted with a scientific attitude of "transcendence" and unbiased description.

描述性现象学，是基于认识论的基础之上而建立起来的，以胡塞尔为代表。这种哲学反映在知识上，就是要探寻一切知识的根源，并由此建构知识的完整体系，而这种根源就存在于"事实"之中，即回到事物本身。描述性现象学认为知识的终极基础是对经历的最基本的认知，因此研究重点在于现象(人所经历的某种经历)，认为一切与研究者有关的文化、背景、历史等间接知识、外部世界的直接知识和个人的成见都会影响研究的客观性。研究时，以"超然"的科学态度进行无偏见描述。

2. Interpretive Phenomenology(解释现象学)

Interpretive phenomenology takes ontology as its philosophical foundation and Heidegger as its main representative. This philosophy is no longer concerned with the origin of knowledge and its construction, but with the question of how the existence of the essence presents itself to people, emphasizing the existence in the world and the essence of objective reality, arguing that the relationship between the individual and the world is co-constructed and interdependent. Moreover, interpretive phenomenology is not purely descriptive; all prior experience and knowledge possessed by the researcher come into play in explaining the nature of an experience, and cannot be completely isolated from the study of its antecedents.

解释性现象学，以本体论为其哲学基础，以海德格尔为主要代表。这种哲学不再关心知识的根源及其建构的问题，而是关注于本质的存在是如何向人们展示其自身的问题，强调世界中的存在和客观实在的本质，认为个体与世界之间是共同建构的且相互依存的。另外，解释性现象学不是纯粹的描述，研究者先前所拥有的一切经验和知识在解释某种经历的本质时会发挥作用，无法与将其先念与研究完全隔离开来。

3. The Application of Phenomenological Research(现象学研究的适用范围)

Phenomenology is a method to understand people's everyday life experiences. As the philosophical view of phenomenology continues to develop, the philosophical approach it implies is widely applied in various fields, such as psychology, nursing, sociology, and education. In the field of nursing, the phenomenological research approach is applied to the subjective perception or lived experience of the subject.

现象学是一种理解人们日常生活经验的方法。随着现象学哲学观的不断发展，其蕴含的哲学方法也被广泛地应用于各个领域，如心理学、护理学、社会学、教育学等。在护理领域中，现象学研究方法适用于对象的主观认识或生活体验。

4. Basic Process of Phenomenological Research(现象学研究的基本步骤)

4.1 Identifying the Research Questions(确定研究问题)

The phenomenological approach is a process of learning and constructing the meaning of human experience through in-depth dialogue.

现象学方法是一个通过与体验者的深入对话来学习和建构人类体验意义的过程。

4.2 Structuring the Study(构建研究)

Phenomenological researchers need to ask the participant about some past or present experience. In general, the researchers set aside their personal biases about the phenomenon to clarify how personal experience and beliefs may color what is reported. Then researchers do not lead participants to discusses the issues that researchers deem important.

现象学研究者需要向参与者询问一些过去或现在的经验。研究者把他们对现象的个人偏见放在一边，以澄清个人经验和信仰如何影响报告的内容。然后，研究人员不引导参与者去探讨研究者认为重要的问题。

4.3 Gathering and Analyzing Data(收集和分析资料)

When using phenomenological methods, written or oral data can be collected. The researcher can ask questions in writing and ask for written responses, or schedule a time to interview participants and record the interaction. Descriptive phenomenological studies often involve the four steps, named bracketing, intuiting, analyzing, and describing. But bracketing does not necessarily occur in an interpretive phenomenological study. Many techniques are available for data analysis when using the phenomenological method, such as Colaizzi's method, Giorgi method and Van Manen data analysis method.

在使用现象学方法时，可以收集书面或口头数据。研究者可以以书面形式提出问题，并要求书面答复，或者安排时间采访参与者，并记录互动过程。描述性的现象学研究通常包括以下四个步骤，即分隔、直觉、分析和描述。但是在解释性现象学研究中，分隔不一

定会出现。在使用现象学方法时，有许多方法可以用于数据分析，如 Colaizzi 法、Giorgi
法和 Van Manen 数据分析方法。

4.4 Describing the Findings(描述结果)

In reports of phenomenological research, detailed descriptive language is used to convey the
complex implications of life experience provides evidence for this qualitative approach. These
reports should help readers think from a different perspective and enrich their understanding of
experience.

在现象学研究的报告中，详细的描述性语言用来表达生活经验的复杂含义，为这种定
性的方法提供了证据。现象学报告帮助读者从不同角度思考事物，丰富他们对经历的理
解。

Section Ⅳ　Grounded Theory
第四节　扎根理论研究

1. Features of Grounded Theory(扎根理论的特点)

Grounded theory is a bottom-up approach to build theory and is an inductive method
involving a systematic set of procedures. The characteristics of rooted theory are as follows:

扎根理论是一种自下而上建立理论的方法，也是涉及一套系统的程序的归纳方法。扎
根理论的特征如下：

- Supported by scenario information
- 有情景资料的支持
- Constant comparative method
- 持续性比较法
- Theoretical sensitivity
- 理论敏感性
- Theoretical sampling
- 理论抽样
- Abstracting new theories from practice
- 从实践中抽象出新的理论
- Discovering major advances in social contexts

- 发现社会情境中的主要进展
- Data collection, data analysis, and sampling of participants occur simultaneously
- 数据收集、数据分析和参与者取样同时进行

2. The Application of Grounded Theory Research(扎根理论研究的适用范围)

Grounded theory attempts to explain the behavior of the substantive domain from the perspective of the object, using participant observation to obtain data, and the resulting theory is characterized by the correlative effect of the explanation, and compactness and integration. The research approach of grounded theory is applicable to:

扎根理论试图从对象的角度解释实质性领域的行为，采用参与性观察法来获得数据资料，所形成的理论具备解释事物的关联作用的特征，和紧凑与整合的特性。扎根理论的研究方法适用于：

- Exploring process-based questions
- 探索过程类问题
- Studying and understanding human behavior
- 研究和理解人类行为
- Social relevance of phenomena
- 现象的社会关联性

Overall, rooted theory research methodology is generally used to study individual processes, interpersonal relationships, and reciprocal interactions between individuals and larger social processes.

总体来说，扎根理论研究方法论一般用于研究个人过程、人际间关系及个人与更大的社会过程之间的互惠作用。

3. Basic Process of Grounded Theory Research(扎根理论研究的基本步骤)

3.1　Identifying the Research Questions(确定研究问题)

When researchers focus on social processes from the perspective of human interaction or behavior patterns, grounded theory approaches are often used. Its main purpose is to give an in-depth explanation of the phenomena in reality and to produce theories.

当研究者关注于人类互动或行为模式的角度的社会过程，通常使用扎根理论方法。其主要目的是对现实中的现象进行深入解释，并产生理论。

3.2　Structuring the Study(构建研究)

The research questions of grounded theory research are those to be focused on by the participants, not by the researcher himself/herself. In the early stages of research, there is usually a generalized exploratory research question or point of interest due to the uncertainty of the research question. The researcher should avoid preconceptions, enter the situation with interest, and conduct interviews with an open mind to focus on the concerns of the research subject. Research questions are refined and clarified as the phenomenon is further explored and collided with, not predetermined before the research.

扎根理论研究的问题是参与者所要关注的问题，而非研究者本人所关注的问题。在研究初期，由于研究问题的不确定性，通常会有一个笼统的探索性的研究问题或兴趣点。研究者应避免预设，带着兴趣进入情景，以开放的态度进行访谈以聚焦研究对象所关注的问题。研究问题是在对现象的探索与碰撞中不断细化和明确，不是在研究之前就事先确定的。

3.3　Gathering and Analyzing Data(收集和分析资料)

Grounded theory applies participant observation, interview, historical and archival data to collect data. The data are collected and analyzed simultaneously, and the comparison and contrast methods are continuously conducted to discover the similarities and differences between things and to combine the fragmented data into a functional overall framework.

扎根理论采用参与性观察法、会谈法、历史资料和档案资料法等去收集数。资料的收集和分析同时进行，并持续不断进行对照与比较法，去发现事物之间的异同之处，将片段资料组合成有功能的整体框架。

Coding forms the initiating link of grounded theory when systematization is carried out. Coding is the process of gradually refining concepts and will refer to summarizing and summarizing real information based on multiple classification criteria. When all coding is present and no new concepts are generated, a state of categorical saturation is said to have been reached from which conceptual frameworks and theories can be inferred. This induction, deduction, and hypothesis testing is repeated in a continuous cycle throughout the study.

在进行系统整理时，编码形成扎根理论的始发环节。编码是逐渐提炼概念的过程，会指根据多个分类标准对真实资料进行归纳与总结。当所有编码都出现，没有新概念产生时，就已经达到分类饱和状态，可以从中推论概念框架和理论。这种归纳、演绎、假设检验贯穿于研究中，不断循环往复。

3.4 Describing the Findings(描述结果)

The report of the grounded theory study is detailed and specific, reflecting the exact steps of the study. In addition, descriptive language and research flowcharts can be presented to document the researcher's process from raw data to new theory.

扎根理论研究的报告详尽而具体，体现出研究中确切的步骤。另外，可以呈现出描述性的语言和研究流程图来记录研究者从原始数据到新理论的过程。

Section V   Other Types of Qualitative Research
第五节   其他类型的质性研究

1. Case Studies(个案研究)

Case studies are naturalistic, descriptive qualitative studies, which is an in-depth study of an entity or a series of entities that is analyzed in a holistic manner. These entities could be an individual, family, institution, community, or other social unit. The case is the center of the study, and can be a single case or multiple cases. The research needs to take into account of the time, place, scope, context, and relevant materials of the case. The focus of the study is on the case itself or on a particular issue that is illustrated by the case. Case studies allow the researcher to dig deeper into the case and are scientific in nature, but subjective bias in the results needs to be avoided as much as possible.

个案研究是自然主义的、描述性的质性研究，是对一个或一系列实体做全貌式的分析的深入研究。这些实体可以是个人、家庭、机构、社区或其他社会单位。个案是研究的中心，可以是单一个案或多重个案。研究需要结合个案的时间、地点、范围、背景，以及相关的材料等。研究关注重点是个案本身或者通过个案所要说明的某个问题。个案研究使研究者对个案有更深层次的挖掘，具有科学性，但需要尽量避免结果的主观偏差。

2. Narrative Analyses(叙事分析)

Narrative analyses are a study of narrative texts based on structuralist methodology, using linguistic analysis models to discover the relationship between surface phenomena and deep structure of texts, revealing the value systems and deep knots behind them. Narrative analyses focus on the story as an object of investigation in order to examine how individuals interpret the events of their lives. The researcher restores the complete story and constructs meaning from the analysis of the patient's corpus. The story serves as an interpretive process that presents a panoramic view of the patient's events and state of being.

叙事分析是以结构主义方法论为基础，运用语言学分析模式对叙事文本开展研究，发现文本表层现象与深层结构之间的关系，揭示背后的价值系统和深层结。叙事分析的重点是将故事作为调查的对象，以研究个人如何对其生活事件做出解释。研究者从对患者的语料分析中还原完整的故事，并建构意义。故事作为一个诠释的过程，全景式展现患者的事件与状态。

Section VI Critiquing Qualitative Designs
第六节　评判质性研究设计

The use of terminology should be avoided as much as possible. There are many ways to evaluate qualitative research, such as the Criteria for Assessment of Literature Quality (CASP) developed by the Centre for Evidence-Based Medicine, University of Oxford, UK, and the Uniform Reporting Standards for Qualitative Research (COREQ) developed by Allison Tong et al. at the School of Public Health, University of Sydney, Australia. Focusing on the personal characteristics of the researcher, understanding whether the research process is normative, the level of contact with participants, whether the sampling method meets the purpose of the study, whether the sample size is saturated, whether the data collection and coding process is reasonable, etc., and it provides a comprehensive and systematic assessment of the design of qualitative studies.

应该尽量避免使用术语。评价质性研究的方法有许多，例如英国牛津大学循证医学中心制定的文献质量评价项目(CASP)、澳大利亚悉尼大学公共卫生学院 Allison Tong 等人制定的质性研究统一报告标准(COREQ)等。关注研究者的个人特征，了解研究者的研究过程是否合乎规范，和参与者的接触程度，抽样方法是否满足研究目的，样本量是否饱和，资料收集与编码过程是否合理，等等，全面和系统地评估质性研究的设计。

🕮 Studies Cited in Chapter 17（第十七章参考文献）

[1]Martsolf, D. S., Draucker, C., Stephenson, P., Patterns of dating violence across adolescence[J]. Qualitative Health Research, 2012, 22: 1271-1283.

[2]Heidegger, M. Being and time[M]. New York: Harper, 1962.

Chapter 18: Sampling in Qualitative Research
第十八章 质性研究中的抽样

In previous chapters, we have learned knowledge related to sampling approaches in quantitative studies. This chapter will describe common sampling approaches used in qualitative studies. Different from that in quantitative research, sampling approaches in qualitative studies have unique characteristics. Firstly, participants are not selected randomly. The participants in qualitative studies are required with rich background, which cannot be achieved by random sampling approaches. Secondly, samples in qualitative studies are small, and each participant provides a wealth of data. Finally, sample sizes in qualitative studies are not determined in advance, but during data collection.

在前面的章节中，我们学习了量性研究的抽样方法。本章将对常规质性研究抽样方法进行概述。不同于量性研究的抽样方法，质性研究抽样方法有着独特的方式。首先，质性研究中的样本不是通过随机抽样而来。质性研究中的样本具有丰富的背景资料，通过随机抽样无法获得。其次，质性研究的样本量都很小，每个样本可提供丰富的数据资料。最后，质性研究中的样本量不是事先确定的，而是在数据收集过程中确定。

Section Ⅰ Types of Qualitative Sampling
第一节 质性抽样的类型

1. Convenience Sampling(便利抽样)

Convenience sampling is often used in qualitative studies, especially when researchers would like to find potential participants. For instance, we would like to explore the living experiences of women with postpartum depression. It is difficult to identify the potential participants, and the recruitment approach, such as having a notice in a newspaper, on a bulletin board, or the Internet, will be used to request women with postpartum depression to contact us. Convenience sampling is an easy and efficient way to begin the sampling process. However, it is not an appropriate way to find participants who can provide the most information-rich data. Therefore, continence sampling is selected with other methods as data are collected.

便利抽样是质性研究中常用的抽样方法，特别是当研究者寻找潜在参与者的时候。例如，我们想探究产后抑郁妇女的生活经历，在现实生活中确认这类潜在参与者很困难，因此，通过在报纸、公告栏、网络上登广告，可以招募到产后抑郁妇女联系研究者。在开始抽样时，便利抽样是一种简捷有效的方法，但它并不能帮助找到提供最多信息的参与者。因此，在数据收集过程中，便利抽样常常与其他抽样方法一起使用。

2. Snowball Sampling(滚雪球抽样)

When qualitative researchers interview some participants, they may ask these early informants to refer other potential participants in the study, which is called snowball sampling. Snowball sampling has some advantages. It is a more cost-efficient and practical way to recruit appropriate participants because of the referring person. Also, it is easy for researchers to establish a trusting relationship with new participants. Further, researchers can find participants with varied backgrounds, such as age, race, and other characteristics. However, snowball sampling has its weakness as well. The participants may be limited in a small network of acquaintances.

当研究者访谈一些参与者时，他们可能会让这些参与者介绍潜在的参与者，我们称这种抽样方法为滚雪球抽样。滚雪球抽样有其优势所在。由于介绍人的存在，可以更有效地招募到适宜的参与者。另外，研究者也容易与新的参与者建立信任关系。再者，研究者可以借此招募到不同背景的参与者，如不同年龄、种族和其他特性等。然而，滚雪球抽样也有其局限性。参与者可能受限于一个小的熟人圈子里。

3. Purposive Sampling(目的抽样)

In qualitative studies, researchers may begin with convenience sampling and snowball sampling, but many of them choose purposive sampling eventually, which is to select participants who are considered to be typical of the population. There are many categories of purposive sampling, including maximum variation sampling, homogeneous sampling, typical case sampling, intensity sampling, opportunistic sampling, and others. Maximum variation sampling is believed as the most widely used method of purposive sampling, which involves participants with diverse backgrounds represented in the sample, such as different genders, ages, and socioeconomic status. If researchers know the factors influencing the studied living experiences in advance (e. g., literature review), it will help them achieve sufficient diversity in the sample. Different from maximum variation sampling, another type of purposive sampling, homogeneous sampling reduces variation and permits a more focused inquiry, which is often used for group interviews.

在质性研究中，研究者往往通过便利抽样及滚雪球抽样开始抽样活动，但很多研究者最终会选择目的抽样方法，也就是选择能够代表研究人群的参与者。目的抽样有很多类型，如最大差异抽样、同质抽样、典型案例抽样、重点抽样、机会抽样等。最大差异抽样被认为是使用最广泛的目的抽样方法。这种抽样方法包含了不同背景参与者，如不同的年龄、性别和社会经济状况。如果研究者能够提前了解到(如通过文献回顾)所研究生活经历的影响因素，这可以帮助他们在抽样中达到足够的多样性。不同于最大差异抽样，另一种目的抽样方法——同质抽样则是减少抽样的多样性，进行一个更聚焦的调研，常常用于小组访谈。

4. Theoretical Sampling(理论抽样)

As one unique type of purposive sampling, theoretical sampling, also called theory-based sampling, is a key process within the grounded theory. Therefore, we will discuss this separately. According to Charmaz, theoretical sampling is defined as "seeking and collecting pertinent data to elaborate and refine categories in your emerging theory". It relies on the concepts developed in data collection and data analysis to guide where, how, and from whom further data should be collected to develop a new theory. Different from other purposive sampling methods, the criteria which guide theoretical sampling decisions change throughout a study. The purpose of theoretical sampling is to develop categories to refine them, explore their boundaries, identify their properties, and discover relationships between them. For example, in a bereaved PICU parent study conducted by Butler, Hall, and Copnell in 2018, the researchers interviewed five participants from a single hospital at the first stage. Based on the initial concepts and tentative categories developed in the interviews, they undertook three theoretical sampling processes to collect further data, including introducing new research sites to understand support during and after hospitalization, adding new interview questions to understand the initial concept of "judging healthcare providers", and seeking new participant characteristics to better understand the concept of the parental role in the PICU.

理论抽样是一种独特的目的抽样方法，又称基于理论的抽样，是扎根理论研究的核心过程，我们将单独讨论。卡麦兹认为，理论抽样是在新形成理论的过程中，寻找和收集相关数据以细化和完善类别。理论抽样依赖于在数据收集和数据分析中形成的概念去决定在哪里、如何，以及从谁那里获得进一步的数据以发展新的理论。不同于其他目的抽样方法，在整个研究中，指导理论抽样决策的标准是变化的。理论抽样的目的在于发展类别，以完善类别，探索类别的边界，确定其属性，并发现类别间的关系。举例而言，例如，在2018 年，Butler 及其同事进行了一项关于在 PICU 失去孩子的家长经历的研究。研究者在研究第一阶段采访了来自同一家医院的 5 名家长。基于访谈得来的最初概念和初步分类，研究者采取了三个理论抽样过程，进一步收集数据：引入新的研究场所以了解家长在住院期间和住院后获得的支持；添加新的访谈问题以理解最初概念"评判医疗保健提供者"；通过寻找具有新特征的家长以丰富对 PICU 父母角色这一概念的理解。

Section II　Sample Size in Qualitative Research
第二节　质性研究中的样本量

Different from quantitative research, the sample size in qualitative research is not identified before the study. Moreover, it is based on informational needs and expected to be small. In qualitative research, there are no fixed rules for sample size. An essential principle in sampling is data saturation, which is the situation of obtaining the full range of information from the participants, and new data no longer emerge when interviewing additional participants. There are several factors influencing sample size in qualitative research.

与量性研究中的样本量不同，质性研究的样本量并不是在研究之前确定的。此外，质性研究样本量一般数量不大，取决于所需要的信息。在质性研究中，决定样本量大小没有固定规则。一个基本的抽样原则就是数据饱和，即从参与者那里已获得全部信息的状态，当采访额外的参与者时不再出现新的信息。在质性研究中，有很多影响样本量的因素。

Firstly, the sample size depends on the scope of the research questions. The broader the scope, the more participants will likely be recruited. Secondly, the sample size is affected by data quality. If participants have rich experiences and can communicate with researchers effectively, data saturation can be easily achieved with a small sample size. So, purposive sampling can help us find good informants. Also, multiple interviews with the same participants are often conducted to obtain rich and in-depth data because of increased trust. Thirdly, the background and experience of the researcher can affect the sample size. Researchers with rich interviewing or observational skills require fewer participants because they can build a trusting relationship with participants easily and encourage candor. For beginning researchers, they may need more participants to achieve data saturation. Finally, the sensitivity of the phenomenon studied also affects sample size. If it is deeply personal or embarrassing, a larger sample size is needed because the participants are more reluctant to fully share their experiences.

首先，样本大小取决于研究问题的范围。范围越广，需要的参与者就越多。其次，样本量受信息质量的影响。如果参与者有着丰富的经验，并能与研究者进行有效沟通，那么在样本量较小的情况下，即可容易达到数据饱和。因此，目的抽样方法可以帮助研究者找到适宜的参与者。此外，随着信任的增加，可对同一参与者进行多次访谈，以获得丰富和深入的信息。再次，研究者的背景和经验会影响样本量大小。具有丰富访谈或观察技能的研究者需要较少的参与者，因为他们可以很容易地与参与者建立信任关系，并鼓励参与者坦诚表述。因此，对于初级研究者，可能需要更多参与者以达到数据饱和。最后，所研究现象的敏感度也会影响样本量的大小。如果研究主题是非常私人化或令人尴尬的内容，参与者往往不愿意完全分享他们的经历，则需要更大的样本量。

Section Ⅲ   Sampling in the Three Main Qualitative Traditions
第三节   三种重要质性研究类型中的抽样

Sampling in varied qualitative traditions has the same characteristics, such as the sample size being small, and data saturation being the essential principle in sampling. However, there are a few differences in different qualitative traditions.

质性研究的抽样具有一些共性特点：如样本量都不大，数据饱和是抽样原则等。然而，不同的质性研究类型抽样也有不同。

1. Sampling in Ethnography(民族志中的抽样)

Ethnographers need to decide both whom to sample and what to sample because of ethnographic characteristics. The first is to select appropriate participants in the study. To do this, ethnographers may need to have conversations with people having the culture under study as many as possible. They eventually decide on a small number of participants who are highly knowledgeable about the culture by using purposive sampling. We call them key informants.

During conversations with people under study, ethnographers develop a pool of potential key informants. Then, they select key informants in the study in terms of their knowledge about culture and willingness to reveal and interpret the culture. Besides key informants, what to sample is unique in ethnography as well. Observing events, activities, places, and artifacts under culture help ethnographers understand the culture comprehensively. There are different observation methods used by ethnographers, such as descriptive observation, focused observation, and selected observation, varied with different research stages.

由于民族志的特点，民族志学者在抽样过程中需要考虑两个问题：谁是样本，以及抽样哪些内容。第一是选择适宜的研究参与者。为了完成这一目标，民族志学者可能需要与尽可能多的研究文化背景下的个体进行交流。最终，他们通过目的抽样法选择出小部分对文化有高度了解的参与者，我们称之为关键知情者。在与研究文化背景下的个体交流时，民族志学者形成一个潜在关键知情者库。并进一步根据这些潜在关键知情者对文化了解程度及是否愿意分享相关文化而确定出本研究的关键知情者。除了关键知情者，抽样内容也是民族志研究中的特色。通过观察文化背景下的活动、事件、场所、文化制品等可以帮助民族志学者全面地理解所研究的文化。随着不同的研究阶段，民族志学者可以使用不同的观察方法，包括描述性观察、焦点观察和选择性观察。

2. Sampling in Phenomenological Studies(现象学研究中的抽样)

Sampling in phenomenological studies is to select participants having experienced the phenomenon to express what it is like to live that experience. Usually, the sample size is 10 or fewer, depending on data saturation eventually. Although the participants have the targeted experiences, researchers in phenomenological studies consider participants with varied demographic characteristics to explore the common experience.

在现象学研究中，抽样是选择有过所研究现象经历的参与者，其能表达对该经历的感受。通常样本量是少于 10 个，最终取决于数据饱和度。虽然研究参与者都具有特定的现象体验，但现象学研究者往往会选择具有不同人口统计学特征的参与者，以探索他们共同的体验。

3. Sampling in Grounded Theory Studies(扎根理论研究中的抽样)

Typically, the sample size in grounded theory studies is about 20 to 30 people recruited by using theoretical sampling. Just like we discussed before, the purpose of theoretical sampling is to develop categories to contribute to the evolving theory. Therefore, sampling, data collection, data analysis, and theory construction occur concurrently. The participants in grounded theory studies are selected contingently, depending on the emerging concepts. For example, in Butler's study of understanding bereaved PICU parents, researchers seek new participant characteristics to better understand the concept of the parental role in the PICU at the late stage of the study. Sampling in grounded theory studies may consider the following steps. The initial participants may be recruited purposively. Following the emerging conceptualizations, participants are adjusted to help better understand the phenomenon. A final sampling includes a search for confirming and disconfirming cases to test, refine, and strengthen the evolving theory.

一般来说，扎根理论研究的样本量为 20~30，通过理论抽样招募而来。正如我们之前讨论过的，理论抽样的目的是发展类别以形成新的理论。因此，抽样、数据收集、数据分析、理论构建同时进行。扎根理论研究中的参与者是依据新出现的概念而进行选择。例如，在 Butler 关于了解失去亲人的 PICU 父母的研究中，研究者寻找具有新特征的家长，以便在研究后期更好地理解父母角色的概念。扎根理论研究中的抽样可参考以下步骤。最初的参与者可能通过目的抽样招募而来。随着概念的出现，参与者标准被调整，以帮助更好理解所研究的现象。最后阶段的抽样包括进行确认和否定的过程，以检验、完善及强化所形成的理论。

Section Ⅳ Generalizability in Qualitative Research
第四节 质性研究的推广性

Different from quantitative research, qualitative studies address people's living experiences in a particular context, and generalization is clearly not the strength of qualitative research. There are always some controversies in the study integrity and validity of qualitative research. In this section, we focus on issues of generalizability related to sampling strategies. Generalizability means the degree to which findings are transferable to other settings or samples. Most qualitative studies are conducted to understand a contextualized human experience by interaction with specific cases. Therefore, qualitative researchers are careful about the possibility of generalizability. However, some researchers believe that in-depth qualitative inquiry is particularly appropriate to reveal higher-level concepts that are not unique to a particular individual or setting, and the findings with rich detailed nature may be more suitable for generalizability. In the current evidence-based practice environment, it is more critical for the applications of research findings into practice. Based on this, researchers develop the meta-synthesis approach to summarizing qualitative findings within varied contexts for extrapolation. Firestone developed a useful typology with three models of generalizability: extrapolation from sample to population, analytic generalization, and case-to-case translation (also called transferability). We will discuss analytic generalization and case-to-case translation that are appropriate in qualitative research.

不同于量性研究，质性研究强调具体情境下人群的经历，而推广性也不是质性研究的优势。质性研究在研究的完整性及效度方面总是存在争论。在这一节，我们重点讨论与抽样相关的推广性问题。所谓推广，是指研究结果可转移应用到其他环境或人群的程度。大多数质性研究是通过对特定案例的深入互动以了解具体情境下的人群生活经历，因此，研究者对质性研究结论推广的可能性持谨慎态度。然而，有部分学者认为，深入的质性调查特别适合用于揭示非特定个人或环境所特有的更高层次的概念。而这些质性研究结果中所呈现的丰富详尽的性质使之更适合推广。尤其是在现在循证实践环境下，将研究结果推广应用于实践更是非常有意义。基于此，学者提出应用荟萃整合方法，整合不同情境下的研究结果以促进推广。费尔斯通发展了一种有用的类型学，描述了三种推广模型：从样本到群体的外推，解析推广，及可转换性。其中解析推广和可转移性适合于质性研究，我们将在此讨论。

1. Analytic Generalization(解析推广)

Analytic generalization does not depend on samples or populations. In analytic generalization, researchers strive to generalize a broader theory from a set of particular research findings. The process of generalizing a theory is to provide evidence to support the theory. Generalizing a theory is different from generalizing to a population, especially when the theory is intended to apply across a wider range of populations and settings. A single study usually provides weak support for a theory. However, the replication of research findings from different conditions contributes to generalizability. Moreover, similar results under varied conditions illustrate the robustness of the finding. In the model of analytic generalization, there are several sampling approaches contributing to conceptualization. For example, critical case sampling helps contrast alternative conceptualizations, and maximum variation sampling can strengthen the generalization of conceptualization by recruiting cases with varied characteristics that affect the conceptualization of the phenomenon.

解析推广不依赖于样本或人群。在解析推广中，研究者努力把一组特定的结果推广成更广泛的理论。而推广成理论的过程即提供支持理论的证据的过程。推广为理论不同于推广到一个人群，尤其是所形成的理论可适用于更广泛层面的群体及场所。单一的研究往往对形成理论的支持力度较弱。但当多个不同条件下的研究结果的重现则有助于推广。而且不同条件下出现的类似结果也恰恰说明了结果的可靠性。在解析推广的模式下，多个抽样方法可用于促进概念化形成。如关键个案抽样可用于比较相关的概念；最大差异抽样通过纳入可能影响概念化的具有不同特性的个案从而强化概念的推广。

2. Transferability(可转换性)

Case-to-case translation, also called transferability, is judgments of information generalization, whether or not findings from one inquiry can be extrapolated to a different group of population or setting. The transferability of findings depends on readers or consumers who transfer the results, instead of researchers. However, researchers are critical to providing high-quality descriptive information to help identify the transferability of their findings. In order to guarantee transferability as much as possible, thick description is often used in qualitative research, which refers to researchers' need to provide a rich and thorough description of the research context, setting, participants, and processes. Based on the thick description, readers can make good judgments about the similarity of the contexts studied and their environment, and then evaluate its importance for practice and research.

可转换性是对资料推广性的判断，即来自一个调研的结果是否可以推广到不同的场所或人群。研究结果的可转换性取决于读者或用户，因为是他们转换研究结果，而非研究者。然而，研究者在提供高质量的描述性资料以帮助判断结果的可转换性中起到关键作用。为尽可能地保证结果的可转换性，经常用到深描，即研究者需要提供丰富全面的描述性资料，包括研究背景、场所、参与者，以及研究过程等。基于深描所提供的信息，读者才能对所研究的情境及自身的情境进行相似性判断，从而评价该研究对其实践及研究的重要性。

Section Ⅴ　Critiquing Sampling Plans in Qualitative Research
第五节　评判质性研究中的抽样计划

In the last section, we discussed the importance of thick descriptions. Researchers provide comprehensive information such as sampling strategies that can help better understand the research process and results. Therefore, researchers have proposed the evaluation criteria of sampling in qualitative research. Morse advocated two criteria, including adequacy and appropriateness. Adequacy refers that samples can provide sufficient and high-quality information. Appropriateness refers to selecting the best participants who can provide the information needed in the study by using an appropriate sampling method. Further, Curtis and colleagues developed six criteria for evaluating sampling strategies in qualitative research:

在上一节中，我们讨论了深描的重要性。研究者提供全面的抽样策略等信息可帮助读者更好地理解研究过程及结果。因此，学者们对质性研究抽样提出了评价标准。其中，摩尔斯提出了足够和适宜两个标准。其中足够是指样本可以提供充足的高质量的信息，而适宜是指恰当的抽样方法以选择出能够提供研究信息的最佳人选。进而，柯蒂斯及同事于2000年提出评价质性抽样策略的六个标准如下：

（1）The sampling strategy should be relevant to the conceptual framework and the research questions addressed by the research. This implies that participants are relevant to categories in the conceptual framework used in the study.

抽样策略应与研究采用的概念框架及研究问题相关。这提示抽样而来的参与者与研究概念框架中涉及的分类相关。

（2）The sample should be likely to generate rich information on the type of phenomena which need to be studied. That is, participants can provide sufficient and high-quality information.

参与者应该能提供与所研究现象相关的丰富信息。即样本可以提供充足的高质量的信息。

（3）The sample should enhance the "generalizability" of the findings. For example, maximum variation sampling can strengthen the generalization of conceptualization by recruiting cases with varied characteristics that affect the conceptualization of the phenomenon.

参与者应能加强研究结果的推广。如最大差异抽样通过纳入可能影响概念化的具有不同特性的个案从而强化概念的推广。

（4）The sample should produce believable descriptions/explanations. Whether or not samples can provide a really convincing explanation of what is observed?

参与者应能够呈现可信的描述或解释。即是否对所观察的现象提供了一个令人信服的解释。

（5）Is the sampling strategy ethical? Such as, is there informed consent during the sampling? are there any ethical issues between researchers and participants?

抽样方法是否有伦理考量？例如，抽样过程中是否有知情同意，研究者与参与者之间是否存在伦理问题？

（6）Is the sampling plan feasible? Such as, considering issues related to the resource costs of money and time, practicals, and competencies of the researcher.

抽样计划是否可行？考虑相关问题，如研究经费及时间、具体操作可行性、研究者的能力等。

Studies Cited in Chapter 18（第十八章参考文献）

[1] Adebayo, O. W., De Santis, J. P., Gattamorta, K. A., et al. Facilitators of self-initiated HIV testing among youths: A qualitative study[J]. The Journal of Nursing Research, 2020, 28(5): 1-10.

[2] Butler, A. E., Copnell, B., Hall, H. The development of theoretical sampling in practice [J]. Collegian, 2018, 25: 561-566.

[3] Butler, A. E., Hall, H., Copnell, B. The changing nature of the relationships between parents and healthcare providers when a child dies in the paediatric intensive care unit[J]. Journal of Advanced Nursing, 2018, 74(1): 89-99.

[4] Charmaz, K. Constructing grounded theory[M]. 2nd ed. London: SAGE Publications, 2014.

[5] Curtis, S., Gesler, W., Smith, G., et al. Approaches to sampling and case selection in qualitative research: examples in the geography of health[J]. Social Science & Medicine, 2000, 50: 1001-1014.

[6] Firestone, W. A. Alternative arguments for generalizing from data as applied to qualitative research[J]. Educational Researcher, 1993, 22: 16-23.

[7] LoBiondo-Wood, G. Haber, J. Nursing research: Methods and critical appraisal for evidence-based practice[M]. 9th ed. St. Louis, Missouri: Elsevier, 2018.

[8] Misco, T. The frustrations of reader generalizability and grounded theory: Alternative considerations for transferability[J]. Journal of Research Practice, 2007, 3: 1-11.

[9] Morse, J. M. Strategies for sampling. In J. M. Morse (Ed.), Qualitative nursing research: A contemporary dialogue[M]. Newbury Park, CA: Sage, 1991.

[10] Polit, D. F. Beck, C. T. Nursing research: Generating and assessing evidence for nursing practice[M]. 9th ed. Philadelphia: Lippincott Williams & Wilkins, 2012.

Chapter 19: Data Collection in Qualitative Research
第十九章 质性研究中的数据收集

Section I Data Collection Issues in Qualitative Studies
第一节 质性研究中的数据收集问题

Compared with that in quantitative research, data collection is more flexible and creative in qualitative research. For example, researchers may add some questions in the further interviews in terms of previous interviews, or consider to attend related activities to better understand the culture under study. That brings challenges in data collection. We concern about common data collection issues in qualitative research.

相较于量性研究，质性研究中的数据收集方法更加灵活且具有创新性，比如根据前期访谈情况可能会增加后面的访谈问题，或考虑增加相关的活动以更好了解所研究的文化等。这给数据收集过程带来了挑战。在这部分，我们将讨论质性研究数据收集中的常见问题。

1. Types of Data for Qualitative Studies(质性研究中的数据类型)

Typically, the method of data collection in qualitative research is to go into the field under study, which is believed as the most likely source of data. At the same time, researchers to master alternative methods of data collection, such as reviewing genealogies and maps in ethnography studies. Interviewing participants and observation are primary methods of collecting qualitative data, but the types of data are varied in terms of different qualitative traditions. In ethnography research, the primary types of data are observation and interviews. Also, artifacts, documents, photographs, genealogies, and social network diagrams are collected to understand the culture under study. In-depth interviews are the main type of data in phenomenology. Phenomenologists use diaries and other written materials as well. Grounded theory researchers primarily rely on in-depth interviews, and also consider group interviews, observation, and so on.

典型的质性研究数据收集方法是进入所研究的实地，即被认为是最可能获取数据的地方。同时，在研究过程中，研究者要掌握收集数据的其他方法，如在民族志研究中查阅宗谱地图等。访谈法和观察法是质性研究中重要的数据收集方法，而所收集到的数据也因为研究类型的不同而有所侧重。在民族志研究中，数据主要是观察及访谈。另外，文化产品、资料、照片、宗谱、社交网络等都可以用于了解所研究的文化。在现象学研究中，深入访谈是主要类型，研究者也会用到日记和其他书面资料。扎根理论研究者主要依赖深入访谈，另外，他们可能也会用到小组访谈、观察等方法。

2. Field Issues in Qualitative Studies(质性研究相关问题)

In qualitative research, researchers work as an instrument in data collection in the field, which brings several important issues that need to be concerned.

质性研究中，研究者是数据收集工具，这一特质带来需要关注的重要问题。

Firstly, graining trust with participants is essential in qualitative research. Researchers need to develop strategies to establish credibility among the participants under study. For example, attending cultural activities or visiting frequently are useful for building a trust relationship, which can help participants feel more comfortable in sharing personal information. During this process, it is important to respect cultural traditions, beliefs, and local customs, and not to take sides on any controversial issues.

第一，在质性研究中，获取参与者的信任至关重要。研究者需要使用有效的策略在参与者当中建立可信度。例如，参与相关文化活动或多次拜访都是建立信任关系的有效方法。这种信任关系可以使参与者在分享个人信息时更放松。在建立信任关系过程中，研究者需要注意尊重相关的文化习惯、传统、信仰等，不要偏袒任何有争议的问题。

Secondly, researchers need to consider the pace of data collection. Data collection in qualitative studies requires deep concentration and energy, which is an intense and exhausting experience. In order to reduce the emotional strain, researchers need to pay attention to the pace of data collection, such as limit interviewing to no more than once a day or debrief with co-researchers about any distress in the study.

第二，研究者要注意数据收集的节奏。质性研究的数据收集需要精力高度集中，这是一种高强度的疲惫体验。为减轻研究所带来的情绪压力，研究者需要控制数据收集的节奏，如限制每天访谈次数不超过一个、和其他课题研究者反馈自己的压力等。

Thirdly, consider emotional involvement with participants. It is important to build a trust relationship with participants in qualitative research. However, researchers need to pay attention to not get too emotionally involved with participants, which compromises their ability to collect trustworthy data. For instance, provide advices to participants, share their own experiences with participants in interviewing.

第三，考虑情感投入。研究者与参与者建立信任关系在质性研究中很重要。然而，研究者需要注意避免太多情感上的融入，这会影响其收集可靠数据的能力。例如，在访谈过程中向参与者提供建议、与参与者分享自己的经历等。

Finally, use reflexivity in data collection. Reflexivity refers to researchers' awareness of themselves as part of the study. They need to be conscious of how their behaviors can affect the data they obtain. For example, Ethnographers must deal with how to keep a balance between "insider" and "outsider" when they explore a new culture. Researchers in phenomenological studies need to become aware of their personal biases about the phenomenon of interest.

最后，在数据收集中使用反思性。反思性是指研究者意识到自己是研究中一部分的反省能力。他们需要意识到自身在研究中的行为将如何影响到所收集的数据。如在探讨新的文化时，民族志研究者必须处理好"局内人"和"局外人"的平衡关系。而现象学研究者需要意识到自身对所研究现象存在的偏见。

3. Recording and Storing Qualitative Data(质性数据的记录和储存)

Data obtained in qualitative research is descriptive, and it is significant to record data comprehensively and truly. Audio recording is a common data-gathering instrument in qualitative interviews. After getting permission from interviewees, researchers tape-record the whole process of interviewing, including the content, tones, and pauses. Moreover, the interview is transcribed verbatim as soon as possible. Audio recording can help researchers focus on interviewees' speaking to gain in-depth information. Also, researchers take notes during the interviewing, including key information and comments, which can help clarify with interviewees and guide to further narration to achieve the most comprehensive and accurate description. Video recording is mostly used in group interviews, providing a complete recording of an individual's statement, group interaction, and individual behaviors. Field notes are used to record data in observations, especially in ethnography research. Field notes provide a rich and thick description of observations, recording behaviors, interactions, and activities seen and heard in the field. Also, field notes record researchers' thoughts, feelings, and confusions during the fieldwork, which can help researchers understand the field from multiple dimensions.

质性研究所获得的是描述性数据，因此如何全面真实地记录数据就显得尤为重要。录音是质性访谈中常用的记录工具。研究者在获得被访谈对象同意后，对整个访谈过程进行录音，包括内容、语调、停顿等。并在访谈结束后尽快将录音内容转录成文字。录音可以帮助研究者专注于被访谈者的陈述，以获得深入的访谈信息。在录音的同时，研究者可配合记录，主要是记录关键信息、评论等，可便于与被访谈对象澄清信息，引导进一步地叙述，从而获得最全面准确的描述信息。录像记录多用于小组访谈，对被访谈对象言论、行为、小组互动提供了全面记录。田野笔记用于记录观察中的数据，尤其是在民族志研究中。田野笔记是详尽的观察笔记，用于记录在观察场所看到的和听到的，如被观察者的行为、相互交流和活动。另外，田野笔记还记录了在观察过程中研究者的思考、感受、疑惑等，这些可以帮助研究者从多角度了解观察场所。

Data need to store in a safe and secure place. All participants were guaranteed confidentiality, and pseudonyms were used. All original tapes and notes need to be locked in a file cabinet in the researcher's office for a period of 3 years, at which time the tapes will be erased.

数据应储存在安全保密的地方。所有被访谈对象的信息保密，在访谈及资料上呈现假名。所有原始访谈录音资料及笔记资料需要保存在研究者办公室上锁的文件柜里，3 年后再销毁。

Section II   Qualitative Self-Report Techniques
第二节   质性自我报告技巧

1. Types of Qualitative Self-Reports(质性自我报告的类型)

Ryan and colleagues described three types of interviews: structured interviews, unstructured interviews and semi-structured interviews. Unstructured interviews and semi-structured interviews are more appropriate for qualitative research than the structured interviews.

瑞恩及其同事描述了三种访谈类型，结构化访谈、非结构化访谈和半结构化访谈。其中，非结构化访谈和半结构化访谈比结构化访谈更适合于质性研究。

1.1 Unstructured Interviews(非结构化访谈)

The unstructured interview is a natural, in-depth, and narrative interviewing method. There is limited structure in the unstructured interview. Researchers do not have a set of preselected questions to interviewees and encourage them tell their stories as much as possible, providing the opportunity for greater latitude in the answers. A broad open-ended question may be asked at the beginning of the interview. For example, in a study of Mensah and colleagues to explore nursing management of gestational diabetes mellitus in Ghana, researchers began the unstructured interview with a main question of "What are your experiences regarding the management/treatment you received from the nurse-midwives related to your diagnosis of GDM?" Further questioning was done regarding the challenges that they reported when having to manage GDM.

非结构化访谈是一种自然的、深入的、叙事式的访谈方法。非结构化访谈给出的提问框架很局限。研究者没有一套预先选择好的问题给受访者，而是鼓励受访者尽可能多地讲述自己的故事，为回答提供了更大的自由度。在访谈开始时，研究者可能会问一个宽泛的开放式问题。例如，门萨和同事在加纳进行了一项探讨妊娠期糖尿病护理管理的研究。研究者以一个主要问题开始其非结构化访谈："对于诊断为妊娠期糖尿病，您从助产士那里得到了哪些治疗和护理?"进而，通过他们所描述的管理糖尿病面临的挑战，做进一步的提问。

1.2 Semi-structured Interviews(半结构化访谈)

Different from an unstructured interview, a semi-structured interview has a clear interview guide which needs to be followed, including related questions in specific topics originated from research questions. However, A semi-structured interview guide is also flexible, which can follow interviewees' opinions or answers to move to further questions. There may be probes in the guide, such as "What happened next?" to elicit more detailed information. Interviewees are encouraged to share their opinions in terms of the topics in the guide. Researchers order the questions in a logical sequence, from general to specific, or be ordered chronologically. At the beginning of the interview, researchers may ask some questions that are easy to answer, and interviewees do not feel nervous. For example, in a study of sharing clinical nursing decision making experiences, the first question asked is "What do you know regarding the concept of shared decision making?" Also, abstracted or complicated questions or sensitive questions may be ordered at the late stage of the interview, when interviewers and interviewees have established rapport.

不同于非结构化访谈，半结构化访谈有明确的需要遵循的访谈指南，里面是基于研究问题而带来的特定话题相关的问题。然而，半结构化访谈指南也很灵活，它可随着受访者的某些观点或意见而转向进一步的问题。访谈指南中可能会有一些引导性问题，如"后面发生了什么?"以期获得详细的信息。受访者被鼓励对访谈指南中的主题畅所欲言。研究者按照一定逻辑关系排列半结构化访谈中的问题，如从一般到特性、随着事件发生的时间顺序等。在访谈刚开始时，访谈者可能会问一些容易回答的问题，使受访者没有那么紧张。如在一个分享临床护理决策经验的研究中，第一个问题是你所了解的分享临床决策是什么。另外，复杂抽象或敏感的问题会放在访谈的后面进行，因为此时访谈者与受访者之间已经建立了融洽关系。

1.3　Structured Interviews(结构化访谈)

The characteristic of structured interview is that questions are standardized and then answered or selected by the interviewee. The interviewer controls the pace of the interview according to the questionnaire, takes the questionnaire as a script, and asks all interviewees with the same questions in the same order. Interviewers record answers according to a pr-designed coding scheme. Structured interviews are often used in telephone interviews, face-to-face interviews, and interviews stopped on the road or in the park. Structured interview is often used as a precursor to open interview, or to confirm whether the assumptions obtained from the qualitative interview can be verified statistically after the completion of open interview. There are two ways of structured interview: one is that the interviewer controls the question outline and raises almost the same question for each interviewee; The other is to print the questions and possible answers on the questionnaire, and interviewees can choose freely. The former is widely used in anthropology, while the latter is widely used in sociology and social psychology.

结构化访谈的特点是把问题标准化，然后由被访谈者回答或选择回答。访谈者根据问卷控制访谈的节奏，将问卷当作剧本，以同样的顺序、同样的问题询问所有的被访谈者。访谈者根据事先设计好的编码方案记录答案。结构化访谈常被应用于电话访谈、面对面访谈、在马路上或公园里拦截的访谈。结构化访谈往往被用于开放式访谈的前导，或者是在开放式访谈完成后用来确认质的访谈所得出的假设能否在统计上得到证实。结构化访谈有两种方式：一种是访谈者控制问题大纲，对每个被访谈者提出差不多的问题；另一种是把问题与可能答案印在问卷上，由被访谈者自由选择。前者在人类学相关研究中应用较多，后者在社会学及社会心理学相关研究中应用较多。

1.4 Focus Group Interviews(焦点小组访谈)

Besides individual interview, focus group interviews are also commonly used to collect data in qualitative research. In a focus group interview, interviewers assemble several individuals with one or more homogeneous characteristics as a group to interview together. People are more at ease expressing their opinions with others having similar backgrounds. Therefore, focus group interviews not only concern each interviewee's feedback, but only encourage interactions among interviewees, especially those who are hesitate to share their own feelings. The number of group members is not standardized. The optimal group size is 6 to 12 persons, suggested by some researchers. The setting of a focus group interview should be comfortable, accessible, and easy to find. The places may not be appropriate if they have specific meanings, for example, if we would like to arrange a focus group interview with patients with HIV, it may not be appropriate in a HIV clinic or having related posters around. An interview guide includes several questions developed from the research topics. Usually, there are about 12 questions discussed in a two-hour focus group interview, moving from the general to the specific questions. The interviewer, also called the moderator, plays a significant role in a focus group interview. At the beginning of the interview, the moderator needs to introduce the ground rules for the group interactions, such as reaffirm that there are no right or wrong answers, explain confidentiality, and discuss taping. Then, during the interview, the moderator engages the involvement of each participant, instead of dominating the discussion by a few vocal interviewees. Also, the moderator needs to realize that personal opinions may be inhibited in the group discussion and "group think" takes hold. At the end of the interview, it is very useful that the moderator has a brief summary of information discussed and to pose a final question, such as "Is there anything else that you would like to talk?

除了个人访谈，在质性研究中还用焦点小组访谈方法收集数据。焦点小组访谈是访谈者组织具有一个或多个同质特点的个体形成一个团队，对他们同时进行访谈。与背景相类似的人在一起，人们会更轻松分享自己的观点，所以焦点小组访谈不仅仅关注小组中每个受访者的反馈，而且鼓励受访者之间的互动，尤其是之前不愿意分享自己观点的被访谈对象。虽然焦点小组的人数没有统一标准，但有学者认为，理想人数为6~12。焦点小组访谈的场所要使受访者感到舒服、便捷、容易找到。带有特殊含义的地点可能不适合，如在艾滋病诊所进行对艾滋病患者的焦点小组访谈，或有类似的活动海报出现。焦点小组访谈提纲包括基于研究主题的一些问题。通常2小时的焦点小组访谈讨论12个问题左右，问题排列从一般到特殊。访谈者，又称主持人，在焦点小组访谈中起到关键作用。在访谈开始时，主持人要介绍访谈互动的规则，如重申讨论没有正常错误答案、保密原则，及全程录音等。在访谈过程中，主持人要关注到每个受访者的参与，而不是由个别受访者主控整个访谈。另外，主持人要意识到在小组访谈中，可能抑制了个人观点的表述，形成一个群体思维。最后，在访谈结束时，主持人对所讨论的内容进行简要总结非常有用，而且，有必要加上最后一个问题："大家还有想补充的吗？

2. Gathering Qualitative Self-Report Data Through Interviews （通过访谈收集质性自我报告数据）

Researchers need to do preparation before, during, and after interviews.

为了获得丰富全面的自我报告数据，研究者在访谈前、访谈中、访谈后需要进行相应准备。

Before the interview. The researcher reviews the purpose and the content of the interview comprehensively. If the researcher has similar experience, it helps easily understand the information obtained from interviewees. For example, a Chinese researcher interviews Chinese Canadian seniors about their dietary practices. However, at the same time, the researcher needs to concern not guide interviewees' expression. It is useful to interview with a stand-in respondent if possible. Moreover, researchers need to decide where the interviews will be conducted with participants, and participants feel comfortable and safe without interruptions. In-home interviews are preferred because researchers can explore more individual information to help better understand their living experiences. The most interview method is in person. Video conferencing is also used for interviewing participants in rural area. Finally, researchers bring some related materials with them before interviewing, such as recording equipment, notebooks and pens, and consent and demographic forms.

访谈前。研究者要充分认识到此次访谈的目的及访谈内容。如果研究者有过类似的经历，有助于对受访者所提供信息的理解。如一位华裔研究者访谈了解加拿大华裔老人的饮食行为。但同时需要注意，研究者不要引导受访者。如果可能，事先找人进行访谈对访谈有帮助。另外，研究者需要和受访者确定访谈地点，一个让受访者感到舒服、不被打扰、安全的地方。受访者家里是研究者希望的访谈地点，因为可以为研究者提供更多受访者个人信息以便更好地了解受访者的经历。面对面个人访谈是最常用的访谈方式，现在视频会议也用于访谈偏远地区的受访者。最后，研究者还需要随身带相关资料，如录音设备、笔记本和笔、知情同意书及一般资料表。

Conduct the interview. Researchers need to provide an environment that interviewees feel at ease during the interview. For example, provide information related to the study to interviewees, ice-breaking exchanges of conversation at the beginning of the interview, etc. Interviewer personality is important to develop rapport, such as, be a good listener, do not interrupt interviewees, do not provide suggestions, facial expressions and nods show that the researcher understands from the respondent's perspective. In closing, interviewers ask interviewees whether they would mind being contacted again to ask additional questions or do member check.

进行访谈。研究者需要关注在访谈中使受访者保持轻松的状态，如向受访者讲述研究的相关信息、访谈开始时的破冰过程等。访谈中研究者的个人特质对建立和谐关系非常重要，如做一个好的倾听者，不打断、不提供建议等；面部表情、点头等表现出与受访者有共鸣。在访谈即将结束时，询问受访者是否可以接受再次访谈，以补充问题或进行成员检查。

Post interview. After interviewing, researchers listen to the interview as soon as possible to check for audibility and completeness. It is suggested that interviewers listen to the tapes by themselves to critique their own interviewing style and conduct better in the further interviews. Transcribers may be hired to transcribe verbatim. Researchers need to concern about the quality of transcriptions, and they may have misspelling words, or not adequately entering information about crying or speech volume.

访谈后。在访谈结束后，尽快听录音，检查录音的质量及完整性。建议访谈者自己听录音，评价自身的访谈风格，从而更好地开展后面的访谈。研究者可能会雇佣转录人员，但需要注意转录的质量，可能会有拼写错误，没有加入哭泣、音量改变等重要信息。

3. Evaluation of Qualitative Self-report Approaches(评估质性自我报告法)

Qualitative self-report approaches, such as in-depth interviews or unstructured self-reports, have distinct advantages. These approaches can provide participants with a great opportunity to express their feelings and ideas freely, which help researchers explore the basic issues, understand individual opinions, and the underlying meanings of a pattern. However, implementation of qualitative self-report approaches is time-consuming and it requires researchers with abilities in data collection and data analysis.

质性自我报告方法，如深入访谈或非结构化的自我报告等，具有独特的研究优势。这些方法可以为受访者提供自由表达自己感受和想法的机会，从而帮助研究者了解事物的本质、个人对事物的理解，及事物的内在含义等。然而，质性自我报告方法实施起来费时，且对研究者在数据收集和分析方面的能力提出要求。

Section Ⅲ　Observation
第三节　观察法

Observation is a common data collection method used in qualitative research through seeing, listening, smelling, and touching. It is a basic method to collect nonverbal information. In qualitative research, unstructured observations are used to comprehend the actions and interactions among people under study.

观察法是质性研究中常见的数据收集方法，通过所看、所听、所嗅、所触而获得信息，是非语言资料的基本收集方法。非结构化观察用于质性研究以理解研究对象的活动及他们之间的互动。

1. Features and Application of Observation(观察法的特点及应用)

Observation is required as objective, intuitive, planned, and sensitive. Observations should display what actions really are, and keep the natural situation. Researchers have a plan how and what they observe in the field, and are sensitive what they see and hear. Participant observation is most used to gather unstructured observational data. Participant observation demands complete commitment to the task of understanding, with intensive social interactions between the researcher and the participants in the field. It is often used in ethnography and grounded theory.

观察法要保持客观性、直观性、有计划的和敏锐性。观察法要展示所观察到活动的真实情况，保持其自然的状态。另外，研究人员要有一个计划，他们在现场如何观察和观察什么，并且对他们看到和听到的东西很敏感。参与式观察是用于收集非结构化观察数据的主要方法。参与式观察是通过研究者和参与者之间在研究实地的密切的社会互动，对所要理解事物的完全投入。常用于民族志研究和扎根理论研究。

2. Types of Observation(观察法的类型)

According to different roles of the researcher in observation, Junker described four types of observation: complete observer, observer as participant, participant as observer, and complete participant. Complete observer is that the researcher is a full observer, without any interactions between the researchers and people under study. Observer as participant means that the majority of the researcher's time is on observation, instead of participation. Sometimes, the researcher may attend some activities in order to fit into the setting, such as local festivals. Participant as observer is that the researcher is most interested in being a member of the group. It brings issues like that the researcher becomes so engrossed in getting involved, he/she forgets the purpose of being with the group. The last one is complete participant, which is, researchers conceal their purposes, and become a member of the group. However, researchers should not become complete participants because of ethics. Most observational field work uses the approaches and shifts over time.

根据研究者在观察中所承担的角色不同，Junker 将观察者分为四种：完全观察者、观察者的参与、参与者的观察、完全参与者。完全观察者是研究者完全观察，与所研究的人们没有任何互动。观察者的参与，是指研究者的大部分时间是用于观察，而不是参与。有时，研究者为了融入环境，可能会参加一些活动，如当地的节日。作为观察者的参与者是指研究者最感兴趣的是成为群体中的一员。但由此带来的问题是研究者对所研究的活动太过沉迷，而忘记融入活动的真正目的。最后是完全参与者，即研究者隐藏他们的目的，成为团体的一员。因为涉及伦理问题，研究者不可能成为完全参与者。大部分的实地研究交替使用上述方法。

3. Gathering Unstructured Observational Data(收集非结构化观察数据)

In qualitative research, researchers often have a broad plan for the types of information observed in the field. There are some aspects that are considered relevant, including the physical setting, the participants, activities and interactions, frequency and duration of activities, organization, precipitating factors. Also, Spradley distinguished three levels of observation during the whole process. First is descriptive observation, which is broad and general to figure out what the field is. Researchers observe as much as possible in the field. Based on descriptive observations, researchers move to key aspects of the setting, and observe selected events and interactions more carefully, which is called focused observation. Finally, researchers use the method of selective observations to most highly focus on activities that help compare categories with each other.

在质性研究中，研究者对实地观察信息的类型有着比较宽泛的计划。但有些方面被认为是相关的，包括物理环境、参与者、人们的活动及其之间的互动、活动的频率和持续时间、组织、事件发生的诱发因素。此外，Spradley 将整个观察过程分成三个层次的观察。首先是描述性观察，这是广泛而笼统的，可以帮助研究者了解实地的概貌。研究者尽可能多地观察实地的各种信息。基于描述性观察，研究者转向对实地中关键部分的观察，更仔细观察选定的事件和人们的互动，称之为焦点观察。最后，研究者使用选择性观察方法，最高度关注相关活动有助于比较不同的类别。

4. Recording Observations(观察的记录)

Systematic recording of observational data is significant after obtaining rich and deep information from participating and observing. It must be recorded as soon after observations as possible. A log and field notes are the most common forms for recording. A log is a daily record of what researchers done in the field, like a checklist. Differently, field notes are broader and more interpretive, including descriptive notes and reflective notes. Descriptive notes are objective descriptions related to observed events, conversations, and behaviors, and need to be recorded as completely, detailed, and objective as possible. While, reflective notes include information about the researcher's experiences, feelings, and expectations in the field, which helps researchers achieve analytic distance from the actual data. Hundreds of pages of field notes will be created in a qualitative study. Therefore, researchers need to mark observational sessions with date, time, or name.

当通过参与和观察获得丰富深入的信息后，对所获得的信息进行系统记录具有重要意义。在观察后，应尽快将观察结果记录下来。日志和田野笔记是最常见的记录形式。日志是研究者对自己在实地所做工作的每日记录，就像一个清单。与之不同，田野笔记涉及内容更为广泛，也更具解释性，包括描述性笔记和反思性笔记两种。描述性笔记是研究者对观察到的事件、人们的对话和行为等的客观描述，需要尽可能完整、详细、客观地进行记录。而反思笔记是研究者在实地的自身经验、感受和期望等信息，这有助于研究者完成对实际数据的解析。在一项质性研究中，会有数百页的实地观察记录。因此，研究者需要用日期、时间或名称等来标记不同的观察内容。

5. Evaluation of Participant Observation(对参与性观察的评价)

Participant observation provides researchers a valuable opportunity to get inside a situation and have a deeper and richer understanding of people's behaviors and the social situation under study. It is a great supplement with interviews because it can help answer questions about phenomena that are taken for granted from insiders' perspectives. However, participants observation has limitations. Observer bias and observer influence are prominent risks. Once researchers participate in a group's activities, emotional involvement becomes a significant concern. Researchers may lose objectivity in recording observations. Also, the ethical dilemmas need to be concerned in participant observation.

参与性观察为研究者提供了一个宝贵的机会，使他们能够进入一个情境，对人们的行为和所研究的社会情境有更深入和更丰富的了解。同时参与性观察也是对访谈的一个重要补充，因为它帮助回答了那些在局内人看来理所当然的问题。然而，参与性观察也有其局限性。观察者的偏见及观察者的影响是显著的危险因素。一旦研究者参与到所观察群体的活动，情感融入会成为问题。研究者可能在记录观察中失去客观性。另外，参与性观察中所涉及的伦理困境也需要考虑。

Section Ⅳ　Critiquing Data Collection in Qualitative Research
第四节　评判质性研究中的数据收集

There is so much rich and deep information obtained in qualitative data collection. It is difficult to critique the decisions made in collecting the data because these decisions are seldom expressed in research report. One critique method used is to involve an appraisal of information provided about the data collection methods. Researchers have responsibilities to display the data collection approaches that readers can assess the quality of evidence. Also, we can evaluate whether or not the types and amount of data are adequate to support an in-depth understanding of the phenomena under study. There is a guideline example for critiquing data collection in qualitative research.

质性数据收集过程中可获得大量丰富而深刻的信息。在现实中，我们很难评价研究者在进行数据收集时所做的决定，因为这些决定很少出现在研究报告中。我们常用的一种评价方法是对数据收集方法的信息进行评估。研究者有责任向读者展示这些数据收集方法，借此，读者可以评估研究所得证据的质量。此外，我们可以评估所获得数据的类型和数量是否足以支持我们对研究中现象的深入理解。下面有些指导评价的例子。

(1) Was the collection of unstructured data appropriate to the study aims?

收集非结构化数据是否适合本研究的研究目的？

(2) Given the research question and the characteristics of study participants, did the researcher use the best method of capturing study phenomena (i. e., self-reports, observation)?

结合研究问题和被研究对象的特点，研究者是否采用了了解研究现象的最佳方法(即自我报告，观察)？

(3) If a topic guide was used, did the report present examples of specific questions? Were the questions appropriate and comprehensive? Did the wording minimize the risk of biases? Did the wording encourage full and rich responses?

如果使用了访谈提纲，提纲中是否提供了具体问题的示例？所提问题是否恰当而全面？问题的措辞是否将偏见风险降到最低？问题的措辞是否鼓励受访对象做出充分而丰富回应？

(4) Were interviews tape-recorded and transcribed? If interviews were not tape-recorded, what steps were taken to ensure the accuracy of the data?

采访被录音及转录了吗？如果没有录音，研究者采取了什么方法以确保数据的准确性？

(5) What did the researcher actually observe, in what types of setting did the observations occur, and how often and over how long a period were observations made? Were risks of observational bias addressed?

研究者实际观察了什么？观察是在什么场所进行的？观察的频率和周期是多少？观察偏差的风险是否被考虑？

(6) What role did the researcher assume in terms of being an observer and a participant? Was this role appropriate?

在作为观察者和参与者方面，研究者具体扮演了什么角色？角色是否合适？

(7) How were observational data recorded? Did the recording method maximize data quality?

观察数据是如何记录的？记录方法是否最大限度保障了数据的质量？

📖 Studies Cited in Chapter 19（第十九章参考文献）

[1] Chung, F. F., Wang, P. Y., Lin, S. C., et al. Shared clinical decision-making experiences in nursing: A qualitative study[J]. BMC Nursing, 2021, 20: 85.

[2] Grove, S. K., Burns, N., Gray, J. R. The practice of nursing research: Appraisal, synthesis, and generation of evidence[M]. 7th ed. St. Louis, Missouri: Elsevier, 2013.

[3] LoBiondo-Wood, G. Haber, J. Nursing research: Methods and critical appraisal for evidence-based practice[M]. 9th ed. St. Louis, Missouri: Elsevier, 2018.

[4] Mensah, G. P., Van Rooyen, D. R. M., Ten Han-Baloyi, W. Nursing management of gestational diabetes mellitus in Ghana: Perspectives of nurse-midwives and women[J]. Midwifery, 2019, 71: 19-26.

[5] Morrison-Beedy, D., Côté-Arsenault, D., Feinstein, N. Maximizing results with focus groups[J]. Applied Nursing Research, 2001, 14: 48-53.

[6] Polit, D. F. Beck, C. T. Nursing research: Generating and assessing evidence for nursing practice[M]. 9th ed. Philadelphia: Lippincott Williams & Wilkins, 2012.

[7] Ryan, F., Coughlan, M., Cronin, P. Interviewing in qualitative research: The one-to-one interview[J]. International Journal of Therapy and Rehabilitation, 2009, 16(6): 309-314.

[8] Spradley, J. P. Participant observation[M]. New York: Holt, Rinehart & Wilson, 1980.

[9] Streubert, H. J. Carpenter, D. R. Qualitative research in nursing: Advancing the humanistic imperative[M]. 5th ed. Philadelphia: Lippincott Williams & Wilkins, 2011.

[10] 李峥, 刘宇. 护理学研究方法: 第 2 版[M]. 北京: 人民卫生出版社, 2018.

Chapter 20: Qualitative Data Management and Analysis
第二十章 质性研究数据的整理分析

Section Ⅰ Introduction to Qualitative Data Analysis
第一节 质性数据分析简介

The purpose of qualitative research data analysis is to organize data, develop a structure in terms of data, and elicit meanings. Different from quantitative research data analysis, qualitative research data analysis usually occurs simultaneously with data collection. Qualitative research data analysis is a process of conjecturing, verifying, modifying, revising, suggesting, and defending, which requires researchers having creativity and conceptual sensitivity. Moreover, researchers often face different challenges in the process of data analysis. The absence of standard qualitative data analysis procedures makes it difficult for researchers to explain how data analysis is performed. In addition, qualitative data analysis is sheer hard work, and researchers need to read a large number of narrative data again and again to organize and understand the intrinsic meanings.

质性研究数据分析的目的在于组织数据，基于数据而发展结构，并引出内在的意义。不同于量性研究数据分析，质性研究数据分析往往是和数据收集同步进行。质性研究数据分析是一个推测、验证、修改、修正、建议和辩护的过程，需要研究者具有创造性及对概念的敏感性。而且，在数据分析过程中，研究者往往面临不同的挑战。由于没有标准的质性数据分析流程，这使研究者很难解释如何进行的数据分析。另外，质性数据分析工作量大，研究者需要反复阅读大量的叙述性资料以组织和理解内在意义。

Section Ⅱ Qualitative Data Management and Organization
第二节 质性数据管理及组织

There are some tasks to help manage qualitative data in qualitative research.
在质性研究过程中，有一些常见的任务可用于帮助进行数据分析。

1. Transcribing Qualitative Data(质性数据的转录)

Prior to data analysis, the qualitative research data need to be transcribed. It is required to transcribed verbatim. When doing transcriptions, researchers or transcribers need to pay attention to not omit any information, such as omitting phones ringing, removing "ums" and "uhs" in the interviews, etc. Also, do not misinterpret words, such as change mute to moot. Maclean and colleagues provide some suggestions for avoiding transcription errors, such as, use speech recognition systems; symbols are used to represent different speakers and nonlinguistic utterances in transcriptions; transcriptionist's effect; emotionally loaded audiotaped material, etc. Moreover, researchers should transcribe the interviews into text as soon as possible in order to prevent from forgetting the related interview information due to a long time.

在进行数据分析前，质性研究数据需要转化为文字转录稿。对访谈资料要求逐字逐句地转录。在进行转录时，需要注意不要遗漏任何录音中的信息，如删除电话铃声、去掉访谈中的"嗯""啊"等。另外，不要误读单词，如错把沉默写成无意义。麦克莱恩及同事提出一些避免转录错误的建议：使用语音识别系统；转录稿中使用符号表示说话者、非语言信息等；转录人员的影响；转录访谈中的情感信息等。研究者在获取访谈资料后应尽可能快地将其转录为文本资料，以防止因时间过长对访谈现场信息遗忘。

2. Developing A Coding Scheme(制定编码方案)

Qualitative analysis starts with data organization, that is, classifying and indexing the data. The most common method used at this stage is to develop a coding scheme and then to code the data in terms of the scheme. Developing a high-quality category scheme requires a careful reading of raw data and concerning identification of underlying concepts and clusters of concepts. At this stage, two researchers are needed to develop a category scheme separately. Then, researchers compare these two coding schemes and reach a consensus. The final category scheme is developed.

质性分析从数据组织开始，即对数据进行分类和索引。在这一阶段最常用的方法就是制定编码方案，然后根据分成的类别对数据进行编码。制定高质量的分类纲要需要仔细阅读原始数据，并有意识地识别潜在的概念和概念群。在这个阶段两个研究者可分别制定编码方案，将各自提出的分类纲要进行比较并达成共识，形成最终的分类纲要。

3. Coding Qualitative Data(质性数据编码)

According to the developed category scheme, the data are read and coded into the corresponding categories. This is a hard task. In order to select an appropriate category, it may be possible to read the data several times to find the nuances. In addition, during the coding process, researchers may realize that the initial categories were incomplete. So, it is necessary to reread all of the previous coding materials to identify categories truly and comprehensively.

根据所制定的分类纲要，数据被读取并编码到相应的类别中。这是一个艰巨的工作。为了选择适宜的类别，可能要阅读好几遍数据资料以发现其中的微小差别。另外，在编码过程中，研究者可能会发现最初的分类不完整。这时，有必要重新阅读所有之前的编码资料，以真正全面地确定类别。

4. Manual Methods of Organizing Qualitative Data(人工整理质性数据的方法)

With the use of computer data management software, traditional manual methods of organizing qualitative data are not popular any more. When a category system is simple, researchers can code different narrative contents by using colored paper clips. Then, select all the material with a certain color clip to determine one issue. In addition, researchers can read the transcriptions and write relevant codes in the margins. Then, cut up a copy of the material with relevant content and put it into a file folder for the appropriate category. All of the content can be arranged in the appropriate file folders.

随着计算机辅助数据管理软件的使用，传统人工整理质性数据的方法已不再是主流。在分类比较简单的情况下，研究者可以使用彩色回形针对不同内容进行编码。然后，整理特定颜色回形针汇总的材料，对单个问题进行探讨。另外，研究者可以阅读转译文稿，并在文稿空白处写下相关代码。然后，按照分类剪切相关内容，并将其放入相应类别的文件夹中。所有内容都可归档于相应文件夹中。

5. Computer Assisted Qualitative Data Management and Analysis
(计算机辅助的质性数据管理分析)

With the development of computer assisted qualitative data analysis software (CAQDAS), more and more qualitative researchers have applied the software in their research. CAQDAS has many advantages, compared with traditional manual methods of organizing qualitative data. CAQDAS can convert audio into text, and make it easier to save and extract materials. In addition, the software can search text and codes. Because it can be shared with others easily, the software also helps conduct a team work. However, CAQDAS has its weakness, such as the lack of consideration of context in the code formation process, which need to be addressed by researchers.

随着计算机辅助的质性数据管理分析软件（CAQDAS）的开发，越来越多的质性研究者在其研究中使用这些软件。与传统人工整理质性数据方法相比，CAQDAS 有很多优势。CAQDAS 可以进行语音转译，使资料的保存及提取变得更加简单。另外，软件有寻找文字和代码功能。因为可以共享，分析软件有助于团队研究的开展。但是，CAQDAS 也有其不足之处，如形成代码过程缺乏对情境的考虑，需要研究者关注。

Section Ⅲ Analytic Procedures
第三节 分析步骤

Qualitative data analysis is a process of putting segments together into meaningful conceptual patterns, which is constructionist. Although the qualitative data analysis methods are varied with different qualitative research theories, they have common characteristics. In this section, we discuss the basic concepts of qualitative content analysis and different content analysis methods used in different qualitative research theories.

质性数据分析是将相关的片段信息组合成有意义的概念模式的过程，是建构主义。虽然不同研究理论下的质性数据分析方法各有不同，但他们有着相同的特点。本节讨论质性内容分析的基本概念，及在不同质性研究下的内容分析方法。

1. An Overview of Qualitative Analysis(质性分析概述)

Qualitative analysis usually begins by looking for broad categories or themes. Scholars believe that a theme is an abstract entity that gives meaning and identity to current experiences and varied manifestations. Themes originates from raw data. According to the similarity principle and the contrast principle, thematic analysis explores patterns and commonalities under study, as well as inconsistencies. Then, it is necessary to verify the developed themes, that is, whether the themes accurately represent interviewees' perspectives. Some methods are used to improve validation, such as a few researchers participate in the study. In the final stage of qualitative analysis, researchers strive to relate the different themes into an integrated whole, providing an overall structure, such as developing a theory.

质性分析通常从寻找广泛类别或主题词开始。学者认为，主题是一个抽象实体，赋予现有体验及不同表现意义和身份。主题词来源于原始数据。遵循相似原则及对比原则，主题分析发现研究中的模式和共性，以及不一致。继而，对形成的主题词进行验证，即主题词是否准确代表受访者的观点。我们常用一些方法来提高主题词的有效性，如多个研究者参与研究。在质性分析的最后阶段，研究者努力将不同主题关联，成为一个完整的整体结构，如形成理论。

2. Qualitative Content Analysis(质性内容分析)

Qualitative content analysis is the analysis of descriptive data content to identify prominent themes and patterns among the themes. In qualitative content analysis process, data are broken down into smaller units, and the units are coded and named in terms of what they represent, and grouped based on similar concepts. When conducting qualitative content analysis, a basic issue is to decide whether the analysis should focus on manifest content (that is, visible things) or latent content (such as the underlying meaning of the text). In addition, it is necessary to decide the unit of analysis to be selected. Usually, scholars suggest that the unit of analysis should be whole interviews or observational protocols, which can be considered as a whole, or also conducted in small codes analysis.

质性内容分析是对描述性数据内容进行分析，以确定突出主题词和主题间的模式。质性内容分析是将数据分解成更小的单元，再根据其表示的内容进行编码和命名，并根据相似概念对编码资料进行分组。在进行质性内容分析时，一个基本问题是决定分析应侧重于显性内容(即可见的事物)还是隐性内容(如事物的潜在意义)。另外，质性内容分析中需要决定所选择的分析单元。通常学者们建议分析单元为整个访谈或观察资料，可以作为一个整体来考虑，或进行小的编码分析。

3. Ethnographic Analysis(民族志分析)

Data collection and analysis in ethnographic research occur simultaneously at the beginning of entering in the field. The data analysis method consists of four phases: domain analysis, taxonomic analysis, componential analysis, and theme analysis. Domains are units of cultural knowledge, containing a broad category of smaller domains. Domain analysis refers to identify relational patterns among terms in domains used by members of the culture. Taxonomic analysis allows researchers to determine how many domains to encompass. After making this decision, a system of classification and organizational terms is developed to describe the internal organization of a field and the relationship between the categories and the whole. The third stage, componential analysis, is to compare the differences and similarities of cultural terms in a field. The last stage is theme analysis, which is the generation of cultural themes. Moreover, the data analysis method of ethnic nursing research developed by Leininger and MacFarland is commonly used in nursing research, including four steps:

民族志研究中的数据收集及分析同时进行，从研究者进入研究场地的那一刻开始。数据分析方法包括四个阶段：领域分析、分类分析、成分分析、主题词分析。领域是文化知识单位统称，包含更小领域的广泛类别。领域分析是指研究者确定所研究文化下人群所运用的领域中术语之间的关系模式。而分类分析是研究者决定研究中包括多少领域。决定后，一个用于分类及组织术语的系统形成，用于说明一个领域里的内部组织及各分类与整体之间的关系。第三阶段，成分分析，是比较一个领域中文化术语的不同及类似点。最后是主题词分析，即文化主题词产生。另外，常用于护理研究的是由莱宁格和麦克法兰发展的人种护理研究数据分析方法，包括四个步骤：

（1）Analyze detailed raw data, including interview records, observations, participation experiences, and field notes;

分析详细的原始数据，包括访谈记录、观察资料、参与经历和田野笔记；

（2）Data coding and classification in terms of research domains and research questions;

基于研究领域及研究问题，将数据编码分类；

（3）Carefully check the data to find repetitive ideas and patterns;

仔细检查数据，发现重复出现的想法及模式；

（4）Interpret and integrate findings.

解读及整合结果。

4. Phenomenological Analysis(现象学分析)

Phenomenologists prefer holistic contextualizing strategies to interpret descriptive data in a whole context. Commonly used in phenomenological analysis are Colaizzi, Giorgi, and Van Kaam data analysis methods. We introduce the Colaizzi data analysis method here. Colaizzi's data analysis method includes seven steps:

现象学关注于整体的情景化的策略，在整体情境下解释描述性资料。常用于现象学分析的有 Colaizzi，Giorgi，及 Van Kaam 资料分析方法。这里，我们对 Colaizzi 资料分析方法进行说明。Colaizzi 资料分析方法包括七个步骤:

（1）Read all the interview data carefully to have a feeling for them;

详细阅读所有访谈资料以期产生印象;

（2）Read each interview and extract meaningful statements consistent with the phenomenon under study;

阅读每一个访谈资料并摘取与所研究现象相吻合有意义的陈述;

（3）Extract the meaning of each significant statement;

从有意义的陈述中提炼意义;

（4）Form meaningful clusters of themes;

形成由主题组成的有意义的主题群;

（5）Integrate results into an exhaustive description of the phenomenon under study;

将结果结合所研究的现象，进行完整叙述;

（6）Formulate an exhaustive description of the phenomenon under study as unequivocal as possible;

形成对研究现象尽可能明确的描述;

（7）Bring the results back to the interviewees to verify the authenticity.

将所得结果返回给受访者，以求证结果的真实性。

5. Grounded Theory Analysis(扎根理论分析)

Grounded theory methods originated in a study conducted by American scholars Glaser and Strauss in 1967. Further, there are three versions of grounded theory with research: Glaser and Strauss's Grounded Theory (also known as Classical Grounded Theory), Strauss and Corbin's Grounded Theory (also called Procedural Grounded Theory), and Charmaz's Grounded Theory (also known as The Constructivist's Approach to Grounded Theory). Strauss and Corbin's Grounded Theory (i. e., Procedural Grounded Theory) is often used in the field of health, so we discuss Strauss and Corbin's Grounded Theory data analysis method here. Procedural

Grounded Theory requires researchers to have sufficient imaginative explanations for the phenomena under study, and develop a complete framework for explaining and predicting objective phenomena by connecting a set of concepts related to each other. In Procedural Grounded Theory, data analysis includes three stages of coding: open coding, axial coding, and selective coding. In open coding, raw data are broken down into parts to form conceptualization and categorization. Then, in the process of axial coding, the paradigm is used to help integrate structure and process, including causal conditions, context, intervening conditions, action and interaction, and consequences. Based on the paradigm, the codes formed in the first stage are classified and reclassified. Finally, in selective coding, the core category is selected, the relationship between the core category and other categories is systematically integrated and verified.

扎根理论起源于美国学者格拉斯和斯特劳斯在 1967 年的研究，之后随着学者们的研究，形成了三大学派：格拉斯风格的扎根理论(又称为经典扎根理论)，斯特劳斯风格的扎根理论(又称为程序化扎根理论)，及卡麦兹风格的扎根理论(又称为建构型扎根理论)。其中，斯特劳斯扎根理论常用于卫生健康领域。所以在这里，我们主要讨论斯特劳斯扎根理论(程序化扎根理论)数据分析方法。程序化扎根理论要求研究者对所研究的现象有足够想象力的解释，在相互联系概念关系中构成一个完整框架，可用来解释和预测客观现象。在程序化扎根理论中，数据分析包括三阶段编码方式：开放式编码、轴心式编码、选择式编码。在开放式编码中，原始数据被打散，形成概念化及范畴化。继而，在轴心式编码中，用范式进行结构和过程的整合，包括因果条件、文脉、干预条件、行为/相互行为的策略、结局等。在此基础之上，对第一阶段形成的代码进行分类和再分类。最后，在选择式编码中，找出核心类属，系统整合核心类属和各类属之间的关系，并验证其关系。

6. Analysis of Focus Group Data(焦点小组数据分析)

Compared with other qualitative research data, focus group data are richer and more complex, bringing challenges for data analysis. Scholars state that analysis of focus group data includes analysis at the individual level, group level and interaction level. Therefore, as discussed before, it is recommended to use videotapes for data collection in focus groups. Also, other researchers except the moderator finish fieldnotes during the interviewing, which can help clarify speakers' sequence, and non-verbal behaviors, such as body language, crying, etc. Krueger developed a continuous analysis method, from the accumulation of raw data to the interpretation of the data. The first stage begins with data collection. Rich data are obtained from interviews, and supplemented by recorded information from field observation. Then, researchers get familiar with the data by listening to the audio tapes, reading the translation records for several times, reading observation notes made during the interview and summary notes formed immediately after the interview. In the second stage, memos are completed in the form of phrases, ideas, or concepts at the margin of the text, and categories are developed to form descriptive statements and data analysis. The third stage is to sift data, extract the original data to be referenced, and compare within and between cases. In the final stage, charts are drawn to extract citations from the original context and rearrange them in the context of the newly developed thematic content.

比较其他质性研究数据，焦点小组数据更丰富及复杂，这给数据分析带来了挑战。学者认为，焦点小组数据分析包括了个体层面、团队层面和人际间的分析。因此，正如前面提到的，焦点小组数据收集时，建议使用录像设备进行配合，并且，除主持人之外的其他研究者在现场进行田野记录，以帮助明确发言者顺序及非语言类动作，如形体语言、哭泣等。克鲁格提出连续分析方法，从原始数据的积累到对数据的解释。第一阶段，从数据收集开始，从访谈中获取丰富数据，并通过田野观察记录信息进行补充。接着，通过听录音磁带，多次完整阅读转译记录资料，阅读访谈过程中的观察笔记和访谈后立即形成的总结笔记，以熟悉数据。第二阶段，通过在转译记录文本边缘以短语、想法、或概念的形式完成备忘，并以此发展类别，形成描述性陈述及数据分析。第三阶段，筛选数据，提取需要引用的原始数据，并在个案内部和个案之间进行比较。最后一个阶段，绘制图表，将引文从原始资料中提取出来，在新发展的主题内容情境下重新排列。

Section Ⅳ Interpretation of Qualitative Findings
第四节 质性研究结果的解读

Data analysis and interpretation in qualitative research occur concurrently, in an iterative process. Interpretation of qualitative findings is defined as a process which involves explaining, reframing, and showing an understanding. Interpretation is a part of recontextualization, moving from the description of the manifest content to the interpretation of the latent content, and developing themes and sub-themes, etc. This requires an incubation process in which researchers make thorough and in-depth reading of the data, try to explore their meanings, discover their essential patterns, and create insightful conclusions. In this process, researchers need to concern their own influence on interpretation, which is reflexivity discussed before. Researchers bring the findings back to the interviewees to verify whether the interpretation of the interviews or observations is true, or whether there is any misunderstanding or omission.

质性研究的数据分析及解读同时发生并交替进行。质性结果的解读被定义为一个包括解释、重新构建及显示理解的过程。解读是进行重新语境化的一部分，从对显性内容的描述转向对潜在内容的解读、发展主题词及副主题词等。这就要求研究者有个孵化的过程，即对数据进行全面深入解读，试图探寻其内在含义，发现基本模式，并创造出合理的结论。在此过程中，研究者要考虑到自身对解读的影响，即我们前面提到的反思性。研究者将形成的结果反馈给受访者，以验证研究者对采访或观察的解释是否真实、有无错误理解或遗漏。

Section V Critiquing Qualitative Data Analysis
第五节 评判质性数据分析

The rich and in-depth data in qualitative research bring challenges for readers to critique the analytical process of qualitative studies, as it is difficult for them to obtain relevant information to determine whether the researchers have made good judgments in coding data, analyzing themes, and integrating the final results. On the other hand, it is not easy for researchers to describe the process by which abstract concepts are developed from raw data. Therefore, an important task of evaluating data analysis is whether the researcher has provided a detailed description of the analysis process, including data analysis approaches, coding systems and refinements made, and so on. For example, is there congruity between the research methodology and analysis of data? In detailed, what methods of data analysis are used? Whether they are appropriate to address the research question? Does the researcher follow the steps described for data analysis? Is there a logical connection between raw data and themes? Is more than one researcher involved in the data analysis process?

质性研究中丰富性的资料给读者评判质性研究的分析过程带来挑战，因为他们很难获得相关信息以判断研究者是否在编码原始数据、主题词分析及整合最后结果时进行了好的判断。另一方面，研究者确实不容易描述从原始数据中形成抽象概念的过程。因此，对数据分析的一个重要评价内容是研究者是否对分析过程进行了详细的陈述，包括数据分析的方法、编码系统及所做的精练等。如研究方法与数据分析过程是否保持了一致性？具体而言，运用了什么样的数据分析方法？数据分析方法对回答研究问题是否适合？研究者是否遵循了相应的数据分析步骤？原始数据与所形成的主题词是否有逻辑相关性？数据分析过程中是否纳入了一个以上的研究者？

Studies Cited in Chapter 20（第二十章参考文献）

[1] Colaizzi, P. F. Psychological research as the phenomenologist views it. In R. Valle & M. King (Eds.), Existential phenomenological alternative for psychology[M]. New York: Oxford University Press, 1978.

[2] Corbin, J., Strauss, A. Basics of qualitative research: Techniques and procedures for developing grounded theory[M]. Los Angeles: Sage, 2008.

[3] Graneheim, U. H., Lundman, B. Qualitative content analysis in nursing research: concepts, procedures and measures to achieve trustworthiness[J]. Nurse Education Today, 2004, 24: 105-112.

[4] Grove, S. K., Burns, N., Gray, J. R. The practice of nursing research: Appraisal, synthesis, and generation of evidence[M]. 7th ed. St. Louis, Missouri: Elsevier, 2013.

[5] Krueger, R. A. Focus groups: A practical guide for applied research[M]. Thousand Oaks: Sage Publications, 1994.

[6] Lindgren, B. M., Lundman, B., Graneheim, U. H. Abstraction and interpretation during the qualitative content analysis process[J]. International Journal of Nursing Studies, 2020, 108: 1-6.

[7] LoBiondo-Wood, G., Haber, J. Nursing research: Methods and critical appraisal for evidence-based practice[M]. 9th ed. St. Louis, Missouri: Elsevier, 2018.

[8] MacLean, L., Meyer, M., Estable, A. Improving accuracy of transcripts in qualitative research[J]. Qualitative Health Research, 2004, 14(1): 113-123.

[9] McFarland, M. R., Mixer, S. J., Webhe-Alamah, H., et al. Ethnonursing: A qualitative research method for studying culturally competent care across disciplines[J]. International Journal of Qualitative Methods, 2012, 11(3): 260-279.

[10] Morse, J. M., Field, P. A. Qualitative research methods for health professionals[M]. 2nd ed. Thousand Oaks: Sage, 1995.

[11] Rabiee, F. Focus-group interview and data analysis[J]. Proceedings of the Nutrition Society, 2004, 63: 655-660.

[12] Streubert, H. J., Carpenter, D. R. Qualitative research in nursing: Advancing the

humanistic imperative[M]. 5th ed. Philadelphia: Lippincott Williams & Wilkins, 2011.

[13] Treloar, C., Champness, S., Simpson, P. L., et al. Critical appraisal checklist for qualitative research[J]. Indian Journal of Pediatrics, 2000, 67(5): 347-351.

Chapter 21：Trustworthiness in Qualitative Research
第二十一章　质性研究的可信度

The philosophical and professional paradigm of qualitative research differs from that of quantitative research and is often challenged by quantitative researchers, for example, regarding the lack of rigor and objectivity in the design of the research and the need to consider the generalizability and generalizability of the results. The design of qualitative research focuses on a deep understanding of its philosophical underpinnings and a true and profound reflection of the inner world of the research subject. The issues discussed in this chapter are important for researchers learning to do qualitative research and can help beginners to clarify how to conduct rigorous qualitative research.

质性研究的哲学观和专业范式与量性研究不同，经常受到来自量性研究者的质疑，例如关于研究设计不够严谨和客观、结果的普适性和推广性有待考量等问题。质性研究的设计聚焦于对其哲学基础深刻的理解，对研究对象内心世界的真实而深刻的反映。本章讨论的问题对于学习做质性研究的研究者来说，是十分重要的，可以帮助初学者明确如何进行严谨的质性研究。

Section Ⅰ　Perspectives on Quality in Qualitative Research
第一节　质性研究的质量

1. Debates About Credibility in Qualitative Research(关于质性研究可信性的争议)

Credibility is one of the important criteria for judging the level of quality of qualitative research. There has been controversy about the credibility of qualitative research, particularly the issues of reliability and validity. Because qualitative research uses words rather than numbers to focus on social facts and constructs of human phenomena, which distinguishes it from quantitative research that uses objective measurement tools, the reliability and validity of qualitative cannot be verified using quantitative criteria. Special evaluation methods are needed for qualitative research that is empirical and experiential.

可信性是评判质性研究质量水平的重要标准之一。关于质性研究的可信性一直存在争议，特别是信度和效度问题。由于质性研究用文字而非数字来关注社会事实和人类现象的建构，这区别于使用客观测量工具的量性研究，因此不能用量性的标准进行验证质性的信度和效度。需要对质性这种经验和体会的研究使用特殊的评价方法。

2. Generic Versus Specific Standards(通用标准及特定标准)

There is an ongoing academic debate about the need for generic or specific criteria for qualitative research. Many scholars have argued that different rubrics should be used in different studies, while others have proposed specific forms of criteria. For example, the ethnographic criteria proposed by Hammersley (1992), and the descriptive qualitative research criteria proposed by Milne & Oberle (2005). However, some researchers argue that certain quality criteria are quite general in the constructivist paradigm. On the other hand, some scholars argue that there are universal standards that apply to all qualitative research, for example, Whittemore et al. (2001) proposed four standards for qualitative generality, and O'Brien et al. (2014) constructed SRQR, a reporting standard that can be used for broad qualitative research.

关于质性研究是否需要通用标准或特定标准，学术界一直在讨论。许多学者认为在不同的研究中应使用不同的评判标准，也有学者提出了具体的标准形式。例如，Hammersley于1992年提出的民族志标准、Milne 和 Oberle 于2005年提出的描述性定性研究标准。然而，一些研究者认为，在建构主义范式中，某些质量标准是相当普遍的。另一方面，有学者认为存在通用标准适用于所有质性研究，例如，Whittemore 等人于2001年提出质性通用四个标准、O'Brien 等(2014)构建了可用于广义质性研究的报告标准 SRQR。

Section Ⅱ Frameworks of Quality Criteria
第二节 质量标准框架

1. Lincoln and Guba's Framework(Lincoln 和 Guba 提出的框架)

Lincoln and Guba propose a framework of quality criteria for qualitative research, which are the most commonly cited by qualitative researchers, namely:

Lincoln 和 Guba 提出了质性研究的质量标准框架，是质性研究者最常引用的标准，即：

（1）Credibility：refers to the authenticity of the data, and the ability to adequately reflect the multi-layered constructs of reality, which is an important part of reflecting the quality of the data.

可信性：指资料的真实性，能否充分体现现实的多层构造，这是反映资料质量的重要部分。

（2）Dependability：refers to the stability of the data over time, place and scenario.

可靠性：指资料随着时间、地点、情景的变化的稳定性。

（3）Confirmability：refers to the degree of objectivity of the information.

可确认性：指资料的客观程度。

（4）Transferability：refers to the generalizability of the findings and the presence of situational similarities.

可转换性：指研究结果的推广性，是否存在情景相似性。

（5）Authenticity：refers to the extent to which the researcher reflects reality fairly and impartially. Only when truthfulness is demonstrated in a research report can the reader gain insight into the true meaning and deeper nature of the text.

真实性：指研究者公平公正地反映现实的程度。只有当研究报告中能体现出真实性时，读者才能深入理解文字所表达的真正含义和深层本质。

2. Whittemore and Colleagues' Framework(Whittemore 及同事提出的框架)

Whittemore and his colleagues （2001） built on Lincoln and Guba's framework by summarizing ten criteria （credibility, dependability, confirmability, transferability） and six secondaries （explicitness, vividness, creativity, thoroughness, congruence, and sensitivity）. In their view, the four primary criteria are essential building blocks, applicable to any qualitative research, and the six secondary criteria provide an effective complementary framework, of which they consider validity to be the primary goal.

Whittemore 和他的同事（2001）在 Lincoln 和 Guba 的框架的基础上，总结了 10 条标准，分别为 4 个主要标准（可信性、可靠性、可确认性和可转换性）和 6 个次要标准（明确性、生动性、创造性、彻底性、一致性和敏感性）。在他们看来，4 个主要标准是必不可少的基石，适用于任何质性研究，6 个次要标准提供了有效的补充框架，其中，他们认为有效性是首要目标。

Section Ⅲ Strategies to Enhance Quality in Qualitative Inquiry
第三节 提升质性研究质量的策略

The quality of qualitative research has always been of concern to researchers and a number of strategies can help to improve the quality of qualitative research. This section will look at quality improvement strategies in collecting data, relating to coding and analysis, or relating to presentation.

质性研究的质量一直受到研究者们的关注，一些策略可以有助于提升质性研究的质量。本节会从数据收集质量提升策略、编码和分析质量提升策略与呈现相关的质量提升策略来介绍。

1. Quality-Enhancement Strategies in Collecting Data(数据收集质量提升策略)

Qualitative researchers use a number of strategies to enhance the quality of data collection, such as prolonged engagement and persistent observation, reflexivity strategies, data and method triangulation, etc. These are explained concretely as follows:

质性研究者为了提升数据收集质量，使用了许多策略，例如长时间的参与和持续性的观察、反射性策略、数据和方法的合众法等，具体解释如下：

1.1 Prolonged Engagement and Persistent Observation(长时间参与和持续性观察)

Long-term participation and continuous observation are important aspects of quality assurance in qualitative research. Long-term participation allows for a good relationship to be established with the research participants, facilitating the conduct of the survey and making it easier to obtain more detailed information. Ongoing observation allows for a deeper understanding of the research situation and the characteristics of the information being collected and recorded.

长时间的参与和持续性的观察是保证质性研究质量的重要环节。长时间的参与可以与研究对象建立良好的关系，便于调查的开展，使信息的获得更为便利、翔实。持续性的观察可以更深入地了解研究的情景与信息的特征，使正在收集和记录的资料更贴近本质。

1.2 Reflexivity Strategies(反省性策略)

Reflexivity requires special attention to the context of the research and the researcher himself. The researcher themselves as research instruments may have an influence on the collection, analysis and interpretation of data. A reflective diary is an ongoing method of ensuring reflexivity, recording details or other elements of the research process on an ongoing basis. Through self-questioning and reflection, the researcher attempts to probe deeply and grasp the experience, cultural context or research process in the study through the lens of the participants.

反省性需要特别关注研究的背景和研究者自身。研究者自己作为研究工具可能对数据的收集、分析和解释有一定的影响。反思日记是保证反身性的持续性方法,将研究过程中的细节或其他内容持续记录下来。通过自问自答和反思,研究者试图通过参与者的视角来深入探究和把握研究中的经验、文化背景或研究过程。

1.3 Data and Method Triangulation(数据和方法的合众法)

The triangulation method is the use of multiple referents to construct the essence and validate the data. Data triangulation refers to the collection of data at multiple points in time, in multiple locations, and for multiple research subjects; the methodological triangulation refers to the use of multiple data collection methods (e. g. interviews, observations, etc.). The pooling method increases the credibility of the data, helps to capture more complete information and obtain a richer context, and avoids the esbiases of a single referent.

合众法是使用多个参照物来构建本质,验证数据。数据合众法是指在多个时间点、多个地点、针对多个研究对象进行数据的收集;方法合众法指运用多种资料收集的方法,例如访谈法、观察法等)。通过合众法,可以提高资料的可信程度,有助于捕捉更完整的信息和获取丰富的背景,避免单一参照物的偏见主义。

1.4 Comprehensive and Vivid Recording of Information(全面而生动地记录信息)

Interviews are the main source of data and the researcher needs to fully document information from the field, provide vivid and comprehensive descriptions of events and processes, provide detailed details and thorough records. The researcher will use an audit trail to collect information systematically, e. g. to record raw data, process descriptions, material relating to the researcher's intentions and other relevant material, etc.

访谈是主要的数据来源，研究者需要充分记录现场的信息，对事情和过程进行生动和全面的描述，提供翔实的细节和彻底的记录。研究者有时会使用跟踪检查来系统地收集资料，如：记录下原始数据、过程说明、研究者的意图和其他有关的材料，等等。

1.5　Member Checking（参与者复核）

Member Checking is important in establishing the credibility of qualitative data. During participant review, the researcher provides feedback to the research participants on emerging interpretations to obtain their reactions, confirm the accuracy of the interpretation and understand whether it reflects their true situation.

参与者复核对于建立定性数据可信度有重要意义。在参与者复核时，研究者向研究对象提供关于新出现的解释的反馈，去获得他们的反应，确认解释的准确程度，以及了解是否体现了他们的真实情况。

2. Quality-Enhancement Strategies Relating to Coding And Analysis（编码和分析质量提升策略）

A qualitative study with good quality must have trustworthiness in its coding and analysis. The following strategies related to the coding and analysis of qualitative study data are shown as follows：

一项高质量的质性研究，它的编码和分析也一定具有可信度。如下是与质性研究数据的编码、分析的策略：

2.1　Investigator and Theory Triangulation（研究者和理论的合众法）

Triangulation explores truth from multiple perspectives. The investigator triangulation, conceptually similar to internal reliability in quantitative research, is commonly used to code qualitative data. Two or more researchers code, analyze and interpret the same data, and the researchers use continuous and iterative data to analyze while continuously comparing the results against the original data. This reduces the risk of bias and idiosyncratic interpretation of results through collaboration. The theory triangulation means that researchers use competing theories or hypotheses to analyze and interpret the data, which can help them rule out competing hypotheses and prevent premature conceptualization.

合众法从多角度探索真相。研究者的合众法，概念上类似于量性研究中的内部信度，常用于编码质性数据。两名或以上研究者编码、分析和解释同一份资料，且研究者在分析资料时，采用连续的、反复的资料分析，并将结果与原资料不断比较对照。这样可以通过合作减少结果的偏倚和特异性解释的风险。理论的合众法是指，研究人员使用相互竞争的理论或假设来分析和解释数据，这可以帮助研究者排除对立的假设，并防止过早的概念化。

2.2　Searching for Confirming or Disconfirming Evidence（寻找确定的或不确定的证据）

Mining external evidence from other research areas for corroboration is a methodological strategy for validating research findings. For example, having someone outside the study review the preliminary results and confirm the accuracy, relevance, and significance of the data. Uncertain evidence cannot be sought when the researchers themselves are not clear about what they need to know, and this is when researchers can discuss the results and seek uncertain or conflicting evidence.

从其他研究领域中挖掘外部证据用于佐证，这是验证研究结果的一种方法策略。例如，让研究以外的人来审查初步的结果，并确认数据的准确性、相关性和意义。当研究人员自己不清楚自己需要知道什么时，就无法寻求不确定证据，这时研究者们可以对结果进行讨论，寻求不确定的或相互矛盾的证据。

2.3　Peer Review and Inquire Audits（同行评议和调查审计）

External review through peer review is an important strategy to improve the quality of research. In a peer review debriefing session, the researcher needs to sort out the study clearly and logically and provide a written explanation or oral summary of the results of the data. Then, the peers analyze the design, process, and results of the study and make comments and recommendations. A more formal approach is to conduct an inquiry audit, which involves a review of the data and supporting documentation by an external reviewer. This requires the researcher to carefully document all aspects of the investigation.

通过同行评议进行外部审查是提高研究质量的重要策略。在同行评议汇报会上，研究者需要对研究内容梳理清晰和有逻辑性，对数据的结果进行书面解释或口头总结。同行分析研究的设计、过程和结果等，提出意见和建议。更正式的方法是进行调查审计，包括由外部审查员对数据和支持性文件进行审查。这需要研究者仔细记录调查的所有方面。

3. Quality-Enhancement Strategies Relating to Presentation （与呈现相关的质量提升策略）

3.1 Disclosure of Quality Enhancement Strategies in Research （披露研究中的质量提升策略）

When writing a report, the writer needs to disclose the quality improvement strategies used in the process and provide a good description of the issues of rigor, integrity and trustworthiness of the study. It is an important part that gives confidence to readers and demonstrates integrity to them. Sharing with readers the efforts made to improve quality in the research process helps to demonstrate the readability and authenticity of the research.

在撰写报告时，作者需要呈现出在过程中涉及的质量提升策略，对研究的严谨性、完整性或可信度的问题进行良好的描述，这是给读者信心，向读者展示诚信的重要部分。与读者分享研究过程中为提高质量所作的努力，有助于证明研究的可读性和真实性。

3.2 Thick and Contextualized Description（详细且语境化的描述）

A thick and contextualized description of the research context, participants, and process of the research is needed. Verbatim quotations of the research subjects can be attached to the thorough inductive analysis of the sequence, structure, or form of the findings to reflect the authenticity of the findings. Meanwhile, the process of the description often calls for the capacity to evoke readers' empathy and inspire them, but one-sided and biased results that can mislead the readers should be avoided.

对研究背景、参与者和研究过程等需要进行详细和生动的描述，对研究结果的顺序、结构或形式进行彻底的归纳分析，可以加上对研究对象的逐字引述，体现研究结果的真实性。同时，描述的过程往往需要具有唤起性和共情的能力，但是避免陷入结果片面、以偏概全的陷阱，而误导读者。

3.3 Researcher Credibility（研究者可信性）

The role of the researcher in qualitative research is crucial. The researcher is the performer of data collection and analytical coding at the same time. The researcher's background, experience, and competence influence the credibility of the findings. When writing a research report, it is sometimes necessary to illustrate the researcher's personal connection to the subject, topic, or setting being studied. To be a good qualitative researcher, one needs to conduct transparent and thorough investigations and have insight.

研究者在质性研究中的作用至关重要。研究者既是数据收集的工具也是分析编码的执行者。研究者的背景、经验和能力等对研究结果的可信性是有影响的。在写研究报告时，有时需要说明研究者与被研究对象、主题或环境的个人联系。要成为一名优秀的质性研究者，需要进行透明、彻底的调查，具备洞察能力。

Section IV Critiquing Overall Quality in Qualitative Studies
第四节 评判质性研究的整体质量

To judge the overall quality of qualitative research is to assess the trustworthiness of qualitative research. The philosophical perspective used in the study, the methodology of the study, the consistency between interpretations of the results, and the researchers themselves, among others, all affect the overall quality of qualitative research. The researcher needs to balance authenticity and wholeness to demonstrate trustworthiness. Therefore, strategies used to improve quality and the standardization of the research process need to be recorded in a detailed and informative manner. However, when it comes to actual research, the length of qualitative research papers is limited by the space of the journal, which conflicts with the requirement of rich verbatim records. Therefore, how to find the balance and compromise also calls for researchers' attention.

评判质性研究的整体质量就是要对质性研究的可信程度做出评估。研究所用的哲学观、研究的方法学、对结果阐释之间的一致性和研究者本身等都会影响到质性研究的整体质量。研究人员需要兼顾到真实性与整体性，证明研究具有可信度。所以，需要用翔实而丰富的文字记录下所使用到的提高质量的策略，以及研究过程的标准化。但是，在实际研究时，质性研究的论文受到期刊页数的限制，与丰富的逐字记录的要求产生冲突。所以，如何进行平衡和妥协，也是研究者需要关注的地方。

📖 Studies Cited in Chapter 21（第二十一章参考文献）

[1]Hammersley, M. What's wrong with ethnography? Methodological explorations [M]. London: Routledge, 1992.

[2]Milne, Obelisk. Enhancing rigor in qualitative description[J]. Journal of Wound, Ostomy,

and Continence Nursing, 2005, 32: 413-420.

[3]Whittemore, R. Chase, S. K., Mandle, C. L. Validity in qualitative research [J]. Qualitative Health Research, 2001, 11: 522-537.

[4]O'Brien, B. C., Harris, I. B., Beckman, T. J., et al. Standards for reporting qualitative research: a synthesis of recommendations[J]. Acad Med, 2014, 89(9) : 1245-1251.

[5]Lincoln, Y. S., Guba, E. G. Naturalistic inquiry[M]. Newbury Park: Sage, 1985.

PART 5：Designing and Conducting Mixed Methods Studies
to Generate Evidence for Nursing

第五部分　设计及开展混合方法研究，
为护理实践提供证据

Chapter 22: Basics of Mixed Methods Research
第二十二章　混合方法研究的基础

Section Ⅰ　Overview of Mixed Methods Research
第一节　混合方法研究概述

The integration of qualitative and quantitative data into a single study or a consistent series of studies is a trend in methodology. This chapter presents basic information about mixed methods research in nursing.

将定性数据和定量数据整合到单个研究或一系列研究中是方法论的一种趋势。本章介绍了护理中混合方法研究的基本信息。

1. Definition of Mixed Methods Research(混合方法研究的概念)

In the first issue of *Journal of Mixed Methods Research*, mixed methods research is defined as research in which researchers collect and analyze data, integrate results, and draw inferences using both qualitative and quantitative methods or approaches in a single study or survey program (Tashakkori, A., & Creswell, J, 2007).

在《混合方法研究杂志》的第一期中，混合方法研究被定义为研究人员收集和分析数据、整合结果，并在单一研究或调查计划中使用定性和定量的方法得出推论的研究 (Tashakkori, A. 和 Creswell, J, 2007)。

2. Background and Development of Mixed Methods Research (混合方法研究产生的背景及发展)

Mixed methods research stems from the debate between the two paradigms, sociology and behavioral science. Sociology is a positivist/empiricist path that emphasizes quantitative research methods, while behavioral science is a constructivist/phenomenological path that advocates qualitative research methods. In the mid-19th century, academics began to take an interest in quantitative methods as having the objectivity and scientific nature of the natural sciences and should be introduced into the field of social science research, and it was not until the 1960s that qualitative research methods became the main paradigm for revealing social phenomena and objective facts. Quantitative research is deductive in nature, tending to reveal the relationship between things, and in the process of research, the researcher maximizes the objectivity of the research, while qualitative research is inductive in nature, believing that the subject and the object are inseparable.

混合方法研究来源于社会学和行为科学这两种范式的争论。社会学是实证主义/经验主义路径，强调的是量性研究方法，而行为科学是建构主义/现象学路径，主张的是质性研究方法。19 世纪中叶，学术界开始对量性方法产生兴趣，认为其具有自然科学的客观性和科学性，应该引入社会科学研究领域，直到 60 年代，质性研究方法才成为揭示社会现象和客观事实的主要范式。量性研究属于演绎性质，倾向于揭示事物之间的关系，在研究过程中，研究者最大限度地追求研究的客观性，而质性研究属于归纳性质，认为主体与客体是不可分割的。

There were initial forms of mixed methods research in the 1930s and 1940s, such as Mayo's study of the Hawthorne effect, which used methods such as interviews and observations in addition to experimental methods. Mixed methods can be applied in sociology, education, psychology, management and organizational research, evaluation research, health sciences, and nursing. 2005 saw the first international symposium on mixed methods held at the University of Cambridge, which led to the widespread acceptance and official recognition of mixed methods by Western scholars. 2007 saw mixed methods research become the third research paradigm after quantitative and qualitative research paradigms, marking the determination of the status of mixed methods in research methodology.

在 20 世纪三四十年代就有最初形式的混合方法研究，如 Mayo 对霍桑效应的研究，除了使用试验方法外还使用了访谈和观察等方法。混合研究方法可以在社会学、教育学、心理学、管理和组织研究、评价研究、健康科学，以及护理学中应用。2005 年剑桥大学首次举行混合方法国际研讨会，混合方法因此得到了西方学者的普遍认同和官方认可；2007 年混合方法研究成为继量性与质性研究范式之后的第三研究范式，标志着混合方法在研究方法学上地位的确定。

3. Rationale for Mixed Methods Studies(混合方法研究的原理)

Some scholars argue that combining quantitative and qualitative data can enrich many areas of investigation and that the advantages of mixed methods research include the following:

一些学者认为将定量和定性数据进行结合，可以丰富许多调查领域，混合方法研究的优点包括以下几点：

（1）Complementarity: quantitative methods and qualitative methods represent constructivism and positivism, respectively, and they are complementary, and the limitations of a single method can be avoided through mixed use.

互补性：定量和定性方法分别代表了建构主义和实证主义，两者是相辅相成的，通过混合使用可以避免单一方法的局限性。

（2）Practicality: since phenomena are complex, it is necessary not to let one method bind itself, and mixed-methods researchers often ask questions that cannot be solved by a single research method.

实用性：由于现象是复杂的，不让一种方法束缚住自己是很有必要的，而且混合方法研究者常提出的问题无法用单一的研究方法解决。

（3）Enhanced validity: when using mixed methods research questions, the researcher has access to complementary types of data support, which leads to enhanced validity of the results.

增强的效度：当运用混合方法研究问题时，研究者可以得到互补类型的数据支持，就会使结果的效度增强。

（4）Collaboration: mixed methods research provides opportunities and possibilities for quantitative and qualitative researchers to collaborate.

协作性：混合研究方法为定量和定性研究人员提供了合作的机会和可能性。

4. Paradigm Issues and Mixed Methods Studies(混合方法研究与范式)

There is much discussion about the appropriate paradigm for mixed methods research, and the pragmatist paradigm is most often associated with mixed methods research. Both induction and deduction are important in the pragmatist paradigm, and pluralistic perspectives are encouraged, with pragmatism providing the basis for what has been called the "dictatorship of the research problem" position. In addition, pragmatism is practical, so any method that leads to a conclusion is appropriate.

关于混合研究方法的合适范式的讨论有很多，而实用主义范式最常与混合方法研究联系在一起。在实用主义的范式中归纳和演绎都很重要，鼓励多元化的观点，实用主义为被称为"研究问题的独裁"的立场提供了基础。此外，实用主义是实用的，因此凡是能得出结论的方法都是合适的。

Section Ⅱ　Getting Started on a Mixed Methods Study
第二节　混合方法研究的入门

In this section, we discuss the mixed methods research questions, purpose, design, and data analysis of the mixed methods.

在本节中我们讨论了混合方法研究的问题、目的、设计及混合方法的数据分析。

1. Purposes and Applications of Mixed Methods Research （混合方法研究的目的及应用）

Mixed methods research is applicable in six situations.

混合方法研究适用于以下六种情况。

（1）Where the concept under study is new and difficult to understand and needs to be explored using qualitative methods prior to the use of formal, structured methods.

研究的概念是新的，很难被理解的，需要在使用正式的、结构化的方法之前使用定性方法进行探索。

（2）Complex problems that cannot be solved by a single quantitative method or a qualitative method.

单一的定量方法或者定性方法不能解决的复杂的问题。

（3）Data obtained by another method（quantitative/qualitative）that can significantly improve the conclusions obtained by the original method（qualitative/quantitative）.

另一种方法(定量/定性)得到的数据，可以极大地改进原始方法(定性/定量)得到的结论。

（4）A quantitative study yields a result that cannot be understood, and a qualitative study can explain exactly that result.

定量研究得到的结果不能被理解，而定性研究正好能够解释这一结果。

（5）A specific theoretical perspective that requires a joint interpretation of quantitative and qualitative data.

需要定量数据和定性数据联合解释的特定的理论观点。

（6）The key objectives require a multi-phase project to achieve.

关键目标需要一个多阶段的项目来实现。

1.1　Instrument Development（发展研究工具）

Researchers typically collect qualitative data as the basis for the development of structured tools for research or clinical use, which are then rigorously tested. In contrast, questions for formal tools come from clinical experience or prior research, but when the structure of a research tool is relatively new, clinical experience or prior research does not encompass all dimensions, so the collection of qualitative data becomes more important.

研究人员通常收集定性的数据作为用于研究或临床的结构化工具开发的基础，然后进行严格的测试。而对于正式工具的问题则来自临床经验或先前的研究，但是当研究工具的结构比较新时，临床经验或者先前的研究并不能包含所有的维度，因此，定性数据的收集就显得较为重要。

1.2　Intervention Development（构建干预措施）

Qualitative research plays a large role in developing interventions and evaluating their effectiveness, and the development of interventions needs to take into account the thoughts of the study population. As a result, intervention studies are increasingly likely to use mixed research methods.

定性研究在构建干预措施和评价其有效性方面发挥很大的作用，制定干预措施时需要考虑到研究对象的想法。因此，干预研究越来越有可能使用混合研究方法。

1.3　Hypothesis Generation and Testing（生成及验证假设）

Qualitative research will provide insights into concepts and the relationships between them, and these findings can be validated on a large scale in quantitative research. But it can often take considerable time to move from qualitative insights to formal testing of hypotheses based on those insights, so researchers can conduct a coordinated set of mixed-methods studies with hypothesis generation and validation as explicit goals.

定性研究会对概念及其之间的关系有深刻的见解，而这些发现可以在定量研究中进行大规模的验证。但是通常从定性的洞察力到基于这些洞察力的假说的正式测试可能需要相当长的时间，因此，研究人员可以进行一组协调一致的混合方法研究，将假设生成和验证作为明确的目标。

1.4 Explication(阐明观点)

Quantitative methods can demonstrate that variables are correlated, but cannot explain why they are correlated, whereas qualitative data are used to explain the quantitative descriptions, and qualitative data can provide a more comprehensive and dynamic view of the phenomenon being studied.

定量的方法可以证明变量是相关的，但是不能解释为什么相关，而定性数据被用来解释定量描述的原因，而且定性数据可以为正在研究的现象提供更全面、更动态的观点。

1.5 Theory Building, Testing and Refinement(理论的构建、验证及改进)

Mixed methods research has promising applications in the field of theory construction, verification, and improvement. The use of multiple methods provides opportunities for potential contradictions in the theory to emerge, and if the theory can withstand the attacks of these contradictions, it can provide a more solid foundation.

混合方法研究在理论的构建、验证及改进领域有广阔的应用前景，多种方法的使用为理论中潜在的矛盾提供了出现的机会，如果理论能够经受住这些矛盾的攻击，它就可以提供更加坚实的基础。

2. Research Questions for Mixed Methods Research(混合方法研究的研究问题)

There is usually an overarching research goal in mixed methods research, but there will be two and more research questions, each of which will use different methods and data. For example, a researcher may ask both exploratory and validation research questions, both to test causality and to elucidate its mechanisms. Also, specific mixed research questions that combine with quantitative and qualitative data may be considered in mixed methods research, e. g., do the two corroborate each other and to what extent?

混合方法研究中通常会有一个总的研究目标，但是会有两个及以上的研究问题，每个研究问题会用不同的方法和数据。例如，研究人员可以同时提出探索性和验证性研究问题，既可以检验因果关系，也可以阐明其机制。同时，混合方法研究中还可以考虑与定量和定性数据结合的特定的混合研究问题，例如，这两种是否可以相互印证，程度如何呢?

Section Ⅲ　Mixed Methods Designs
第三节　混合方法研究设计

1. Key Decisions in Mixed Methods Designs(混合方法研究中的关键问题)

When designing a mixed-methods study, researchers consider whether to use a fixed design or allow prior results to guide subsequent designs, and other key decisions include sequencing, prioritization, and integration.

在设计混合方法研究时，研究人员会考虑使用固定的设计还是允许先前的结果指导随后的设计，其他的关键决定包括顺序、优先级别和整合。

1.1　Sequencing in Mixed Methods Designs(混合方法研究中的顺序)

The sequence of mixed-methods research is divided into two main parts: sequential mixed research, in which the researcher conducts a qualitative study followed by a quantitative study or vice versa; and simultaneous mixed research, in which the researcher collects data using both quantitative and qualitative methods and analyzes the collected data by complementing both.

混合方法研究的顺序主要分为两个部分，一是顺序性混合研究，即研究者先进行质性研究然后再进行量性研究，或者顺序相反；二是同时性混合研究，即研究者同时使用量性和质性的方法收集资料，通过两者互补的方式对收集到的资料进行分析。

1.2　Prioritization in Mixed Methods Designs(混合方法研究中的优先级别)

In a mixed methods study, researchers usually determine the priority level of the methods, and if the researcher uses both qualitative and quantitative research methods equally to explore the topic, it is called an equal status mixed methods design. However, in a typical study, researchers will use qualitative or quantitative methods as the dominant method, adding a small number of the other research design, referred to as a primary-secondary mixed methods design. The choice of mixed methods priority may be influenced by the researcher and the audience. Researchers will prefer positivism or constructivism, and in addition, target audiences such as funders and journal editors are accustomed to qualitative or quantitative research.

在混合方法研究中，研究人员通常会确定方法的优先级别，如果研究者平等地使用质性和量性研究的方法来探索主题，则称为同等地位混合方法设计。但在通常的研究中，研究人员会以质性或量性方法为主导方法，加入少部分的另一种研究设计，称为主次混合方法设计。混合方法的优先级别的选择可能会受到研究人员和受众的影响。研究人员会倾向于实证主义或者建构主义，另外，目标受众如资助者、期刊编辑等习惯定性或者定量研究。

1.3　Integration in Mixed Methods Designs（混合方法研究中的整合）

There are several strategies for integrating mixed methods research：first，the type of data can be integrated when interpreting quantitative and qualitative results；second，integration can take place during data analysis；and third，integration can take place during data collection.

混合方法研究的整合有以下几种策略：一是在解释定量和定性的结果时，数据的类型可以整合；二是可以在数据分析过程中进行整合；三是可以在数据收集期间进行整合。

2. Notation and Diagramming in Mixed Methods Designs
（混合方法研究中的符号和图表）

Morse（Morse et al.，1991）proposed a system of notation，which involves order and priority levels，that has contributed greatly to mixed methods research and is suitable for quickly summarizing mixed methods research designs. In Morse's notation system，case is used to distinguish priorities. QUAL/quan indicates that the main method in a mixed methods study is qualitative，while qual/QUAN indicates that the main method is quantitative，or QUAL/QUAN if the two methods are equal. The order is indicated by + or →，QUAL→quan indicates that the main method is a quantitative study，while the qualitative data collection is in the second stage；if both methods are present at the same time then QUAL+quan is indicated.

Morse 等提出了一套符号系统，其中涉及顺序和优先级别，对混合方法研究做出了很大的贡献，适用于快速总结混合方法研究设计。在莫尔斯的符号系统中，用大小写来区分优先级，QUAL/quan 表示混合方法研究中主要方法是定性的，而 qual/QUAN 则表示主要方法是定量的，若两种方法是平等的则用 QUAL/QUAN 表示。顺序用"+"或"→"表示，QUAL→quan 表示主要是定量方法的研究，而定性数据的收集则在第二阶段；若两种方法同时出现则用 QUAL+quan 表示。

In addition to the symbolic system，mixed-methods research designs can be mapped as diagrams. For example，the process of tool development can be divided into two phases，with the first phase being qualitative research and the second phase being quantitative research. In the first stage, the results are obtained through qualitative data collection and analysis to develop the instrument, while in the second stage, quantitative data is collected and analyzed, and the qualitative data informs the development of the quantitative instrument.

　　除了符号系统外，混合方法研究设计还可以绘制成为图表。例如，在工具的开发过程就可以分为两个阶段，第一阶段是定性研究，第二阶段是定量研究。第一阶段通过定性数据收集、分析，得到结果，从而开发出工具；而在第二阶段收集、分析定量的数据，定性数据为定量工具的开发提供了信息。

3. Basic Mixed Methods Designs(基本混合方法研究设计)

Creswell (Creswell et al., 2015) proposed three basic mixed methods research designs, namely, convergent parallel research design, interpretive sequential research design, and exploratory sequential research design.

　　Creswell 等提出了三种基本的混合方法研究设计，分别是会聚平行研究设计、解释性顺序研究设计和探索性顺序研究设计。

3.1　Convergent Parallel Design(会聚平行研究设计)

A convergent parallel research design is a research design in which quantitative and qualitative data are collected simultaneously and analyzed separately, and the results of the two independent analyses are compared and contrasted to confirm whether the results corroborate each other. The advantage of a convergent design is that it allows for efficient collection of both qualitative and quantitative data, but it is difficult for researchers to give equal weight to both qualitative and quantitative data.

　　会聚平行研究设计是指在研究设计中将定量和定性数据同时收集，分开分析，将两个独立分析的结果进行了比较和对比，确认结果之间是否相互印证。会聚设计的优势在于它可以高效地收集定性资料和定量资料，但是研究人员很难做到给予定性数据和定量数据同等的权重。

3.2　Interpretive Sequential Designs(解释性顺序研究设计)

The interpretive sequential research design involves collecting quantitative data in the first phase and qualitative data in the second phase. The data collected in the second phase are used to interpret the data in the initial phase, while the quantitative research in the first phase is used to formulate the qualitative research questions in the second phase. The advantage of an interpretive sequential study is that it is simple to conduct and can be completed by a single researcher, but it can be limited in that the second phase cannot begin until the results of the first phase are available.

解释性顺序研究设计是指在第一阶段收集定量数据，在第二阶段收集定性数据。第二阶段收集的数据用于解释初始阶段的数据，而第一阶段定量的研究用于第二阶段定性研究问题的提出。解释性顺序研究的优点在于操作简单，可由一名研究人员完成，但是会受到限制，第一阶段得出结果之前，第二阶段无法开始。

3.3　Exploratory Sequential Designs(探索性顺序研究设计)

An exploratory sequential research design is used when a phenomenon needs to be initially explored, first in detail using qualitative methods, and the results obtained are used in quantitative research to measure or classify it. In an exploratory sequential research design there can be either a qualitative or a quantitative approach dominant. Exploratory sequential research designs are designed to develop better measurements and have similar advantages and disadvantages to interpretive sequential research designs.

探索性顺序研究设计用于需要对一种现象进行初步的探究，首先用定性的方法对现象进行详细的探索，得到的结果被用于定量研究对其进行测量或分类。在探索性顺序研究设计中可以由定性方法主导，也可以由定量方法主导。探索性顺序研究设计的目的是发展更好的测量，它的优点和缺点与解释性顺序研究设计相似。

4. Selecting a Mixed Methods Designs(混合方法研究设计的选择)

The key to mixed methods research design selection is suitability for the research problem, and it is difficult for researchers to be equally skilled in qualitative and quantitative methods, while the best solution for new researchers is to choose one familiar method to predominate. In addition, practical issues such as resources and time can influence the choice of mixed methods research design. Teddlie and Tashakkori suggest that the most appropriate research design should be selected in relation to the realities of the research situation, or new designs should be created in combination with existing designs.

混合方法研究设计选择的关键在于是否适合于研究问题，而且对于研究人员来说，对定性和定量方法同样熟练是很难的，而对于刚开始做研究的人而言，最好的解决方法是选择一种熟悉的方法占主导地位。另外，资源和时间等的实际问题也会影响混合方法研究设计的选择。Teddlie 和 Tashakkori 建议在研究时应该结合现实情况选取最合适的研究设计，或者结合现有的设计创造新的设计。

Section Ⅳ Sampling and Data Collection in Mixed Methods Designs
第四节 混合方法研究设计中的抽样及数据收集

Sampling and data collection methods in Mixed Methods（MM）research are a mixture of the methods for quantitative and qualitative data described in the previous sections, and there are its own special sampling and data collection problems in mixed methods research.

混合方法研究中的抽样和数据采集方法是前面章节中介绍的定量和定性数据的方法的混合，同时，混合方法研究中也存在自身特殊的抽样和数据收集问题。

1. Sampling in a Mixed Methods Study(混合方法研究中的抽样)

MM researchers can combine sampling methods in different ways depending on the needs of the study. In order to obtain a more representative sample, the quantitative part of a mixed methods study usually uses probability sampling, but sometimes continuous or quota sampling is needed to enhance representativeness, and the qualitative part usually uses purposive sampling in order to obtain cases with typical and rich information.

混合方法研究者可以根据研究的需要对抽样方法以不同的方式进行组合。为了获得更具有代表性的样本，混合研究方法的定量部分通常采用的是概率抽样，但有时也需要采用连续抽样或配额抽样来增强代表性，定性部分通常采用的是目的抽样，以便获得具有典型和丰富信息的案例。

The sample size requirements for the quantitative and qualitative components of a MM study are different. The quantitative component requires a larger sample size, in addition, the sample size number for quantitative studies is usually calculated under the guidance of power analysis in order to reduce Type Ⅱ errors in statistical analysis. The qualitative part requires a smaller sample size, and the saturation of the data is used as an indicator to stop sampling.

混合方法研究中的定量和定性部分对样本量的要求是不同的。定量部分要求的样本量更大，此外，为了减少统计分析中的Ⅱ型错误，定量研究的样本量数目通常在功率分析的指导下进行计算。定性部分要求的样本量较少，以数据的饱和度作为停止抽样的指标。

Researchers in MM studies often face a special sampling problem of whether to include the same sample in both the quantitative and qualitative portions of the study, which usually depends on the study purpose and study design, but it is also advantageous to use overlapping samples to allow aggregation and comparison of the two data sets.

混合方法研究的研究者通常面临一个特殊的抽样问题，即是否将相同的样本同时纳入定量和定性部分的研究中，这通常取决于研究目的和研究设计，但使用重叠的样本也是有利的，可以对两个数据集进行汇总和比较。

The study of Onwuegbuzie and Collins have indicated the MM sampling design is divided according to the relationship between the quantitative and qualitative components of the MM study. The relationship between the quantitative and qualitative components consisted of four main categories: identical, parallel, nested, or multilayered.

Onwuegbuzie 和 Collins 的研究表明混合方法抽样设计是根据混合研究中定量部分和定性部分的关系进行划分的，定量和定性部分之间的关系主要包括四类：相同的、平行的、嵌套的或多层的。

Identical sampling means that the quantitative and qualitative portions of a MM study use exactly the same sample; parallel sampling means that the quantitative and qualitative portions of a MM study use exactly different samples, although the samples in these two portions come from the same or similar groups, and parallel sampling can be used in parallel or sequential designs or any other prioritization design as well as identical sampling. In a nested relationship, the qualitative study part of the sample comes from the sample in the quantitative study, nested sampling is a very common sampling method in MM studies, especially when there is an explanatory design in the study, and nested sampling facilitates the researcher to delve into the phenomena and relationships captured in the quantitative study in the qualitative study. The opposite is often true for MM studies where an exploratory design exists, which require the use of completely different samples in the two research phases in order to ensure the reliability and accuracy of the findings. Multilayer sampling refers to the selection of samples from different levels of the hierarchy, which usually means sampling from different but related population. (e. g., nursing department managers, clinical nurses, and patients).

相同抽样指的是混合研究中的定量和定性部分使用的是完全相同的样本；平行抽样指的是混合研究中的定量和定性部分使用的是完全不相同的样本，虽然这两部分的样本来自相同或相似的群体，平行抽样和相同抽样都可以用于并行设计、顺序设计或其他任何优先次序设计中。在嵌套关系中，定性研究部分的样本来自定量研究中的样本，嵌套抽样是混合型研究中很常用的一种抽样方法，尤其是研究中存在解释性设计，嵌套抽样便于研究者在定性研究中对定量研究中捕获的现象和关系进行深入研究。而存在探索性设计的混合研究往往相反，它需要在两个研究阶段使用完全不同的样本，以便确保研究结果的可靠性和准确性。多层抽样指的是从层次结构的不同等级中选择样本，通常指从不同但相关的总体中进行抽样。（例如，护理部管理者、临床护理人员和病人）。

2. Data Collection in a Mixed Methods Study(混合方法研究中的数据收集)

Data collection methods in MM research can creatively combine data collection methods from both quantitative and qualitative studies；therefore，data collection methods in MM research include group or individual interviews，biomedical measurements，questionnaires，scales，observations，and diaries. Data collection methods in MM research fall into two main categories（Johnson & Turner，2003），intra-methods mixes，e. g.，biomedical measures and questionnaires，and inter-methods mixes，e. g.，scales and interviews.

混合方法研究中的数据收集方法可以将定量研究和定性研究中的数据收集方法创造性地结合起来，因此，混合研究的数据收集方法包括小组或个人访谈、生物医学测量法、问卷法、量表法、观察法和日记等。混合方法研究的数据收集方法主要分为两大类(Johnson & Turner，2003)，一类是方法内混合，如，生物医学测量法和问卷法，另一类是方法间混合，如，量表法和访谈法。

In selecting data collection methods，the MM researcher is guided by the principle that each data collection method is the most appropriate method to address the research question. MM researchers should fully understand the advantages and disadvantages of each data collection method before choosing a data collection method，and consider the strengths and weaknesses between these methods to facilitate complementarity between methods.

在选择数据收集方法时，混合方法研究者要遵循每种数据收集方法都是最合适的解决研究问题的方法的原则。混合研究者在选择数据收集方法之前要充分了解每种数据收集方法的优缺点，考虑这些方法间的优缺点，便于方法间的互补。

In parallel study designs，data collection methods for MM studies must be developed in advance，but in sequential study designs，the choice of data collection methods for the second phase usually depends on the methods and results of the first phase.

在并行研究设计中，混合方法研究的数据收集方法必须提前制定，但在顺序研究设计中，第二阶段的数据收集方法的选择通常取决于第一阶段的方法和结果。

When developing a data collection plan, the researcher should also consider whether one of the methods is also an "intervention" that influences the views and behaviors of the study participants, thereby biasing the results, e. g., an unstructured interview about a phenomenon may influence the participants' perceptions of the phenomenon in subsequent structured questions.

在制定数据收集计划时，研究者还应考虑其中一种方法是否也属于一种"干预"，影响研究对象的观点和行为，从而造成结果偏倚，如关于某一现象的非结构化访谈可能会影响研究对象在之后的结构化问题中对该现象的看法。

The final data collection issue for the researcher to consider is the collection of additional data, as it sometimes involves the problem of collecting data that do not adequately analyze and interpret the findings, in addition to the problem of conflicting quantitative and qualitative findings that sometimes exist, for which the collection of additional data may be an effective solution.

最后，研究者要考虑的数据收集问题是额外数据的收集，因为有时涉及收集的数据不能充分分析和解释研究结果的问题，此外，有时也存在定量和定性研究结果冲突的问题，而收集补充数据可能是有效的解决办法。

Section V   Analysis of Mixed Methods Data
第五节   混合方法研究数据分析

Integrating the analysis and interpretation of data from quantitative and qualitative studies is one of the biggest challenges faced by MM researchers. MM researchers often analyze and interpret data from both components independently, which fails to demonstrate the significance of MM research, but there are no formulas or rules for analyzing and integrating data from MM research, and there are many factors that influence the integration of data sets, such as study design and sampling plan.

综合分析及解释定量和定性研究的数据是混合方法研究者面临的最大挑战之一。混合方法研究者通常对两部分的数据进行独立的分析和解释，这无法显示出混合方法研究的意义，但混合方法研究的数据分析和整合没有公式或规则，有很多因素影响数据集的整合，如研究设计和抽样计划。

1. Interpretive Integration(解释整合)

1.1　Mixed Methods Designs and Interpretive Integration(混合方法设计和解释整合)

In interpretive integration, quantitative data are analyzed statistically and qualitative data are analyzed qualitatively, and then the researcher brings the two results together for a comprehensive interpretation, focusing on comparing the findings of the two results, which may involve "constructing a meta-matrix" in the next section. MM studies of parallel design often use interpretive integration. The interpretive integration is narrative only and is summarized in the subsequent discussion section of the study. Interpretive integration can also be used in MM studies with sequential designs and is often referred to by Bazely (2009) as "integration 'on the way'", meaning that it is not a formal integration at the end of the study, meaning that the design and analysis of the second dataset can be based on the analysis of the first dataset and its interpretation, and providing an overall interpretative integration of the two datasets is not usually possible.

在解释整合中，利用定量数据进行统计学分析，利用定性数据进行定性方法分析，然后，研究者将两者的结果汇总在一起，进行全面的解释，重点是比较两种结果的发现，可能会涉及下一部分中的"构建元矩阵"。并行设计的混合方法研究经常采用解释整合方法。解释整合只停留在叙述方面，在之后的研究讨论部分会进行总结。解释性整合也可用于顺序设计的混合方法研究中，通常被 Bazely (2009)称为"在途中的集成"，意味着不是研究结束时的正式集成，而是指一个数据集的分析被解释并用于告知第二个数据集的设计和分析，通常不能对两个数据集进行总体的解释整合。

Iterative analysis involves an evolving interpretative feedback loop in which knowledge learned in one phase of the study is applied in the next phase for data collection or analysis, and then refined or developed through subsequent iterations Bazely (2009). For example, a researcher using a mixed methods study for the development of a questionnaire requires literature reading and qualitative interviews for the development of questionnaire items, followed by a quantitative study to test the reliability of the questionnaire.

迭代分析包括不断发展的解释反馈循环，将在研究的一个阶段学到的知识运用在下一阶段，以进行数据收集或分析，然后通过后续迭代进行完善或开发(Bazely，2009)。如，研究者利用混合方法研究进行一个问卷的开发，需要先进行文献阅读和质性访谈进行问卷条目的开发，之后再进行量性研究对问卷的信效度进行检验。

1.2　Nature of Results from Interpretive Integration(解释整合结果的性质)

Interpretive integration focuses on the comparison of two datasets and can lead to convergent, divergent, or nuanced results. The ideal outcome of a mixed methods study is that the results of the two datasets are consistent or complementary to each other. However, many mixed methods researchers believe that different results can also help advance the research (e. g., by further exploring the reasons for divergent results).

解释性整合侧重于两种数据集的比较，可以导致收敛的、分歧的或具有细微差别的结果。混合方法研究的理想结果是两种数据集的结果一致或互相补充。但许多混合方法研究者认为不同的结果也有助于推动研究的发展(如进一步探索结果分歧的原因)。

Moffatt and colleagues (2006) proposed a method for resolving divergent results consisting of six steps：(1) treating the methods as fundamentally different, (2) checking the rigor of the respective methods, (3) exploring the comparability of the data sets, (4) collecting additional data, (5) exploring the intervention process, and (6) exploring whether the results of the two components actually match.

Moffatt 和其同事(2006)提出了解决分歧结果的方法，包括六个步骤：(1)将这些方法视为根本不同的，(2)检查各自方法的严谨性，(3)探索数据集的可比性，(4)收集额外的数据，(5)探索干预过程，(6)探索两部分的结果是否真的匹配。

2. Converting Quantitative and Qualitative Data(量性和质性数据的转换)

Depending on the purpose of the study, quantitative and qualitative data can be transformed into each other. However, there are conflicting arguments regarding the quantification of qualitative data, which some qualitative researchers consider inappropriate, but Sandelowski (2001) argues that it is inevitable because some descriptors in qualitative research (e. g., large number, partial, minimal) are themselves quantifications of the frequency of a behavior or a phenomenon, and in addition, there are many benefits to quantifying qualitative data. This is because quantitative data are easier to document and more intuitive, more convincing, and help the mixed methods researcher to develop a higher level of understanding of a phenomenon.

根据研究目的，定量数据和定性数据之间可以互相转化。但是有关定性数据量化的说法不一，有些定性研究者认为这是不合适的，但 Sandelowski (2001)则认为这是不可避免的，因为定性研究中的一些描述词(如大量的、部分的、极少部分的)本身就是对某种行为或某种现象出现频率的量化。此外，定性数据量化也有许多好处，因为量化的数据更容易记录且更直观，更有说服力，也有助于混合方法研究者对某一现象进行更高层次的理解。

3. Constructing Meta-matrices(构建元矩阵)

A matrix is a common method used by MM researchers to compare data from different sources. In a meta-matrix, MM researchers arrange quantitative and qualitative data, generally with rows corresponding to a situation, i. e., individual participants, and columns corresponding to information collected by the study, such as participants' anxiety scores, depression scores, and the researcher's observation notes. Researchers can detect patterns or anomalies in the study results by examining the meta-matrix in detail. Meta-matrices have the advantage of allowing researchers to examine all data sources simultaneously and comprehensively, and also help researchers explore whether quantitative statistical findings are supported by qualitative data from participants, or whether qualitative findings are supported by quantitative statistics from participants. In addition, meta-matrices can be used to integrate data and findings after data analysis has been completed, such as can be used in data analysis for qualitative interview studies.

矩阵是混合方法研究者用来比较不同来源数据的一种常用方法。在元矩阵中，混合方法研究者对定量和定性数据进行排列，一般来说，行对应于某种情况，也就是单个参与者，列对应于研究搜集到的信息，如参与者的焦虑得分、抑郁得分和研究人员的观察记录。研究人员可以通过对元矩阵的详细检查发现研究结果的规律或异常。元矩阵的优点在于允许研究人员同时且全面地检查所有数据源，同时也有助于研究人员探索定量的统计结论是否由参与者的定性数据支持，或探索定性结论是否由参与者的定量统计数据支持。此外，元矩阵还可以用于在完成数据分析后整合数据和结果，如可用于质性访谈研究的数据分析中。

4. Displaying Data in Mixed Methods Analysis(混合方法研究数据展示)

In addition to meta-matrices, there are other visualization tools that display information from multiple data sources. The article of Happ and his colleagues (2006) shows an example of using bar charts to quantify the frequency of qualitative data. In addition, they employ a modified stem-and-leaf plot to quantify qualitative data, with unstructured data sources on one side and the identification numbers of those data on the other. Scatter plots are also an important visualization tool, with the vertical axis representing the interiority score and the horizontal axis representing the exteriority score. Scatter plots allow researchers to clearly identify clusters and "outliers" that are difficult to detect through quantitative analysis only. Further suggestions for visual displays of mixed-methods analysis information can be found in Onwuegbuzie and Dickinson's (2008) study.

除了元矩阵外，还有其他可视化工具显示来自多个数据源的信息。Happ 和他的同事 (2006)的文章中展示了用柱状图来量化定性数据频率的例子，此外，他们还运用了改良茎叶图来量化定性数据，一侧为非结构化的数据源，一侧为这些数据的识别号。散点图也是一个重要的可视化工具，纵轴代表内部性得分，横轴代表外部性得分。散点图使研究人员可以清楚地识别只通过定量分析难以发现的聚类和"异常值"。关于混合方法分析信息的可视化显示更多的建议可以在 Onwuegbuzie 和 Dickinson（2008）的研究中找到。

5. Meta-inferences in Mixed Methods Research(混合方法研究中的元推断)

The most important and challenging step in MM research is the integration of quantitative and qualitative results into a holistic concept. In a MM study, the researcher has to consider the quality of the study, such as the quality of the design, data, and analysis, in order to draw meta-inferences. More guidelines on making appropriate inferences in the interpretation phase of a MM study can be found in Teddy and Tashakkori (2009).

混合方法研究中的最重要也是最具有挑战性的一步是将定量和定性的结果整合到一个整体概念中。在混合研究方法中，研究者要想得到元推断就要考虑研究的质量，如设计、数据和分析等的质量。更多有关在混合方法研究的解释阶段做出适当推论的指导方针可以在 Teddy 和 Tashakkori（2009）的研究中找到。

Section Ⅵ   Quality Criteria in Mixed Methods Research
第六节   混合方法研究的质量标准

Regarding the quality criteria of MM research, a prominent research team has introduced the terms "inferential quality" and "inferential transferability", in which inferential quality is the primary criterion for assessing MM research. Inferential quality includes internal validity and statistical validity of findings in quantitative research quality standards and credibility in qualitative research quality standards, so that inferential quality refers to the credibility and accuracy of MM research findings. Inferential transferability includes external validity in quantitative research quality criteria and transferability in qualitative research, and inferential transferability refers to the extent to which the findings of MM studies can be applied to other similar populations, settings, time periods, etc.

关于混合方法研究的质量标准，有著名研究团队推出了"推断质量"和"推断可转移性"两个专业术语，其中，推断质量是评估混合方法研究的首要标准。推断质量包括量性研究质量标准中的内部有效性和统计结论有效性，以及质性研究质量标准中的可信度，因此，推断质量指混合方法研究结论的可信度和准确性。推断可转移性包括量性研究质量标准中的外部有效性和质性研究中的可转移性，推断可转移性指混合方法研究的结论可以应用于其他类似的人群、环境、时间段等的程度。

Section Ⅶ Critiquing Mixed Methods Research
第七节 评判混合方法研究

Teddy and Tashakkori (2009) proposed a comprehensive framework for judging inferential quality that contains many criteria for evaluating the quality of quantitative and qualitative studies, including two main categories of quality assessment criteria：design quality and interpretive rigor. Criteria for design quality include design applicability, accuracy, internal consistency, and analytical adequacy, while criteria for interpretive rigor include interpretive consistency, theoretical consistency, interpretive agreement, interpretive uniqueness, integrative validity, and interpretive correspondence. The most important factor for mixed methods researchers to consider is whether valid integration has taken place and whether it facilitates the drawing of accurate and reliable meta-inferences. In addition, more information about the assessment framework developed to evaluate mixed methods research can be found in the study by Heyvaert and colleagues (2013).

Teddy 和 Tashakkori (2009)提出了一个评判推断质量的综合框架，包含了很多评价量性研究和质性研究质量的标准，主要包括设计质量和解释严谨性两大类质量评估标准。设计质量的标准包括设计适用性、准确度、内部一致性和分析充分性；解释严谨性的标准包括解释一致性、理论一致性、解释的同意度、解释独特性、整合的有效性和解释的对应性。混合方法研究者要考虑的最重要的因素是是否进行了有效整合，是否有利于得出准确可靠的元推断。此外，更多有关评估混合方法研究而开发的评估框架可以在 Heyvaert 及其同事（2013）的研究中找到。

🔖 Studies Cited in Chapter 22（第二十二章参考文献）

［1］Tashakkori, A., Creswell, J. The new era of mixed methods［J］. Journal of Mixed Methods Research, 2007, 1：3-7.

［2］Morse, J. M. Approaches to qualitative-quantitative methodological triangulation［J］. Nursing Research, 1991, 40：120-123.

［3］Creswell, J. W. A concise introduction to mixed methods research［M］. Thousand Oaks：Sage, 2015.

［4］Onwuegbuzie, A., Collins, K. A typology of mixed methods sampling designs in social science research［J］. The Qualitative Report, 2007, 12(2)：281-316.

［5］Johnson, B., Turner, L. Data collection strategies in mixed methods research. In A. Tashakkori & C. Teddlie (Eds.), Handbook of mixed methods in social and behavioral research［M］. Thousand Oaks：Sage, 2003：297-319.

［6］Bazely, P. Analysing mixed methods data. In S. Andrew & E. Halcomb (Eds.), Mixed methods research for nursing and the health sciences［M］. Oxford：Blackwell-Wiley, 2009：84-117.

［7］Moffatt, S., White, M., Mackintosh, J., et al. Using quantitative and qualitative data in health services research—What happens when mixed method findings conflict? ［J］. BMC Health Services Research, 2006, 6：28.

［8］Sandelowski, M. Real qualitative researchers do not count：The use of numbers in qualitative research［J］. Research in Nursing & Health, 2001, 24：230-240.

［9］Happ, M., Dabbs, A., Tate, J., et al. Exemplars of mixed methods data combination and analysis［J］. Nursing Research, 2006, 55：S43-S49.

［10］Onwuegbuzie, A. J., Dickinson, W. Mixed methods analysis and information visualization：Graphical display for effective communication of research results［J］. The Qualitative Report, 2008, 13：204-225.

［11］Heyvaert, M., Hannes, K., Maes, B., et al. Critical appraisal of mixed methods studies［J］. Journal of Mixed Methods Research, 2013, 7：302-327.

Chapter 23: Feasibility Assessments and Pilot Tests of Interventions Using Mixed Methods
第二十三章　使用混合方法研究进行干预的可行性评估及开展预实验

Clinical research is to carry out simple scientific research in a complex clinical environment, and the contradiction between science and feasibility is prominent. It is particularly important to obtain theoretical, methodological and technical support from the perspective of research methods. Although the existing quantitative research methods have solved many problems in clinical research, some problems cannot be solved well by quantitative or qualitative research alone, and there are still limitations. Mixed Methods Research (MMR) is the third Research paradigm that organically combines quantitative and qualitative Research. This method can help researchers to solve some problems that cannot be completely, reasonably and comprehensively explained by qualitative or quantitative methods alone.

临床研究是在复杂的临床环境中开展简单的科学研究, 科学性与可行性之间矛盾突出。从研究方法角度获得理论、方法和技术支持尤为重要。虽然目前现有的定量研究方法在临床研究中解决了很多问题, 但有些问题单用定量研究或定性研究仍不能很好地解决, 仍存在局限性。混合方法研究 (Mixed Methods Research, MMR) 是将定量研究与定性研究这两大主要研究范式有机结合的第三种研究范式。这种方法可以帮助研究者解决一些单用定性或定量无法完整、合理、全面解释的问题。

In 2007, the first dedicated to international academic mixed methods research in the inaugural issue of the journal of the "mixed methods research" broadly defined as "the researchers in a single study or a scheme to use both qualitative and quantitative research methods to collect, analyze data, integrated study and make inference".

2007 年, 国际学术界第一本专门针对混合方法研究的杂志在其创刊号上把"混合方法研究"宽泛地定义为"研究者在单个研究或者某个研究方案中同时使用定性和定量研究方法来收集、分析数据资料，整合研究发现，以及做出推断"。

Section I　Basic Issues in Piloting Interventions
第一节　预实验的基本问题

1. Definition of Pilot Tests and Feasibility Assessment
（预实验和可行性评估的定义）

Feasibility study is research completed prior to a main intervention study to test specific and discrete aspects of an emerging intervention or the anticipated trial. For example, a feasibility study might assess whether a 10-week intervention is feasible and acceptable or whether a shorter intervention would be preferable. Or, a feasibility study might be undertaken to assess whether a sufficient number of sites could be enlisted to participate in a multisite trial.

可行性研究是在主要干预研究之前完成的研究，以测试新干预或预期试验的具体和离散方面。例如，可行性研究可能会评估 10 周的干预是否可行和可接受，或者更短的干预是否更可取。或者，通过进行可行性研究，以评估是否可以征募足够数量的站点参加多中心试验。

Pilot study is considered small-scale versions of a full trial. Thabane and colleagues (Thabane et al., 2010) defined a pilot study as an investigation designed to test the feasibility of, and to support refinements of, the protocols, methods, and procedures to be used in a larger scale trial of an intervention. Feasibility is also a major issue in a pilot study, but the emphasis is on assessing the feasibility of an entire set of procedures for a randomized assessment, including recruitment (participants' willingness to be randomized), protocol implementation, data collection procedures, outcome measurement, blinding, and the ability to avoid contamination across treatment groups. Thus, according to the NETSCC definition, a pilot study for a full trial typically requires a randomized design.

预实验被认为是全面试验的小规模版本。预实验被定义为一项旨在测试在更大规模干预试验中使用的方案、方法和程序的可行性，并支持其改进的调查（Thabane 等，2010）。可行性也是预实验的一个主要问题，但重点是评估随机评估的一整套程序的可行性，包括招募(参与者是否愿意随机化)、方案实施、数据收集程序、结局测量、盲法，以及在治疗组间避免污染的能力。因此，根据 NETSCC 的定义，一个完整试验的预实验通常需要一个随机设计。

2. Overall Purpose of Pilot Work(预实验的总目的)

The overall purpose of pilot work is simply this : to avoid a costly fiasco. Fully powered RCTs are extremely expensive. Without adequate piloting, a full-scale trial can result in wasted resources and erroneous conclusions. A strong pilot can enhance the likelihood that a full test will be methodologically and conceptually sound, ethical, and informative. Large-scale trials typically cannot get funded unless adequate pilot work has been undertaken.

预实验的总体目的很简单：避免代价高昂的失败。全要素随机对照试验非常昂贵。如果没有充分的试点，全面的试验可能导致资源浪费和错误的结论。一个强有力的预实验可以提高完整测试在方法和概念上是合理的、合乎伦理的和信息丰富的可能性。除非开展足够的预实验，否则大规模试验通常无法获得资助。

3. Lessons from Pilot Work(预实验发现的问题)

An important product of pilot work is the description of the "lessons learned." Almost inevitably, the pilot will reveal that the intervention did not play out in "real life" the way it was intended "on paper".

预实验的一个重要成果是对"经验教训"的描述。几乎不可避免地，预实验将揭示，干预在"现实生活"中并没有按照"纸面上"的方式进行。

A review of published reports on lessons learned in pilot studies reveals that some lessons are recurrent—which in theory should make them easier to avoid. The following are among the most frequently mentioned lessons from pilot intervention studies :

对已发表的关于预实验中总结经验的报告的回顾表明，有些经验教训是反复出现的——这在理论上应该使它们更容易被避免。以下是预实验中最常提到的经验教训：

(1)Fewer people meet the eligibility criteria than anticipated.

符合资格标准的人数比预期的要少。

(2)Recruitment of participants is more difficult and takes longer than anticipated.

招募参与者比预期得更困难，花费的时间也更长。

(3) Materials intended for direct use by participants (e. g., pamphlets, educational materials) need to be simplified.

供参加者直接使用的材料(例如小册子、教育材料)必须简化。

(4)Participant burden, especially with regard to data collection, needs to be reduced.

需要减轻参与者的负担，特别是在数据收集方面。

(5)Effect sizes tend to be larger in the pilot than in the main trial.

预实验中的效应量往往大于主实验中的效应量。

(6)Key ingredients of the intervention should be front-loaded—that is, delivered early—because greater attention and higher attendance occurs early.

干预的关键因素应该是提前实施的——也就是说，要尽早实施——因为更大的注意力和更高的出席率发生在早期。

(7)When there is a control condition, diffusion and contamination are recurrent problems.

当有对照条件时，扩散和污染是反复出现的问题。

(8)Even expert interventionists need to be trained (and this includes the researchers themselves).

即使是专业的干预人员也需要接受培训(这包括研究人员自己)。

(9)Relationships with others need to be continuously nurtured.

与他人的关系需要不断培养。

Researchers who undertake pilot work should keep these lessons in mind and try to design their study in such a way that frequently occurring problems are avoided.

从事预实验的研究人员应牢记这些教训，并尽量完善研究设计，以避免经常发生的这些问题。

Section Ⅱ　Objectives and Criteria in Pilot Work
第二节　预实验的目标及标准

Writers who offer advice about the conduct of feasibility and pilot studies almost invariably encourage researchers to carefully articulate explicit objectives. Vagueness in delineating what exactly needs to be known in pilot work is likely to result in gaps in the lessons that need to be learned.

为可行性和预实验提供建议的作者总是鼓励研究人员仔细阐明明确的目标。在预实验中需要具体了解哪些方面的不明确性，可能导致注意不到需要吸取的教训。

1. Process-related Objectives(流程相关目标)

Process-related objectives focus on the feasibility of planned procedures for launching and maintaining the study. These include such issues as eligibility criteria, recruitment, retention, comprehension, adherence, acceptability, and human subjects' concerns. Each objective can be addressed by gathering data to answer a variety of questions. Pilot and feasibility assessments are a good way of investigating potential problems in putting an intervention into place—and exploring ways to remedy those problems.

与流程相关的目标集中于启动和维持研究的计划程序的可行性。这些问题包括资格标准、招募、保留、理解、遵守、可接受性和人类受试者关注的问题。每一个目标都可以通过收集数据回答各种问题来实现。预实验和可行性评估是一种很好的方法，可以调查干预措施实施过程中可能出现的问题，并探索解决这些问题的方法。

Pilot work can be useful in revealing the adequacy of the initial eligibility criteria and in suggesting how eligibility criteria affect recruitment, retention, and protocol adherence. Defining the eligibility criteria must take numerous concerns into account, including substantive ones (Should some people be excluded because they might not benefit?), ethical ones (Might certain people be harmed?), methodologic ones (Can eligibility criteria be readily measured? Will the criteria result in an adequate pool for the full-scale trial?), and scientific ones (Will eligibility criteria constrain the generalizability of the findings?). Pilot data can be used to fine-tune decisions about eligibility and about the length of time needed to recruit a sufficiently large sample.

预实验在揭示初始资格标准的充分性和说明资格标准如何影响招募、保留和遵守协议方面是有用的。确定资格标准必须考虑到许多问题，包括实质性问题(一些人是否应该因为他们可能不会受益而被排除在外?)，伦理方面的(某些人是否会受到伤害?)，方法学方面的(资格标准是否容易测量? 这些标准能否为全面实验提供足够的样本池?)和科学的样本池(资格标准是否会限制研究结果的普遍性?)。试点数据可以用来微调有关资格的决定，以及招募足够大的样本所需的时间长度。

A particularly important process issue concerns recruitment—not only of study participants but also of sites and research staff. If a multisite trial is envisioned for the full RCT, feasibility of enlisting cooperative sites should be explored early. It is not just an issue of getting enough sites to achieve an adequate sample size but also of making sure that there are sites that represent the diversity of the target population of participants. Also, if exploration of sites suggests a very high rate of refusals, researchers might want to explore what factors led to refusals by site administrators, especially if those factors are relevant for the eventual uptake of the intervention, should the RCT reveal promising results. For example, if concerns about staff time are a key consideration, the intervention may have little hope of being translated on a large scale.

涉及招募的流程问题至关重要——不仅是研究参与者，还包括场地和研究人员。如果为全面随机对照试验设想进行多中心试验，应尽早探讨征募合作地点的可行性。这不仅仅是一个获得足够的中心来实现足够的样本规模的问题，而且也是一个确保有能够代表参与者目标人群多样性的中心的问题。此外，如果对中心的考察表明有很高的拒绝率，研究人员需要探索是什么因素导致了中心管理者的拒绝——特别是如果这些因素与最终要采取的干预措施有关，随机对照试验是否能显示较好的结果。例如，如果管理者对其工作人员时间的担忧是一个关键的考虑因素，那么这种干预可能没有多大希望被大规模地推广。

Recruitment of participants is a perennial problem in clinical trials, and recruitment is becoming increasingly more challenging. A review of funded trials in the United Kingdom revealed that fewer than one out of three clinical trials successfully recruited the targeted number of participants (Campbell et al., 2007). Quantitative data from the pilot work will answer questions about the feasibility of recruiting a sufficient number for a full trial, but qualitative data may suggest how key barriers can be eliminated or how additional recruitment techniques could be pursued.

在临床试验中，招募参与者是一个长期存在的问题，而且招募变得越来越具有挑战性。一项对英国资助的试验的审查显示，不到 1/3 的临床试验成功招募了目标数量的参与者（Campbell 等，2007）。来自预实验的定量数据将回答关于招募足够数量的人进行全面试验的可行性问题，但定性数据可能会表明如何消除关键障碍或如何采用额外的招募技术。

Poor retention of participants in the study and low protocol adherence (on the part of participants or intervention agents) are two other problems that are strong candidates for scrutiny in pilot work. Attrition can reduce the final sample size for analyses and can also lead to biases in estimating the intervention's potential benefits. High attrition, low adherence to protocols, and low levels of satisfaction suggest that an intervention is not yet ready for a full RCT.

在预实验中，参与者的留存率较低和方案遵守度较低（就参与者或干预执行者而言）是另外两个需要严格审查的问题。流失会减少最终分析样本量，也会导致在评估干预措施的潜在效益时产生偏差。高流失、低遵守方案和低满意度表明，干预措施还没有准备好可以进行全面的随机对照试验。

Human subjects' issues also can be explored during the pilot phase. In particular, researchers need to be vigilant during a pilot regarding any unanticipated human subjects' protection transgressions that would need to be remedied before a main trial could be undertaken. Pilots are also a good place to get feedback about the consent process. Several commentators have pointed out the absence of any special guidelines for the ethical conduct of pilot studies. There is some agreement, however, that researchers have an obligation to disclose the feasibility nature of pilot studies during informed consent procedures (Thabane et al., 2010).

人类受试者问题也可以在预实验进行探讨。特别是，在试验期间，研究人员需要警惕任何预料之外的对人类受试者的保护违规行为，这些行为需要在全面试验进行之前加以纠正。预实验也是一个获得关于知情同意过程反馈的好环节。一些评论人士指出，对于预实验的道德操行，没有任何特别的指导方针。然而，也有一些共识，即研究人员有义务在知情同意程序中披露预实验的可行性（Thabane 等，2010）。

2. Resource-related Objectives(资源相关目标)

Pilots are often a useful way to get a handle on the resources that would be needed in a full-scale trial. Resource objectives typically concern questions about the following aspects of a study:

预实验通常是掌握全面试验所需资源的有效途径。资源目标通常涉及研究的以下方面的问题：

(1)Monetary costs;

货币成本；

(2)Time demands;

时间要求；

(3)Institutional capacity;

机构能力；

(4)Personnel requirements and availability;

人员需求和可用性；

(5)Other resource needs such as equipment, technology, and lab facilities.

其他资源需求，如设备、技术和实验室设施。

3. Management-related Objectives(管理相关目标)

Another category of objectives for pilot work are ones that concern the ability for the research team to manage the effort and for research staff to work productively as a team. Pilot work can help to identify management "glitches" that should be addressed before moving on to a full-scale trial. The management-related objectives in pilot work include assessing feasibility in terms of the following:

预实验的另一类目标涉及研究小组管理工作的能力和研究工作人员作为一个团队进行富有成效的工作的能力。预实验可以帮助确定在进行全面试验之前应该解决的管理"故障"。预实验中与管理有关的目标包括从下列方面评估可行性：

(1) Viability of the site or sites;

一个或多中心的可行性；

(2) Motivation and competence of project staff;

项目员工的积极性和能力；

(3) Adequacy of reporting, monitoring, technologic, and other systems;

报告、监控、技术和其他系统的充分性；

(4) Ability to manage or nurture interpersonal relationships.

管理或培养人际关系的能力。

4. Scientific-Related Objectives: Substantive Issues (科学相关目标——实质性问题)

4.1　Intervention Attributes(干预属性)

A pilot test provides an opportunity to make judgments about whether the decisions made during the development phase regarding intervention content, dose, timing, setting, sequencing, and so on, were sensible ones. A pilot study is an ideal time to make final revisions to the intervention protocols, based on feedback from participants and intervention staff and such other indicators as attendance and feedback about satisfaction.

预实验提供了一个机会来判断在开发阶段所做的关于干预内容、剂量、时间、设置、顺序等决策是否明智。根据参与者和干预人员的反馈，以及出勤率和满意度反馈等其他指标，预实验是对干预方案进行最终修订的理想时机。

4.2   Safety and Tolerability(安全性和耐受性)

Assessing the safety of patients in trials of a new intervention and the tolerability of the intervention are crucial objectives of many pilot studies. Unfortunately, it is widely acknowledged that pilots do a poor job of providing reliable safety and tolerability data because of their small sample size. For example, in a pilot with 30 patients, zero adverse events do not necessarily mean that there are no safety risks.

评估患者在新干预试验中的安全性和干预的耐受性是许多预实验的关键目标。不幸的是，人们普遍认为预实验在提供可靠的安全和耐受性数据方面做得很差，因为他们的样本太小了。例如，在一个有 30 名患者的预实验中，零不良事件并不一定意味着没有安全风险。

4.3   Intervention Efficacy(干预效力)

Most pilot studies are undertaken with the objective of gaining preliminary evidence of the intervention's potential to be efficacious. As previously noted, hypothesis testing is not considered appropriate in pilot tests because of the high risk of making a Type Ⅱ error—that is, falsely concluding that the intervention is not more beneficial than the control treatment, even when it was.

大多数预实验的目的是获得干预的潜在有效性的初步证据。如前所述，假设检验被认为不适合在先导试验中进行，因为它有犯第二类错误的高风险——即错误地得出干预并不比对照治疗更有益的结论，即使干预确实比对照治疗更有益。

4.4   Clinical Significance(临床意义)

Another possible objective for pilot work is an assessment of the likelihood that the intervention will be clinically significant. At the group level, ES estimates are often used to draw conclusions about clinical significance of positive effects. This means that the researchers should establish in advance the size of the effect that would be regarded as clinically significant. For example, the criterion could be based on a consensus reached by an advisory panel of experts. Arnold and colleagues (Arnold et al., 2009) advised that an intervention can be declared to have potential efficacy if the 95% CI around the estimated effect size includes a predesignated minimal for clinical significance. However, given the width of 95% CIs when the sample is small, this may be too liberal a standard. For example, with a sample of 50 pilot participants (25 per group), and a criterion of .50 for a clinically significant d, even an obtained d of 0.0 would meet this criterion (95% CI = −0.57 to 0.57). Thus, it might be more prudent for the advisory group to establish not only the criterion for clinical significance but also the acceptable range. For example, if the criterion were 0.50, experts might set the lower bound at 0.20.

　　预实验的另一个可能目标是评估干预将具有临床意义的可能性。在组水平上，ES 估计经常被用来得出关于积极效应的临床意义的结论。这意味着研究人员应该提前确定被认为具有临床意义的效应的大小。例如，该标准可以根据专家咨询小组达成的共识。Arnold 和他的同事（Arnold 等，2009）建议，如果估计效应量附近的 95% CI 包含一个预先指定的临床意义最小值，就可以宣布干预具有潜在疗效。然而，当样本很小时，考虑到 95% CI 的宽度，这可能是一个过于宽松的标准。例如，对于 50 个试点参与者(每组 25 人)的样本，临床显著 d 的标准为 0.50，即使获得的 d 为 0.0 也符合该标准(95% CI = −0.57 ～ 0.57)。因此，咨询小组不仅要确定临床意义的标准，还要确定可接受的范围，这可能会更加谨慎。例如，如果标准是 0.50，专家可能会将下限设为 0.20。

4.5　Research Design(研究设计)

Preliminary evidence about feasibility can be obtained in feasibility studies using fairly simple designs, such as a one-group pretest-posttest design. However, for a pilot study, the design ideally should be a trial run of the full-scale test. It is precisely because of the need to be confident that an RCT of the full trial is feasible that experts recommend that a pilot study use a randomized design rather than a quasi-experimental one (Conn et al., 2010; Lancaster et al., 2004; Thabane et al., 2010). As noted by Leon and colleagues (Leon et al., 2011), the inclusion of a randomized control group in a pilot study "allows for a more realistic examination of recruitment, randomization, implementation of intervention, blinded assessment procedures, and retention".

　　可行性的初步证据可以在可行性研究中使用相当简单的设计，如单组前-后测设计。然而，对于预实验，理想的设计应该是全面试验的试运行。正是因为需要对整个试验的随机对照试验（RCT）的可行性有信心，专家们才建议预实验采用随机设计而不是准实验设计（Conn 等，2010; Lancaster 等，2004; Thabane 等，2010）。Leon 和他的同事（Leon 等，2011）指出，在一项试点研究中纳入随机对照组"可以对招募、随机化、干预实施、盲法评估程序和保留情况进行更现实的检查"。

4.6　Intervention Fidelity(干预真实性)

Pilots offer researchers the opportunity to examine whether the intervention agents can successfully implement the intervention as planned. In addition, pilots offer an opportunity to assess the adequacy of intervention fidelity procedures. As with other objectives, both quantitative and qualitative data play an important role in helping researchers understand how successful the implementation of the intervention was and identify barriers to full enactment of the intervention protocols. Quantitative data can be used to calculate actual rates of achieving fidelity, and qualitative data can help researchers understand factors that made fidelity difficult to accomplish.

预实验为研究人员提供了检查干预剂是否能按计划成功实施干预的机会。此外，预实验提供了一个机会来评估干预真实度的充分性。与其他目标一样，定量和定性数据在帮助研究人员了解干预实施的成功程度和确定全面制定干预方案的障碍方面发挥着重要作用。定量数据能够用于计算达到真实度的实际比率，定性数据帮助研究者理解导致真实度难以实现的因素。

4.7　Data Collection Protocols and Instruments(数据收集方法及工具)

Researchers make many decisions about data collection instruments and procedures for intervention studies, and a pilot trial offers researchers an opportunity to assess those decisions. Data quality and participant burden are two key areas of inquiry. A pilot provides an opportunity to examine patterns of missing data, to evaluate internal consistency of any scales, to assess comprehension, to explore variability in responses, and to estimate how much time is required to administer the package of instruments. Given the evidence that people often drop out of studies because of a burdensome schedule of data collection, it is important to understand the practicability of the data collection methods. A lengthy data collection instrument is not only risky in terms of attrition but also has cost implications for data collection staff, data entry, and analysis. The pilot might lead researchers to eliminate one or more outcome, to select shorter instruments, or to alter the schedule for measuring outcomes.

研究人员就数据收集工具和干预研究程序做出了许多决定，而预实验为研究人员提供了评估这些决定的机会。数据质量和参与者负担是调查的两个关键领域。预实验提供了一个机会来检查缺失数据的模式，评估任何量表的内部一致性，评估理解，探索反应的变异性，并估计管理工具包需要多少时间。有证据表明，人们经常因为繁重的数据收集计划而放弃学习，理解数据收集方法的实用性是很重要的。冗长的数据收集工具不仅在失访方面有风险，而且对数据收集人员、数据输入和分析也有成本影响。预实验可能会导致研究人员取消一个或多个结果，选择更短的测量工具，或改变测量结果的时间表。

It should be noted that instruments for measuring outcomes should not be developed and evaluated for reliability, validity, and responsiveness in the context of a pilot trial of an intervention, because such evaluations require large samples. Researchers should select instruments with prior evidence of high quality, and then these instruments can be assessed for their adequacy in the context of the pilot.

测量结果的工具不应该在干预试验的背景下开发和评估可靠性、有效性和响应性，因为这样的评估需要大量的样本。研究人员应该选择具有高质量证据的工具，然后可以评估这些工具在试点环境中的充分性。

4.8　Sample Size(样本量)

An objective that is among the most commonly cited reasons for conducting a pilot study is to inform sample size decisions for the main trial. However, performing a power analysis using ES estimates from a pilot is risky because, as we have seen, pilot ES estimates are not reliable.

开展预实验的一个最常见的原因是：为主要试验的样本量决定提供信息。然而，使用预实验的 ES 估计进行效力分析是有风险的，因为，正如我们所看到的，预实验的 ES 估计是不可靠的。

Using the pilot study ES estimate to calculate sample size for a full trial can result in both types of errors in statistical decision making. A large pilot effect size (e. g., d = 0. 80) could reflect an inflated positive result, and possibly a Type I error. In turn, this inflated value would likely result in an underpowered full-scale trial because the sample size projection based on a large ES estimate would be too small. On the other hand, pilot ES estimates can result in a Type II error if the estimate is unduly small. This could lead to a decision to abandon a potentially promising intervention. Several approaches to this dilemma have been proposed. One is to calculate confidence intervals around the ES estimate and then use the lower limit of the CI in the power calculations. However, because the 95% CI results in a range that is unreasonably large with small pilot samples, less conservative CIs have been suggested, such as an 80% CI (Lancaster et al., 2004) or a 68% CI (Hertzog, 2008).

使用预实验 ES 估计值来计算完整试验的样本量可能导致统计决策中的两种类型的错误。一个大的预实验 ES 估计值(例如，d = 0. 80)可以反映一个夸大的积极结果，并可能是第一类错误。反过来，这个夸大的值可能会导致动力不足的全面试验，因为基于大 ES 估计的样本量预测会太小。另一方面，如果预估过小，先导 ES 估计值可能导致第二类误差。这可能导致决定放弃一项可能大有希望的干预行动。已经提出了几种解决这一困境的方法。一种是计算 ES 估计值周围的置信区间，然后在效力计算中使用 CI 的下限。然而，由于在小规模试点样本中，95% CI 导致的范围大得不合理，因此建议采用不太保守的 CI，如 80% CI（Lancaster 等，2004）或 68% CI（Hertzog，2008）。

In short, the most defensible strategy for sample size calculation is to consider a totality of evidence to estimate the size of the effect that is plausibly attainable and clinically meaningful in a main test.

简而言之，对于样本量计算，最合理的策略是考虑全部证据，以估计在主要试验中可能达到且有临床意义的效果的大小。

5. Criteria and Pilot Objectives(预实验目标及标准)

We recommend that researchers select pilot objectives based on several considerations. First, choose objectives for which information is genuinely lacking—that is, objectives that address key uncertainties. You may already have a good estimate of how much attrition to expect, for example, based on your own previous work with the target population or based on attrition rates in other similar trials. Second, select objectives that impinge most significantly on the feasibility of a full-scale trial. For example, if you cannot recruit a sufficient number of participants, a large trial may be impossible, so assessing and enhancing recruitment would be important objectives. Lastly, focus on objectives about which funders will be particularly vigilant. These might include recruitment and efficacy, for example, and might also include resource requirements.

我们建议研究人员根据几个考虑因素选择预实验目标。首先，选择真正缺乏信息的目标——也就是解决关键不确定性的目标。例如，根据你自己之前对目标人群所做的工作，或者根据其他类似试验中的流失率，你可能已经对预期的流失率有了一个很好的估计。第二，选择对全面试验的可行性影响最大的目标。例如，如果你不能招募到足够数量的参与者，大规模的试验可能是不可能实现的，因此评估和加强招募将是重要的目标。最后，把重点放在那些资助者将特别警惕的目标上。例如，这些可能包括招募和效果，也可能包括所需资源。

The importance of articulating key pilot objectives stems from the fact that pilot work should lead to a decision about "next steps." Essentially, there are three options. One decision would be to proceed to a full clinical trial. A second decision would be to make revisions to the intervention protocols, the methodologic protocols, or the procedural processes. The decision to make changes might lead to further Phase I (developmental) work and perhaps to a second pilot, if the needed revisions are major. A third decision would be to abandon the entire effort because of poor prospects of feasibility or acceptability, or lack of adequate evidence that the intervention could be effective.

明确关键的预实验目标之所以重要，是因为预实验工作应决定"下一步"。本质上，有三种选择。第一个决定是进行全面的临床试验。第二个决定是对干预方案、方法方案或程序过程进行修订。做出更改的决定可能会导致进一步的第一阶段(开发)工作，如果需要进行的修改是主要的，可能会导致第二个试点。第三个决定将是放弃整个努力，因为可行性或可接受性前景不佳，或缺乏足够的证据表明干预可能有效。

Most often, researchers who establish criteria look for opportunities to take corrective actions. The decision about "next steps" is likely to depend on how many criteria are not met and the degree of deficiency in meeting them. For example, a 30% recruitment rate when 60% or higher was the benchmark might lead to abandoning the project, but a 50% recruitment rate might lead to making adjustments to enhance recruitment. If identified problems cannot readily be rectified, then researchers might be forced to "go back to the drawing board" in efforts to solve a clinical problem.

大多数情况下，制订标准的研究人员会寻找机会采取纠正措施。关于"下一步"的决定很可能取决于有多少标准未得到满足，以及在满足这些标准方面的不足程度。例如，当基准为60%或更高时，30%的招募率可能会导致放弃该项目，而50%的招聘率可能会导致进行调整以加强招募。如果发现的问题不能轻易得到纠正，那么研究人员可能会被迫"重新开始"，努力解决临床问题。

The decision to move forward to a full trial should be a carefully considered one. In preparing a proposal to fund a rigorous RCT, the research team should be persuaded:

进行全面审判的决定应该经过仔细考虑。在准备资助严格的随机对照试验的提案时，应说服研究团队：

(1) the intervention and the research methods have been found to be feasible;

干预措施和研究方法已被发现是可行的；

(2) any pitfalls for a rigorous test have been identified and solutions to potential problems have been identified;

严格试验的任何缺陷已被发现，潜在问题的解决方案已被确定；

（3）there is preliminary evidence that the intervention will be effective；

有初步证据表明干预将是有效的；

（4）important stakeholders are "on board".

重要的利益相关者已"加入"。

Section Ⅲ　The Design and Methods of Pilot and Feasibility Studies
第三节　预实验的设计及方法

1. Research Design in Pilot Work(预实验研究设计)

As previously noted, we strongly encourage using a randomized design for a pilot trial, especially if the plan is to use the pilot as the basis for requesting funding for a full-scale trial. To the extent possible, all of the design features for the full trial should be tested, including the control group strategy, procedures for blinding, outcome measures, and the schedule of data collection.

如前所述，我们强烈鼓励在预实验中采用随机设计，特别是如果计划将预实验作为申请全面试验资金的基础。在可能的情况下，应测试整个试验的所有设计特征，包括对照组策略、盲法程序、结局测量和数据收集时间表。

In a feasibility study, simpler designs are usually sufficient. Simple descriptive designs may suffice—for example, if a major goal is to assess the number of eligible or to estimate how many sites could be recruited. One-group designs are often used to assess aspects of the intervention itself, such as whether the content is adequate or whether participants find the intervention acceptable.

在可行性研究中，简单的设计通常就足够了。简单的描述性设计可能就足够了——例如，如果主要目标是评估符合条件的数目或估计可以在多少个地点进行招募。单组设计经常被用来评估干预本身的各个方面，例如内容是否足够或参与者是否认为干预是可接受的。

2. Sampling in Pilot Work(预实验抽样)

The sample used in pilot work should be drawn from the same population as the population for the main trial. This means that the eligibility criteria should be the same—although these criteria might be adjusted during the course of the pilot if researchers run into unanticipated problems.

预实验的样本应与主体试验的样本在同一总体中抽取。这意味着资格标准应该是相同的——如果研究人员在试点过程中遇到意想不到的问题,这些标准可能会被调整。

Conventional power calculations are not appropriate for pilot studies because the study purpose is not to test hypotheses about intervention outcomes. However, several experts have suggested that researchers could use confidence intervals to estimate the sample size needed to establish feasibility (e.g., Arnold 等, 2009; Hertzog, 2008; Thabane 等, 2010). For example, suppose we decided a priori that a full-scale trial would be feasible if the rate of attrition from the study was no more than 20% at a 3-month follow-up. Based on evidence from other similar trials (or Phase I development work), we predict that the actual rate of attrition will be 12%. If we used a confidence interval of 95% around the expected attrition rate of 12%, we would need a total sample size of 64 for the upper bound of the confidence interval not to exceed the criterion of 20% attrition (95% CI around 12% = 4% to 20% for N=64). If we relaxed our standard to a less stringent 90% CI for the same scenario, the needed total sample size would be 46 (90% CI around 12%=4% to 20% for N=46).

传统的效力计算不适合预实验,因为预实验的目的不是测试关于干预结果的假设。然而,一些专家建议,研究人员可以使用置信区间来估计建立可行性所需的样本大小(e.g., Arnold 等, 2009; Hertzog, 2008; Thabane 等, 2010)。例如,假设我们预先决定,在3个月的随访中,研究的损失率不超过20%,则全面试验是可行的。根据其他类似试验(或第一阶段开发工作)的证据,我们预测实际的人员流失率将为12%。如果我们使用95%的置信区间的预期流失率12%,我们需要一个总样本量为64且置信区间的上限不超过20%的标准失访(95% CI 约 12%=4%~20%, N=64)。对于相同的情况,如果我们将标准放宽到不那么严格的90% CI,则需要的总样本量为46(90% CI 约为12%=4%~20%, N=46)。

The ideal sample size for a pilot will vary from study to study because of differences in objectives and populations. Hertzog (2008), however, has recommended a pilot size of at least 30-40 per group if funding for the pilot is being sought.

由于目标和人群的不同,理想的预实验样本量将因研究而异。然而,Hertzog (2008)建议,如果寻求预实验的资金,每个小组的试点规模至少为30~40人。

486

3. Data Collection in Pilot Work(预实验数据收集)

The data collection plan for pilots is typically complex because the pilot data serve two purposes: to test the viability of the instruments that would be used in the main trial and to address the various objectives of the pilot itself.

预实验的数据收集计划通常很复杂，因为预实验有两个目的：测试将用于主要试验的工具的可行性，以及解决试验本身的各种目标。

In terms of the second purpose, the type of data to be collected depends on what the specific objectives are. For example, if one objective is to assess the acceptability of the intervention, then a quantitative measure of patient satisfaction should probably be used. If an objective is to ascertain success in screening for eligibility, then forms for extracting information from records are required.

至于第二个目的，要收集的数据类型取决于具体的目标。例如，如果一个目标是评估干预的可接受性，那么可能应该使用患者满意度的定量测量。如果目标是确定是否成功筛选合格，则需要从记录中提取信息的表格。

Thought needs to be given to how best to "get inside" the workings of the pilot through the collection of in-depth data. This is likely to include unstructured observations of various intervention activities (e.g., recruitment, consent procedures, intervention sessions). Participants in both the intervention and control group could be asked to complete exit interviews. Focus group interviews could also be conducted with various stakeholders, including participants, family members, and pilot study staff.

我们需要思考如何通过收集深入的数据来"了解"预实验的工作。这可能包括各种干预活动的非结构化观察(例如，招募、同意程序、干预会议)。干预组和对照组的参与者都可以被要求完成退出研究的访谈。焦点小组访谈也可以与各种利益相关者进行，包括参与者、家庭成员和预实验工作人员。

4. Data Analysis in Pilot Work(预实验数据分析)

The analysis of quantitative data from a pilot study should be driven by the pilot study objectives and therefore tends to involve mainly descriptive statistics. For example, the analysis might indicate what percentage of eligible people agreed to participate or were randomized.

Means and standard deviations are likely to be computed (e.g., mean number of sessions completed, mean length of time to complete the data collection forms). ES estimates may also be computed. For obtaining preliminary evidence about clinical significance, some researchers compute the number needed to treat (NNT).

对预实验的定量数据的分析应受预实验目标的推动，因此往往主要涉及描述性统计。例如，分析可能表明同意参与或随机参与的合格人群的百分比。可能计算平均值和标准偏差(例如，完成会话的平均次数，完成数据收集表格的平均时间长度)。也可以计算 ES 估计值。为了获得临床意义的初步证据，一些研究人员计算了需治疗的人数 (NNT)。

In most of these cases, it is a good idea to compute confidence intervals around estimates. An up-front decision should be made about the desired level of precision (e.g., 68%, 90%). These analyses should yield information that would be compared to the criteria established at the outset and then to a decision about how best to proceed.

在大多数情况下，计算估计值的置信区间是一个好主意。应该预先决定所需的精度水平(例如，68%、90%)。这些分析应提供资料，与开始时确定的标准进行比较，然后就如何最好地进行作出决定。

The analysis of the quantitative data from pilots can be used to guide decisions about how to proceed based on a comparison of the results to the preestablished criteria. Thematic analysis of the qualitative can confirm the wisdom of that decision and can also help researchers make adjustments to improve the likelihood that a full trial will be successful in giving the intervention a fair test.

对预实验的定量数据的分析可用于指导如何根据结果与预先确定的标准进行比较的决定。定性的主题分析可以证实这一决定是明智的，也可以帮助研究人员做出调整，以提高整个审判成功的可能性，从而给予干预一个公平的测试。

Section Ⅳ Products of Pilot Work
第四节 预实验的结果

Pilot work should result in several products. As previously noted, one product should be a compilation of "lessons learned," which ideally should be drafted and reviewed by the research team, advisory panel, and key stakeholders for accuracy and completeness. Other products may include the following:

预实验应产生若干成果。如前所述，一个成果应该是"经验教训"的汇编，理想情况下应该由研究团队、顾问小组和关键利益相关者起草和审查，以确保准确性和完整性。其他成果可能包括：

（1）Revised protocols for the intervention and the research plan（or, if major revisions are needed, a plan for further descriptive and exploratory research）;

修订干预方案和研究计划（或，如果需要重大修订，进一步描述性和探索性研究计划）;

（2）A finalized list of proposed outcomes;

建议结局的最终清单;

（3）A formal proposal for a full Phase Ⅲ trial（or for another pilot）and a plan for seeking funding;

完整的三期试验（或另一个预实验）的正式提案和寻求资金的计划;

（4）A written manuscript for publication in a professional journal.

在专业期刊上发表的书面手稿。

Even if a pilot trial suggests that the intervention has little hope of being effective, that knowledge should be shared. Others working on the same or a similar problem can benefit from learning about failures as well as successes. A related issue is the importance of including findings from pilots in meta-analyses and systematic reviews, especially if the pilot does not translate into a full trial. Meta-analysts must struggle with the issue of publication bias—that is, the tendency to publish studies only when there are statistically significant results. Such a tendency does a disservice to evidence-based practitioners who are then using a biased subset of the evidence.

即使预实验表明，干预措施收效甚微，知识也应该共享。其他处理相同或类似问题的人可以从失败和成功中受益。一个相关的问题是，在 Meta 分析和系统回顾中纳入预实验结果的重要性，特别是在预实验没有转化为全面试验的情况下。Meta 分析必须努力解决发表偏倚的问题，即只在统计上有显著结果时才发表研究的倾向。这种倾向对循证从业者是一种伤害，他们使用的是有偏见的证据子集。

Section Ⅴ　Critiquing Feasibility and Pilot Studies
第五节　评判可行性研究及预实验

Reports of pilot studies should adhere to many of the guidelines described in earlier chapters. For example, the report should provide descriptions of sample characteristics, design elements, instruments, and so on. The intervention theory and development of the intervention should be described or a reference should be provided to any previously published papers on intervention development work. Readers should be able to draw their own conclusions about the potential feasibility and efficacy of the intervention, and so information about the key features of intervention itself needs to be included.

预实验的报告应遵循前几章所述的许多准则。例如，报告应该提供样本特性、设计元素、工具等的描述。应描述干预理论和干预的发展，或提供任何以前发表的关于干预发展工作的论文的参考资料。读者应该能够对干预的潜在可行性和有效性得出自己的结论，因此需要包括干预本身的关键特征的信息。

A critique of pilot work should focus on the researchers' description of the pilot objectives, the criteria used to make decisions about feasibility, and the methods associated with feasibility assessments. Of course, if objectives and criteria were not articulated, readers should be critical of these omissions. If objectives and criteria were stated, readers can assess their reasonableness and judge whether the methods used to assess them were adequate.

对预实验的评价应集中在研究人员对预实验目标的描述，用于作出可行性决定的标准，以及与可行性评估相关的方法。当然，如果没有明确说明目标和标准，读者应该对这些遗漏提出批评。如果有明确的目标和标准，读者可以评估这些目标和标准的合理性，并判断用来评估这些目标和标准的方法是否适当。

📖 Studies Cited in Chapter 23（第二十三章参考文献）

[1] Arnold, D. M., Meade, M. O., Cook, D. J., et al. The design and interpretation of pilot trials in clinical research in critical care[J]. Critical Care Medicine, 2009, 37: S69-S74.

[2] Campbell, M. K., Snowdon, C., Francis, D., et al. Recruitment to randomised trials: strategies for trial enrollment and participation study[J]. Health Technology Assessment (Winchester, England), 2007, 11(48).

[3] Conn, V. S., Algase, D. L., Rawl, et al. Publishing Pilot Intervention Work[J]. Western Journal of Nursing Research, 2010, 32(8): 994-1010.

[4] Hertzog, M. A. Considerations in determining sample size for pilot studies[J]. Research in Nursing and Health, 2008, 31(2): 180-191.

[5] Lancaster, G. A., Dodd, S., Williamson, P. R. Design and analysis of pilot studies: recommendations for good practice[J]. Journal of Evaluation in Clinical Practice, 2004, 10

（2）：307-312.

［6］Leon, A. C., Davis, L. L., Kraemer, H. C. The role and interpretation of pilot studies in clinical research［J］. Journal of Psychiatric Research, 2011, 45（5）：626-629.

［7］Thabane, L., Ma, J., Chu, R., et al. A tutorial on pilot studies：the what, why and how ［J］. BMC Medical Research Methodology, 2010, 10：1.

Chapter 24: Writing Proposals to Generate Evidence
第二十四章 撰写研究计划书以形成证据

Section I Overview of a Research Proposal
第一节 研究计划书概述

1. Concept of a Research Proposal(研究计划书的概念)

A research proposal is a document proposing a research idea, which generally requests for funding to complete that research project. A research proposal is initiated to solve specific research problems with proposed methods of solving the problems. A research proposal can be written by a variety of individuals, such as doctoral students, post-doctoral scholars, faculty, and research scientists.

研究计划书是一份提出研究想法的文件，通常是为了完成研究课题寻求资金资助。研究计划书是为了解决具体的研究问题而提出的，并提出解决问题的方法。一份研究计划书可以由各种人撰写，如博士、博士后、教师和研究科学家。

2. Functions of a Research Proposal(研究计划书的作用)

2.1 Communication of Research Ideas and Concepts(研究想法和概念的交流)

A research proposal is used to communicate research ideas and concepts among various groups, including researchers, reviewers, funding agencies, and policymakers. The researchers are responsible for proposing their research ideas to funding agencies, which either accept the proposal with financial sponsorship of the projects or reject the proposed proposal without financial sponsorship. The researchers have opportunities to revise and resubmit the proposal based on the reviewers' comments and critiques. Most research proposals require revision and resubmission to get funded. After a research proposal is funded, the principal investigator(s) is responsible for reporting progress to the funding agency. The funding agency may require continuous review and monitoring of the project based on specific research policies and annual review criteria.

　　研究计划书通常用来在不同的团体之间交流研究想法和概念，包括研究者、评审员、资助机构和政策制定者。研究者负责向资助机构提出研究想法，资助机构可以接受这个计划书并为课题提供资金资助，也可以拒绝提出的计划书，不提供资金资助。研究者通常有机会基于评审员的意见和建议来修改和重新提交计划书。大多数研究计划书都需要修改和重新提交才能获得资助。在这些受资助的研究项目中，研究者负责向资助机构报告进展情况。资助机构可能需要根据其研究政策和年度审查标准对项目进行持续的审查和监测。

2.2　Action Plans of Research Projects(研究课题的实施计划)

A research proposal lists the detailed action plan of the researchers' ideas and thoughts. This action plan is a step-by-step guide for the researchers on how to conduct the study. From research ideas to grant writing, ambiguities must be addressed at an early stage. Grant reviewers from a specific funding panel make comments and critiques to improve the research proposal. The research proposal helps the research team understand how to proceed with the study as well as keep everyone on the same page.

　　研究计划书列举了关于研究者的想法和思考的详细行动计划。这个行动计划是研究者如何一步步进行研究的指南。从研究思路到基金写作，歧义必须在早期阶段得到解决。来自特定资助小组的基金评审员会提出意见和建议，以改进计划书。研究计划书可以帮助研究团队理解如何进行研究，并让每个成员达成共识。

2.3　Agreement Between Different Parties(不同团体之间的合约)

A research proposal is the foundation to negotiate with other parties (e.g., funding agencies, reviewers, and policy makers). A proposal must be shared with administrators (e.g., the program officers from the National Institute of Health (NIH)) when seeking institutional approval for funding to sponsor a study. Prior to initiating the study, the research proposal is required to be reviewed by different review committees, such as Institutional Review Boards (IRBs) for human subjects or Institutional Animal Care and Use Committee (IACUC) for use of animal models.

　　计划书是研究者和其他团体之间协商的基础(如资助机构、评审员和政策制定者)。当寻求机构的批准来赞助一项研究的资金时，研究计划书必须和管理者共享（如来自美国国立卫生研究院（NIH）的项目管理官员）。在开始研究之前，所有的研究计划书都被要求由不同的评审委员会进行审查，如针对人类受试者的机构评审委员会（IRBs）或针对动物模型使用的机构动物保护和使用委员会（IACUC）。

3. Proposal Content(研究计划书的内容)

In the research proposal, reviewers want to understand what is planned to be studied, why this concept is needed, what methods will be adopted to accomplish the research goals, how, when, and what tasks will be completed, and whether the research team has the resources, manpower, and capabilities to successfully complete the study. According to the NIH, one research proposal is generally evaluated based on several primary merit-review criteria, such as significance (i. e., the importance of the question), innovation (i. e., the new contributions to the literature), approach (i. e., the adequacy of the methods), investigator(s) (i. e., the team's skills and capabilities), and environment (i. e., appropriate environment with needed support and resources). The content and structure of a research proposal are generally similar to those for a research report, but the proposal is written in the future tense and does not have results and conclusions. A proposal uses specific structures based on the instructions from different institutions and funding agencies. Funding agencies provide application guidelines with specific forms to be completed and specify how to organize the proposal content. For a student thesis or dissertation, universities issue detailed guidelines for degree-related proposal.

在研究计划书中，评审员想要了解计划研究什么，为什么这个概念是必须的，完成研究目标需要采取什么方法，如何、何时、将完成什么任务，以及研究团队是否有资源、人力和能力来成功地完成研究。根据美国国立卫生研究院的要求，通常基于几个主要的价值审查标准来评价研究计划书，如重要性（即问题的重要性）、创新性（即对研究的新贡献）、研究方法（即方法的准确性）、调查者（即团队的技术和能力），以及环境（即具有所需支持和资源的适当环境）。大多数研究计划书的内容和结构与研究报告的内容和结构大致相似，但计划书是用将来时态撰写，没有结果和结论。计划书根据不同的所属机构和资助机构的说明使用特定结构。资助机构会提供申请指南，包括需要填写的具体表格，并具体说明如何组织计划书的内容。对于学生的毕业论文和学位论文，学校会发布详细的开题报告模板。

The process of planning and writing a proposal begins with the planning phase, in which the researcher should consider several questions (Bai et al., 2021) (see Table 24.1.1). After the planning phase, the researcher starts writing the proposal and specifically addresses the following contents, including (1) background and importance; (2) specific aims; (3) research design; (4) approaches (i.e., participants, settings, ethical consideration, measures, data collection, data processing and analysis, and time plan).

规划和撰写计划书的过程从规划阶段开始，在规划阶段研究者应该考虑几个问题（Bai 等，2021）（见表 24.1.1）。规划阶段结束后，研究人员开始撰写计划书，并具体阐述以下内容：（1）背景和重要性；（2）具体目标；（3）研究设计；（4）方法（即参与者、环境、伦理考虑、措施、数据收集、数据处理和分析，以及时间计划）。

Table 24.1.1　**Questions in the Planning Phase 规划阶段的问题**

Questions	问题
What is the research question?	研究问题是什么?
What is innovative that expands the science?	拓展科学研究的什么创新性?
Why is answering this question necessary?	为什么回答这个问题是必须的?
How can the question best be answered?	怎样可以更好地回答这个问题?
What resources are needed to answer the question?	回答这个问题需要什么资源?
Who is capable to conduct this study?	谁有能力开展这个研究?

Section Ⅱ　Types of Research Proposals
第二节　研究计划书的类型

1. Writing Research Proposals for Quantitative Studies(量性研究计划书的撰写)

A proposal for quantitative research has specific structures according to different funding agencies. For example, both the NIH from the United States and the Natural Science Foundation of China (NSFC) have posted specific requirements and example of how to write a quantitative proposal. These standardized and successful examples not only help researchers write their own proposal based on their research interest, but also help the proposal reviewers evaluate the quality of the proposal based on specific criteria as mentioned above. Both the NIH and NSFC have specific criteria for grant review and detailed information can be found on the NIH and NSFC websites.

量性研究的计划书根据不同的资助机构的要求有特定的结构。例如美国国立卫生研究院和中国国家自然科学基金委员会(NSFC)已经发布了关于如何撰写量性研究计划书的具体要求和示例。这些标准的和成功的示例不仅有助于研究人员根据他们感兴趣的研究撰写自己的计划书，还有助于计划书评审员根据上述具体的标准评估计划书的质量。美国国立卫生研究院和中国国家自然科学基金委员会都有特定的拨款审查标准，详细的信息可在官方网站上找到。

Table 24. 2. 1 describes some detailed components for a quantitative proposal based on the NIH and NSFC criteria. The researchers should pay attention to each component carefully when writing the proposal. Writing a compelling quantitative proposal is one skill that must be cultivated by working with other experienced researchers and mentors. Taking time to learn from the setbacks and successes of others can increase the rate of successful grant proposals (Gholipour, Lee, & Warfield, 2014; Sohn, 2020). Detailed information about each step is presented in the following section entitled "Writing Research Proposals for Theses and Dissertations".

根据美国国立卫生研究院和中国国家自然科学基金委员会的标准，表 24.2.1 描述了量性研究计划书的一些详细组成内容。研究人员在撰写计划书时应仔细注意每个部分。撰写令人信服的量性研究计划书是必须通过与其他有经验的研究人员和导师合作来培养的一项技能。花时间从别人的挫折和成功中学习，可以提高计划书获得资助的成功率(Gholipour, Lee & Warfield, 2014; Sohn, 2020)。每个步骤的详细信息将在下面"开题报告的撰写"部分中介绍。

Table 24. 2. 1　　**Components of Quantitative Research Proposals**

(量性研究计划书的结构)

	NIH	NSFC	NSSF
Background(背景)	✓	✓	✓
Background of the selected research problem(选题背景)	✓	✓	✓
Significant problem, solving problem aligned with mission of sponsor(重要问题，解决与资助者的任务一样的问题)	✓	✓	✓
Research purpose(研究目的)	✓	✓	✓

续表

	NIH	NSFC	NSSF
Presents solutions to the problem(给出问题的解决方案)	✓	✓	✓
Outlines key steps to address a critical need(概述解决关键需求的关键步骤)	✓	✓	✓
Overall impact(总体影响)	✓	✓	✓
Literature review(文献回顾)	✓	✓	✓
Significance(意义)	✓	✓	✓
Significance of the study(研究的意义)	✓	✓	✓
Innovations of the proposal(计划书的创新点)	✓	✓	✓
Specific aims(具体目标)	✓	✓	✓
Approach(方法)	✓	✓	✓
Research questions(研究问题)	✓	✓	✓
Theoretical framework(理论框架)	✓	✓	✓
Research ideas/Technical route(研究思路/技术路线)	✓	✓	✓
Setting(研究场所)	✓	✓	✓
Population or data sources(人群或数据来源)	✓	✓	✓
Ethical considerations(伦理考虑)	✓	✓	✓
Research design(研究设计)	✓	✓	✓
Intervention protocol（if applicable）(干预协约)（如果适用)	✓	✓	✓
Survey instruments or measures(调查工具或措施)	✓	✓	✓
Collection procedures(收集程序)	✓	✓	✓
Power calculation(功率计算)	✓	✓	✓
Data analysis(数据分析)	✓	✓	✓
Annual research plan and expected results(年度研究计划和预期结果)	✓	✓	✓
Feasibility analysis of the study(研究的可行性分析)	✓	✓	✓
Funding budget(资金预算)	✓	✓	✓
Other problems to clarify(其他需要阐明的问题)	✓	✓	✓
References(参考文献)	✓	✓	✓

2. Writing Research Proposals for Qualitative Studies(质性研究计划书的撰写)

There are specific challenges to prepare a proposal for qualitative research (Klopper, 2008). As the methodological decisions keep evolving in the field, it is rarely possible to provide detailed information for the qualitative proposal, particularly when discussing sample size or data collection strategies. Sufficient details are generally provided in the proposal so that the reviewers understand that the researcher will collect the appropriate data with rigorous collection methods. Qualitative researchers must ensure that the research topic is important, innovative, and worth investigating. Some detailed information regarding the approaches should be provided, even it is different from a quantitative proposal. Knafl and Deatrick (2005) offer 10 tips for a successful qualitative grant writing and application. These tips advise qualitative researchers to (1) use examples to clarify the research design; (2) justify the sample design and sample size for specific studies; and (3) identify qualitative approaches based on the study topic.

准备质性研究计划书有一些特殊的挑战（Klopper, 2008）。由于该领域的方法论决策不断演变，质性研究计划书的撰写过程中很少能提供详细的信息，特别是在讨论样本大小或数据收集策略时。一般来说，计划书中会提供足够的细节，以便评审员了解研究者将以严格的收集方法收集适当的数据。质性研究者必须确保研究主题是重要的、创新的和值得调查的。即使质性研究的计划书与量性研究计划书不同，它也应该提供一些关于研究方法的详细信息。Knafl 和 Deatrick（2005）提供了成功撰写和申请质性研究基金的十大技巧。这些技巧建议质性研究者：（1）使用示例来阐明研究设计；（2）证明具体研究的样本设计和样本量的合理性；（3）根据研究主题确定质性研究方法。

A variety of rich resources are available to guide qualitative researchers in proposal writing and application. For example, the *Journal Qualitative Health Research* published an entire issue (Volume 13, Issue 6) in 2003 devoted to qualitative proposal preparing and writing. Some other useful resources are Carey and Swanson (2003), Padgett and Henwood (2009), and Sandelowski and Barroso (2003). In addition, Sandelowski (2015) provides advice for evaluating the quality of qualitative research.

有各种丰富的资源可用于指导质性研究者的计划书写作和申请。例如，《质性健康研究》杂志在 2003 年出版了整整一期(第 13 卷第 6 期)关于质性研究计划书的准备和写作的内容。其他一些有用的资源也可以在 Carey 和 Swanson（2003），Padgett 和 Henwood

（2009），以及 Sandelowski 和 Barroso（2003）中找到。此外，Sandelowski（2015）为评估质性研究计划书的质量提供建议。

3. Writing Research Proposals for Thesis and Dissertation Proposals （开题报告的撰写）

Thesis and dissertation proposals are sometimes more difficult than theses and dissertations themselves. Students (e.g., master or doctoral degrees) use knowledge from their research training and prepare the proposals under the mentorship of the thesis or dissertation committee, which is generally comprised of 3-4 experts in the field. A great mentorship team is crucial during this proposal writing phase (Bai et al., 2021). The master or doctoral candidates need to actively pursue feedback and comments from the thesis or dissertation committee at the proposal development stage. A well-prepared proposal builds a solid basis for the thesis or dissertation writing and defense. The proposal for a thesis or dissertation primarily includes the following chapters: Introduction; Literature Review; Methodology; and References (Creswell & Creswell, 2018). Creswell and Creswell (2018) provide detailed information regarding the research design of quantitative, qualitative, and mixed studies, with additional research proposal tools and sample student proposals.

毕业论文和学位论文的开题报告有时比论文本身更难。学生(如硕士或博士)利用研究训练中的知识，在学位论文委员会的指导下准备开题报告，该委员会一般由该领域的3~4名专家组成。在这个计划书撰写阶段，一个优秀的指导团队非常重要（Bai 等，2021）。攻读硕士或博士学位的人需要在计划书制订阶段积极征求学位论文委员会的反馈和意见。一份精心准备的计划书为毕业论文和学位论文的写作和答辩打下坚实的基础。计划书主要包括以下几部分：前言，文献综述，方法论，以及参考文献（Creswell 和 Creswell，2018）。Creswell 和 Creswell（2018）提供了有关量性、质性和混合研究的研究设计的详细信息，附加研究计划的工具和开题报告示例。

3.1 Introduction（前言）

One to two paragraphs are used to discuss the general context of the research topic or question. Sometimes it may be recognized as the background to the study. The introduction is an expansion of the abstract and sets the stage for the literature review. This introduction chapter determines the outline of the body of the literature review. Since it is a synthesis and summary of previous work, the student must appropriately cite the sources at the end of the text or as needed within the paragraphs. Specifically, the student should plan on one to two paragraphs of general context regarding the research topic. Then, the student provides one to two paragraphs of more specific context regarding the research topic. These paragraphs prepare the audience to understand the statement of the research problem.

用 1~2 段来讨论研究主题或问题的一般背景。有时，前言可能被认为是研究的背景。前言是摘要的扩展，也为文献回顾做铺垫。前言章节确定了文献综述主体的大纲。因为文献回顾是对之前工作的综合和总结，学生必须在段落的末尾或根据需要在段落内适当地引用文献。具体来说，学生应该计划用 1~2 段话来介绍有关研究主题的一般背景。然后，学生再提供 1~2 段关于研究主题的更具体的背景。这些段落为读者理解研究问题的陈述做好准备。

3.1.1　Statement of the Research Problem(研究问题的陈述)

Following the general introduction, one concise paragraph should be developed to discuss the research problem. Specific information is needed when describing the research problem. For example, a student is interested in investigating the factors associated with the high prevalence of pain in women with breast cancer receiving chemotherapy.

在介绍大概背景之后，将用一个简洁的段落来讨论研究问题。在描述研究问题时，需要具体的信息。例如，一个学生有兴趣调查与接受化疗的乳腺癌妇女的疼痛高发率有关的因素。

3.1.2　Purpose of the Study(研究目的)

One paragraph should discuss what the research proposal is doing. This is made obvious in the argument of the literature review. This is a brief statement of how the research problem is investigated. For example, the purpose of this study is to examine the prevalence of pain in women with breast cancer receiving chemotherapy and the risk factors of pain development and severity in this population.

用一个段落来讨论研究计划书将要做什么。这一点在文献回顾的论证中是很明显的。这是对如何调查研究问题的简要陈述。例如，本研究的目的是研究接受化疗的乳腺癌妇女的疼痛发生率，以及这一人群中疼痛发生和严重疼痛的风险因素。

3.1.3　Significance of the Study(研究的意义)

The significance of the study is very critical in the research proposal. It plays an important role to determine the quality of the proposal. It discusses the benefits of addressing the research problem for the population of the proposal or even the academic community. It is one major review criteria for NIH funding. For example, this study will provide evidence to health professionals, educators, staff members, and policymakers to design an intervention to decrease women's suffering from pain when receiving chemotherapy.

研究的意义在研究计划书中非常关键，它决定着计划书的质量、讨论解决该研究问题对研究人群甚至学术界的好处，是美国国立卫生研究院的一个主要资助审查标准。例如，这项研究将为卫生专业人员、教育者、工作人员和政策制定者提供证据，以设计一种干预措施来减少妇女在接受化疗时经历的疼痛。

3.1.4 Theory or Theoretical Perspective(理论或理论视角)

A brief discussion of the theory the quantitative research study is investigating or a brief discussion of the theoretical perspective of the qualitative research should be provided.

简要讨论量性研究正在调查的理论，或简要讨论质性研究应该提供的理论视角。

3.1.5 Research Method(研究方法)

A concise paragraph is needed to describe the research method used to investigate the problem. This can be expanded into the preamble of your research methods chapter.

用一个简洁的段落来描述用于调查这个问题的研究方法。这可以在后面研究方法那部分进行扩展。

3.1.6 Limitations of the Study(研究的局限性)

A brief description of what your research design cannot accomplish due to the scope of the project or limitations of time/resources.

简要说明你的研究设计由于课题的范围或时间/资源的限制而无法完成的内容。

3.1.7 Summary(总结)

A summary paragraph is generally developed to wrap up the introduction chapter with the summarization of the chapter and a transition to the next section.

通常用一个总结段落来对前言章节进行总结并过渡到下一章节。

3.2 Literature Review(文献回顾)

The literature review starts with a preamble, which does not need a heading. Following the brief introduction, two to four paragraphs set the context for the literature review and discuss what is covered in the literature review chapter.

文献回顾以序言开始，不需要有标题。在简要介绍之后，用2~4段为文献回顾设定背景，并讨论文献回顾部分将涵盖或完成的内容。

3.2.1 Review of Related Research(回顾相关研究)

The literature review provides a synthesis and summary of previous related research targeting the research problem, the strengths and weaknesses, and a justification of the research — What is already known or has been done by others? Why this research is still necessary? And What is new in this proposal? It is important that the researchers conduct a systematic search of the literature associated with the study topic, identify relevant studies, synthesize, and summarize the findings. The literature synthesis and conclusion will address the significance of the study and guide the researchers to understand the current research gap (i. e., What is still missing or needs further study?). A well-written literature review also directly or indirectly addresses the innovation of the proposal (i. e., What is new in the proposal and what will be added to current literature?).

文献回顾对之前针对该研究问题的研究进行了综合和总结，包括优点和不足，也使你的研究合理化——别人已知或已经做过什么？为什么你的研究仍然是必要的？你的计划书有哪些创新点？重要的是研究者必须系统地检索与研究主题相关的文献，确定相关的研究，综合和总结研究结果。文献回顾和结论将强调研究的重要性并指导研究者了解目前的研究空白点(即还缺少或需要什么研究？)。一个写得好的文献综述部分还能直接或间接地强调计划书的创新之处(即研究计划书中有哪些新内容，以及对目前的文献将有哪些补充？)。

3.2.2 Theoretical Framework(理论框架)

In a quantitative proposal, a theoretical framework is generally adopted to guide the research proposal and provide rationales to operationalize the study variables. At minimum, this should include the dependent variable (i. e., constant), the independent variable (i. e., factors that affect the dependent variable), and the moderating and intervening variables. Sometimes, a figure is designed to describe the relationships between all these study variables and explain the abstract concepts of the theoretical construct or framework.

在量性研究中，通常采用一个理论框架来指导研究计划书，并为研究变量的操作化提供依据。这至少应包括因变量（即常数）、自变量（即影响因变量的因素），以及调节变量和干预变量。有时，会设计一个图来描述所有这些研究变量之间的关系，并解释理论结构或框架的抽象概念。

3.2.3　Summary(总结)

A summary paragraph is provided for a brief discussion of what has covered in the chapter and a transition to the next chapter.

提供一个总结段落来简要讨论本章中介绍的内容，也为下一章的内容做铺垫。

3.3　Methodology(方法学)

The methodology chapter describes the worldview of the proposal, the research design (e. g., observation, randomized controlled trials (RCTs), quasi-experiments, or systematic review and meta-analysis), the underpinning practices, and procedures for conducting and replicating the research study. It informs the scholars and practitioners regarding the rigor and the appropriateness of the methodology in relation to the scholarly community in which the research proposal belongs.

方法学一章描述了计划书的世界观、研究设计（如观察、随机对照试验(RCTs)、类实验或系统综述和元分析）、基础实践，以及进行和复制研究的程序，它让学者和从业人员了解到研究方案所属的学术界方法的严谨性和适当性。

3.3.1　Research Questions(研究问题)

Developing a research question is one of the most challenging tasks when proposing a project. The research questions are clearly stated in the argument of the literature review. The researchers need to list, and then discuss each of the general questions that determine what methods will be used and what type of data will be collected. All research questions are indicated by the research problem and bound by the theoretical perspective and the research methodology. The PICO(T) (Population, Intervention, Control, Outcomes, and Time) format is a widely used strategy for framing a research question (Aslam & Emmanuel, 2010). Breaking the research question into five components will facilitate the identification of relevant information

（Figure 24.2.1）. The PICO（T） format will help with searching databases, uncovering evidence, and refining the purpose statement.

　　在提出一个项目时，制订一个研究问题是具有挑战性的任务之一。研究问题在文献综述的论证中被清楚地陈述。研究者需要列出并讨论每一个决定你将使用什么方法和收集什么类型数据的一般问题。所有的研究问题都以范围较大的研究问题为指示，并受到理论视角和研究方法约束。PICO(T)（人群，干预，控制，结果，时间）格式是一种广泛使用的构建研究问题的策略（Aslam 和 Emmanuel，2010）。PICO(T)将研究问题分成五个部分，将有利于识别相关信息（见图 24.2.1）。PICO(T)将有助于推进数据库的搜索，发现证据，并精简研究目的的陈述。

P—Patient, population, or problem
I—Intervention
C—Comparison with other groups, interventions, etiologies, prognosis
O—Outcomes：what outcome or result do you anticipate or may look for
T（optional）—Time period for observation/investigation
P—病人、人群、或问题
I—干预
C—与其他组、干预措施、病因、预后的比较
O—结果：你预计或可能得到什么结果或成果
T（可选）—观察/调查的时间段

Figure 24.2.1　The PICO(T) Components for Research Question(研究问题的 PICO(T)组成部分)

3.3.2　Research Design(研究设计)

　　The research design indicates the overall strategy that the researchers will use to integrate the different components of the study in a coherent and logical way, therefore ensuring an effective addressment of the research problem. It constitutes the blueprint for the data collection, measurement, and analysis of data. Specific research designs include quantitative research, qualitative research, and mixed-method research. There are four main types of quantitative research：descriptive, correlational, causal comparative/quasi-experimental, and experimental research（see Chapter 8 for Quantitative Research Design and Chapter 17 for Qualitative Research Design）.

　　研究设计表明研究人员以连贯和合理的方式整合研究的不同组成部分而采用的总体战略，从而确保有效解决研究问题。它建立了数据收集、测量和数据分析的蓝图。具体的研究设计包括量性研究、质性研究和混合方法研究。量性研究主要有四种类型：描述性研

究、相关性研究、因果比较/类实验性研究和实验性研究(量性研究设计见第 8 章,质性研究设计见第 17 章)。

3.3.3　Setting(研究场所)

For studies involving human participants, it is very important to discuss where potential research participants are enrolled. For example, if an observational study is conducted in an outpatient clinic with patients with breast cancer, location and environment need to be described. Rationales are needed to describe why this is an appropriate setting for recruiting this population.

对于涉及人类参与者的研究,讨论潜在的研究参与者将在哪里被招募是非常重要的。例如,如果观察研究将在乳腺癌患者的门诊中进行,则需要描述地点和环境,需要说明为什么这是一个适合招募这一人群的环境。

3.3.4　Population or Data Source(人群或数据来源)

For studies involving human subjects, the researchers need to calculate and discuss the suggested demographics (e. g., age, gender, and race) and the sample size of the population. Detailed inclusion and exclusion criteria must be set for the selected population. Specifically, the researchers need to determine the sample, the rationales of the population choice, and the type of sampling. The population's size and the calculation of your representative sample should be provided.

在涉及人类受试者的研究中,研究人员需要计算和讨论建议的人口统计学数据(如年龄、性别和种族)和人群的样本量,必须为所选人群制订详细的纳入和排除标准。具体来说,研究者需要确定样本、选择该人群的理由和抽样的类型。研究人群的规模和代表性样本的计算也应被提供。

The secondary data analysis involves the researchers using the information that someone else has gathered for their own purposes. The researchers leverage secondary data analysis to answer a new research question, or to examine an alternative perspective on the original question of the previous study. If any form of secondary data is used, including documents or other non-human intervention methods, specific inclusion and exclusion criteria are needed to determine who, how many, and what variables should be included in the study. Secondary data analysis may have some limitations (e. g., missing some major confounders or lacking a control group) that must be clearly addressed.

二手数据分析包括研究者使用的别人为他/她自己的目的而收集的信息。研究人员利用二次数据分析来回答一个新的研究问题，或者从另一个角度研究之前研究的原始问题。如果使用任何形式的二手数据，包括文件或其他非人类干预方法，都需要有具体的纳入和排除标准，以确定谁、多少、哪些变量要纳入研究。二手数据分析可能有一些局限性(如缺少一些主要的混杂因素或缺少对照组)，必须被明确地解决。

3.3.5　Ethical Considerations(伦理考虑)

There are always ethical considerations, to a greater or lesser degree, depending on whether you are using human subjects and the level of invasiveness of your intervention or data collection instrument. In the proposal, the researchers need to discuss what is required of the participants, what their rights are, what risks the participants might encounter, and what benefits the participants might accrue (Ayer, 1994). For most studies involving human subjects, an approval should be obtained from the Institutional Review Boards (IRBs) or other similar committees.

　　研究总是存在或多或少的伦理考虑，根据你是否使用人类受试者和你的干预或数据收集工具的侵入程度而定。在计划书中，研究人员需要讨论对受试者的要求、他们的权利、受试者可能遇到的风险，以及受试者可能获得的利益(Ayer, 1994)。对于大多数涉及人体的研究，应从机构审查委员会或其他类似的委员会获得批准。

3.3.6　Intervention Protocol(干预计划)

Specific guidelines have been developed to guide the design of intervention studies, including the CONSORT checklist (Grant et al., 2018). The researchers need to discuss the objectives of the intervention, how the intervention is developed, and how it proceeds. Then, supporting materials are provided as necessary (e.g., agenda, handouts, and brochures).

　　已经有了具体的指南来指导干预研究的设计，包括 CONSORT 检查表 (Grant 等，2018)。研究人员需要讨论干预的目标，如何制定干预措施，以及如何进行干预。然后，根据需要提供支持材料(例如，议程、讲义和小册子)。

3.3.7　Instruments or Measures(工具或措施)

Detailed information on all the instruments should be provided. The researchers need to discuss how the instruments are used and provide the supporting materials. The researchers need to describe how the survey was developed, what the logic was behind the determination of specific questions, what information to gain from the use of the survey in the protocol. In addition, discussing the types of questions and the types of data provides good information for the readers. Also, be certain to give an example of each response type the researchers might use, for example, multiple choice, fill in, true/false, yes/no, scaled response (Likert or otherwise).

应提供所有工具的详细信息。研究人员需要讨论如何使用这些工具，并提供支持材料。研究人员需要描述如何进行调查，确定具体问题背后的逻辑是什么，能从调查计划的使用中获得什么信息。此外，讨论问题的类型和数据的类型可以为读者提供更多的信息。另外，一定要举例说明研究人员可能使用的每种回答类型，例如，多选题、填空题、真/假题、是/否题、量表式回答(李克特或其他)。

3.3.8 Summary(总结)

A summary of the chapter reminds the audience of what is covered, reinforces it in their memory, and then transition to the next chapter.

对该章的总结将提醒读者所涉及的内容，并加强他们的记忆，也为下一章内容做铺垫。

3.4 References(参考文献)

The reference section should include every work cited in the paper. Based on the thesis and dissertation requirements, the researchers must follow specific citation styles, such as APA. The reference section should only include what the researchers have cited.

参考文献部分应包括论文中引用的每一个参考文献。根据毕业论文和学位论文的要求，研究人员必须遵循特定的引用格式，如 APA。参考文献部分应该只包括研究人员所引用的内容。

3.5 Appendix(附录)

The appendix provides all the supplementary documents, such as definitions of terms, surveys, and supplementary Tables and Figures.

附录提供所有的补充文档，如术语的定义、调查问卷、补充的表格和图表。

Section Ⅲ   Science Fund
第三节   科学基金

Obtaining funding for research projects is becoming increasing difficult due to growing competition. Successful proposal writers must know the potential funders and the specific requirements according to the funding mechanisms. Proposal writers must also have good proposal-writing skills and read the funding requests (e. g., Request for Applications (RFAs) and Notice of Special Interest (NOSI)) carefully before submitting the research proposals.

由于竞争日益激烈，为研究项目获取资金正变得越来越困难。成功的计划书撰写者必须根据资助机制了解潜在的资助者和具体的要求。在提交研究计划书之前，撰写人必须有良好的计划书撰写技巧，并在提交研究计划书之前仔细阅读资助要求（例如，申请书（RFAs）和特殊利益通知（NOSI））。

The research funding generally includes any funding for scientific research projects. Research funding is primarily categorized into two types: private funds (e. g., professional societies, organizations, or foundations) and federal funding (e. g., specialized government agencies, such as the National Institutes of Health (NIH) and the National Natural Science Foundation of China (NSFC)). A smaller number of scientific programs are funded by charitable foundations, especially in relation to developing cures for diseases, including cancer, HIV/AIDS, and rare diseases.

研究经费一般涵盖任何用于科学研究项目的资金。研究资金主要分为两类：私人资金（如专业协会、组织或基金会）和政府资金（如专门的政府机构，如美国国立卫生研究院和中国国家自然科学基金委员会）。少量的科学项目是由慈善基金会资助的，特别是与开发疾病的治疗方法有关，包括癌症、艾滋病和罕见疾病。

1. The National Natural Science Foundation of China (NSFC)
（国家自然科学基金委员会）

The NSFC is the primary national funding agency for the natural science researchers. The NSFC is an institution directly under the jurisdiction of the State Council, tasked with the administration of the National Natural Science Fund from the Government (Liu et al., 2019). The NSFC has established a rigorous and objective merit-review system to fulfill its mission of supporting basic research, fostering talented researchers, developing international cooperation, and promoting socioeconomic development (Liu et al., 2019). The NSFC is focused on three categories of programs: research promotion, talent fostering, and infrastructure construction for basic research. Each program has its own specific research topics, priorities, and requirements for application. More details can be found on the NSFC website.

国家自然科学基金委员会是针对自然科学研究人员的主要国家资助机构。国家自然科学基金委员会是国务院直接管辖的机构，负责管理政府的国家自然科学基金（Liu 等，2019）。国家自然科学基金委员会建立了严格和客观的评优制度，以履行其支持基础研究、培养优秀研究人员、发展国际合作和促进社会经济发展的使命（Liu 等，2019）。国家自然科学基金委员会重点关注三类项目：研究促进、人才培养和基础研究的基础设施建设。每个项目都有其特定的研究课题、研究重点和申请要求。更多细节可以在国家自然科学基金委员会的网站上找到。

1.1 Funding Programs(资助项目)

At present, the project setting of the NSFC contains several programs, including the General Program, Key Program, Major Research Plan, Youth Scientist Fund, and International (Regional) Cooperation and Exchange Programs.

目前，国家自然科学基金委员会的项目设置包括一般项目、重点项目、重大项目、青年项目和国际(地区)合作与交流项目。

1.1.1 **General Program**(一般项目)

Supporting researchers to conduct innovative and explorative research on open topics within certain areas. The average funding per project is 500K-600K RMB.

支持研究人员对特定领域内的开放课题进行创新和探索性研究。每个项目的平均资助金额为 50 万~60 万元人民币。

1.1.2 **Key Program**(重点项目)

This program focuses on medium-sized projects that support prospective and frontier studies aiming to achieve major breakthroughs in priority industries and technologies. The average funding per project is 2.5-3 million RMB.

支持前瞻性和前沿性研究的中等规模项目，以实现重点产业和技术的重大突破。每个项目的平均资助金额为 250 万~300 万元人民币。

1.1.3 **Major Research Plan**(重大研究计划)

Medium- and large-sized projects of strategic value to economic and social development in national priority areas, featuring a strong top-down design.

在国家重点领域对经济和社会发展具有战略价值的大中型项目，具有较强的自上而下的设计特点。

1.1.4 Young Scientist Fund(青年科学家基金)

Similar to the General Program, but exclusively targeting young scientists. The average funding per project is 200K-250K RMB.

与一般项目相似，但专门针对青年科学家。每个项目的平均资助金额为20万~25万元人民币。

1.1.5 International (Regional) Cooperation and Exchange Programs (国际(地区)合作与交流项目)

Supporting joint research with top researchers and institutions world-wide. It is divided into three sub-groups of projects, one of which targets exclusively international young scientists (see below for more details).

支持与世界顶级研究人员和机构的联合研究。它被分为三个子项目组，其中一个专门针对国际青年科学家(详见下文)。

1.2 International Programs(国际项目)

The NSFC encourages international collaboration in basic research programs. It has signed over 80 Cooperative Agreements with partners from 44 countries and regions worldwide. Specifically, these programs are designed to support joint research programs between Chinese scientists and top researchers and institutions around the world. These programs are divided into three main sub-programs:

国家自然科学基金鼓励国际合作的基础研究项目，它已经与全世界44个国家和地区的合作伙伴签署了80多项合作协议。具体而言，这些项目旨在支持中国科学家与世界顶级研究人员和机构之间的联合研究项目。这些项目被分为三个主要的子项目：

1.2.1 Key International (Regional) Joint Research Projects (重点国际(地区)联合研究项目)

Encouraging and supporting innovative China-based researchers to conduct basic research in priority areas in cooperation with international research structures and scientists based abroad.

鼓励和支持中国的创新研究人员与国际研究机构和国外科学家合作在重点领域开展基础研究。

1. 2. 2　International（Regional）Cooperation and Exchange Programs under framework agreements. （框架协议下的国际(地区)合作与交流项目）

Encouraging and supporting excellent Chinese scientists to conduct joint research in the partner's country and facility, or to organize international conferences in China or abroad.

鼓励和支持优秀的中国科学家在合作伙伴的国家和设施内开展联合研究，或在中国或国外组织国际会议。

1. 2. 3　Research Fund for International Young Scientists（国际青年科学家研究基金）

Encouraging excellent international young scientistsbased abroad to come to mainland of China to conduct basic research in natural sciences. The aim is to promote sustainable academic collaboration and exchanges between Chinese scholars and foreign young scientists.

鼓励国外优秀国际青年科学家来中国大陆开展自然科学基础研究。其目的是促进中国学者与国外青年科学家之间可持续的学术合作与交流。

1. 3　Application（申请）

The programs included in the NSFC annual guidelines follow a "centralized application" mechanism, namely all applications must be submitted by 20 March each year (may change sometimes). Applications must be submitted by the Principal Investigator (PI) through the NSFC's system but must be pre-examined and pre-approved by the institution to which the PI is affiliated ("host institution"). The applications are expected to be completed by the PI before the deadline indicated in the annual project guidelines, as host institutions often set their internal deadlines to review the applications before final submission.

国家自然科学基金年度指南中的项目遵循"集中申请"机制，即所有申请必须在每年的3月20日前提交(有时也可能改变)。申请必须由首席研究员(PI)通过国家自然科学基金的系统提交，但必须由首席研究员所属的机构("主办机构")进行预审和预批准。首席研究员应在年度项目指南中标明的截止日期前完成申请，因为主办机构通常会在最终提交前设定其内部审查截止日期。

2. The National Social Science Fund of China（NSSF）（国家社会科学基金）

The NSSF was established under the guidance of the National Planning Office of

Philosophical and Social Sciences. The NSSF is one of China's main channels to support basic scientific research（Hui, 2015）.

国家社会科学基金是在国家哲学社会科学规划办公室的指导下设立的。国家社会科学基金是中国支持基础科学研究的主要渠道之一（Hui, 2015）。

2.1 Requirements for the Applicants（申请者要求）

All the applicants must（1）have the abilities to conduct studies independently;（2）have doctoral prepared degrees（e. g., MD and PhD）or professional title above associate level. For these without doctoral degree or with professional title below associate level, the Young Scientist program can be applied with the support of two experts with professional title of senior level. The applicants of the Young Scientists Program must be below 35 years old.

所有申请者必须：（1）具有独立进行研究的能力；（2）具有博士学位（如医学博士和哲学博士）或副高级以上职称。对于没有博士学位或职称低于副高的人，可以在两名具有高级职称的专家支持下申请青年科学家项目。青年科学家项目的申请人必须在 35 岁以下。

2.2 Requirements for the Application Institutes（申请机构要求）

All the grant application institutes must（1）have rich resources and research environment;（2）have an office of research management; and（3）have all the prerequisites for research with promising commitment.

所有申请机构必须：（1）有丰富的资源和研究环境；（2）有研究管理办公室；（3）具备所有承诺的研究的前提条件。

2.3 Grant Length（资助时长）

Basic scientific research is generally funded 3-5 years. Translational and policy-related research is generally funded 2-3 years.

基础科学研究的资助时长一般为 3~5 年。转化和政策相关的研究的资助时长一般为 2~3 年。

Section Ⅳ Preparing Applications for Research Funding
第四节 基金申请书的撰写

Before the submission of a research proposal to NSFC and NSSF, it is crucial to carefully review up-to-date instructions for grant application submission. Following the instructions, the researchers need to obtain the standard forms for each component of the proposal, such as proposal structure, bio-sketches of the team, budget form, and other support forms. All this information is available on the NSFC and NSSF websites. Advanced planning is essential to the development of a successful proposal for these funding opportunities. This section offers suggestions for things you can do to prepare for the actual writing and grant application (Polit & Beck, 2017).

在向国家自然科学基金和国家社会科学基金的提交研究计划书之前，仔细查看最新的基金申请提交说明是至关重要的。根据说明，研究人员需要获得计划书各部分的标准表格，如计划书结构、团队简介、预算表和其他支持表格。所有这些信息都可以在国家自然科学基金和国家社会科学基金的网站上找到。提前计划对于为这些资助机会撰写一个成功的计划书是至关重要的。本节提供了为实际写作和资助申请做准备的建议（Polit 和 Beck，2017）。

1. Building a Collaborative Research Team(建立一个合作研究团队)

Building a collaborative research team is the first step for writing and submitting a proposal that will be competitive for funding (Bai et al., 2021). The research team members may function as advisers, advocates, and/or critics. They mostly guide the research project development and help with the implementation of the project upon receiving funding. A successful collaborative team is likely to be more creative, foster beneficial collaborations, share resources, and ensure integrity in research endeavors. If the researchers have had little or no experience with research, non-research projects, and/or writing, the research team likely plays a significant part in mentoring the researcher during proposal writing and submission.

建立一个合作研究团队是撰写和提交有资金竞争力的计划书的第一步（Bai 等，2021）。研究团队成员可以作为顾问、倡导者和/或批评者，他们大多指导研究项目的发展，并在获得资助后帮助项目的实施。一个成功的合作团队可能会更有创造力，促进有益的合作，共享资源，并确保研究工作的完整性。如果研究者在研究、非研究项目和/或写作方面没有经验或经验不足，研究团队很可能在指导研究者撰写和提交计划书方面发挥重要作用。

2. Understanding the Proposal Components(了解研究计划书的要素)

A research proposal requires the research team to address the following areas: research purpose, significance, objectives (i. e., written as specific aims, research questions, hypotheses, or PICOT questions), literature review, theoretical framework, and methods (i. e., design, sample, setting, variables, measures, data collection procedure, and analysis) (Bai et al., 2021; Polit & Beck, 2017). The researchers need to be attentive to every detail in the submission requirements. It is advisable that the mentor(s) and the research team reads and provides constructive feedback on the proposal. Regularly scheduled meetings are recommended. If time permits, asking other nursing researchers with research and grant writing expertise to read the proposal and provide feedback may strengthen the final proposal. Once the grant proposal is written, it is time to submit it for review by the funding agency.

研究计划书要求研究团队解决以下方面的问题：研究目的、意义、目标(写成具体目的、研究问题、假设或 PICOT 问题)、文献回顾、理论框架和方法(即设计、样本、环境、变量、措施、数据收集程序和分析)(Bai 等, 2021; Polit 和 Beck, 2017)。研究者需要注意提交要求中的每个细节。建议导师和团队成员阅读提案并提供建设性的反馈意见，以及定期开会。如果时间允许，请其他具有研究和基金写作专长的护理研究人员阅读计划书并提供反馈，这可能会加强最终的计划书。一旦基金申请书写好，就应该提交给资助机构审查。

3. Selecting an Important and Significant Problem
   (选择一个重要又有意义的问题)

Selecting a problem with clinical or theoretical significance determines the success of funding for a proposal. The proposal must make a persuasive argument that the research could make a significant contribution to a clinical topic that is important to the reviewers and funders.

选择一个具有临床或理论意义的问题决定着计划书的成功资助。计划书必须提出有说服力的论据，说明该研究可以对那些评审员和资助者所重视的临床课题做出重大贡献。

4. Knowing the Audience(了解读者)

The researchers must learn about the audience who may read the proposal. For theses or dissertations, this means getting to know your committee members and learning about their interests, expertise, and expectations. If you are writing a proposal for funding, you should obtain information about the funding organization's priorities and recently funded projects. Funding agencies (e. g., NIH and NSFC) often publish the review criteria for proposals. These criteria should be used to guide the proposal writing.

研究者必须了解将阅读计划书的读者。对于毕业论文或学位论文，这意味着要试图了解你的委员会成员，了解他们的兴趣、专长和期望。如果你要写一份资助计划书，你应该获得有关资助机构的重点项目和最近资助的项目。资助机构(如美国国立卫生研究院和中国国家自然科学基金委员会)通常会公布计划书的审查标准。这些标准应用来指导计划书的撰写。

5. Building a Time Plan for the Proposal Writing
（制订研究计划书撰写的时间计划）

Writing a proposal is time-consuming and usually takes longer than originally planned. The researchers need to build in enough time so that the proposal can be reviewed by members of the team, willing colleagues, and potentially the internal or external mock review committees. The researchers also need to build in adequate time for administrative issues, such as getting budgets approved and securing all the supporting documents.

撰写计划书是很耗时的，而且总是比原来计划的时间要长。研究人员需要留出足够的时间，以便团队成员、愿意合作的同事和内部或外部的模拟审查委员会能够审查该计划书。研究人员还需要为行政问题留出足够的时间，如获得预算批准和所有的支持文件。

6. Reading Successful Proposals as Examples(阅读作为成功示例的计划书)

Many funding agencies (e. g., NIH) have published successfully funded proposals, which can be used as examples for researchers, especially novice proposal writers. It is also likely that some of your colleagues or fellow students have written a proposal that has been accepted (either by a funding sponsor or by a dissertation committee), and many people are happy to share their successful efforts with others. Reviewing and learning from successful proposals increase the success rate of grant applications.

很多资助机构(如美国国立卫生研究院)已经公布了被成功资助的计划书，这些计划书可以作为研究人员，特别是计划书撰写新手撰写计划书的范例。很可能有些同事或同学写的计划书已经被接受了(要么被资助者接受，要么被论文委员会接受)，很多人很乐意与他人分享他们成功的努力。回顾和学习成功的计划书将提高基金申请的成功率。

7. Building a Persuasive Case (建立一个有说服力的案例)

In a research proposal, the researchers need to persuade the reviewers or the audience that the right questions are asked, that you are the right person to ask those questions, and that you can get those questions answered appropriately. The researchers must also convince them that the answers will make a difference to nursing science and nursing practice. The proposal should be written in a positive and confident tone. It is unwise to promise what cannot be achieved, but you should think about ways to put the proposed project in a positive light.

在一个研究计划书中，研究人员需要说服评审员或读者提出的问题是正确的，你是提出这些问题的合适人选，并且你会让这些问题得到适当的回答。研究人员必须说服他们，这些成果将对护理科学和护理实践产生影响。计划书应以积极和自信的语气来写。承诺不可能实现的事情是不明智的，但应该积极看待立项的项目。

8. Justifying Methodologic Decisions(证明方法学决定的合理性)

Methodologic decisions should be made carefully, keeping in mind the benefits and drawbacks of alternatives, and a compelling justification should be provided. To the extent possible, make evidence-based decisions and defend the proposed methods with citations demonstrating their utility. Insufficient detail and inadequate explanation of methodologic choices can weaken the proposal, although page constraints often make full elaboration impossible.

应该谨慎地选择研究方法，牢记替代方法的优点和缺点，并提供令人信服的理由。在可能的范围内，做出基于证据的决定，并通过引用证明来证明方法的合理性。虽然页数限制难以充分阐述，但方法选择的细节不完善和解释不明晰会削弱计划书的合理性。

9. Adhering to Instructions(遵守说明)

Funding agencies provide instructions on what is required in a research proposal. It is important to read these instructions carefully and to follow them precisely. Proposals are sometimes rejected without review if they do not adhere to guidelines, such as minimum font size or page limitations.

资助机构提供关于研究计划书所需内容的说明。仔细阅读这些说明并严格遵守是很重要的。如果计划书没有遵守准则有时会不经审查而被拒绝，如最小字体大小或页数限制。

10. Paying Attention to Presentation(注重表述)

Proposals should be visually appealing, well organized, grammatically sound, and easy to read. The presentation of the proposal should be professional and show respect for the reviewers. It is invaluable to ask professional editors to edit the proposal before submission.

计划书应具有视觉吸引力，组织良好，语法合理，易于阅读。计划书的表述应该是专业的，并表现出对评审员的尊重。请专业编辑在提交前对计划书进行编辑是非常重要的。

11. Participating in Mock Review(参加模拟审查)

The proposal draft should be reviewed by others before formal submission of the proposal. Reviewers should be selected for both substantive and methodologic expertise. If the proposal is being submitted for funding, one reviewer ideally would have first-hand knowledge of the funding source. If a consultant has been proposed because of their specialized expertise, they should be asked to review the draft and make recommendations for its improvement. In universities, mock review panels are often held before submitting a proposal to a funding agency. Faculty and students are invited to these mock reviews and provide valuable feedback for enhancing a proposal.

在正式提交计划书之前，计划书草案应该由其他人审查。应根据实证性和方法学方面的专业知识选择评审员。如果提案是为了资金而提交的，最好有一位评审员对资金来源有第一手的了解。如果顾问因为他们的专业知识而被推荐，应该请他们审查草案并提出改进建议。在大学里，在向资助机构提交计划书之前，通常会举行模拟审查会议。教师和学生被邀请参加这些模拟审查，为加强计划书提供宝贵的反馈意见。

📖 Studies Cited in Chapter 24（第二十四章参考文献）

[1] Bai, J., Booker, S. Q., Saravanan, A., et al. Grant writing doesn't have to be a pain: Tips for preparation, writing and dissemination[J]. Pain Management Nursing, 2021, 22(5): 561-564.

[2] Gholipour, A., Lee, E. Y., Warfield, S. K. The anatomy and art of writing a successful grant application: a practical step-by-step approach[J]. Pediatric Radiology, 2014, 44 (12): 1512-1517.

[3] Sohn, E. Secrets to writing a winning grant[J]. Nature, 2020, 577(7788): 133-135.

[4] Klopper, H. The qualitative research proposal[J]. Curationis, 2008, 31(4): 62-72.

[5] Knafl, K. A., Deatrick, J. A. Top 10 tips for successful qualitative grantsmanship[J]. Research in Nursing & Health, 2005, 28(6): 441-443.

[6] Carey, M. A., Swanson, J. Funding for qualitative research[J]. Qualitative Health Research, 2003, 13(6): 852-856.

[7] Padgett, D. K., Henwood, B. F. Obtaining large-scale funding for empowerment-oriented qualitative research: a report from personal experience[J]. Qualitative Health Research, 2009, 19(6): 868-874.

[8] Sandelowski, M., Barroso, J. Writing the proposal for a qualitative research methodology project[J]. Qualitative Health Research, 2003, 13(6): 781-820.

[9] Sandelowski, M. A. matter of taste: evaluating the quality of qualitative research[J]. Nursing Inquiry, 2015, 22(2): 86-94.

[10] Creswell, J. W., Creswell, J. D. Research design: qualitative, quantitative, and mixed methods approaches[M]. Los Angeles: Sage, 2018.

[11] Aslam, S., Emmanuel, P. Formulating a researchable question: A critical step for facilitating good clinical research[J]. Indian Journal of Sexually Transmitted Diseases and AIDS, 2010, 31(1): 47-50.

[12] Ayer S. Submitting a research proposal for ethical approval[J]. Professional Nurse (London, England), 1994, 9(12): 805-806.

[13] Grant, S., Mayo-Wilson, E., Montgomery, P. et al. CONSORT-SPI 2018 Explanation and Elaboration: guidance for reporting social and psychological intervention trials[J].

Trials, 2018, 19: 406.

[14]Liu, Y., Gao, Z., Wang, H., et al. Analysis of projects funded by the National Natural Science Foundation of China during the years of 2014-2018[J]. Annals of Translational Medicine, 2019, 7(12): 267.

[15]Hui, W. From National Social Science Foundation Projects to Knowledge Production of Library and Information[J]. Proceedings of the International Conference on Management, Computer and Education Informatization, 2015, 06.

[16] Polit, D. F. Beck, C. T. Nursing Research: Generating and Assessing Evidence for Nursing Practice[M]. 10th ed. Philadelphia: Wolters Kluwer Health, 2017.

Chapter 25: Reporting Research Findings
第二十五章　报告研究结果

No study is considered complete until its results have been shared with other professionals. This chapter provides effective methods for reporting research findings, and it will discuss various issues that researchers should consider when reporting research findings.

任何一项研究直到其研究结果与其他专业人员分享才被认为是完整的。本章节为报告研究结果提供有效的方法，我们将会讨论研究人员在报告研究结果时需要考虑的各项问题。

Section Ⅰ　Overview of Research Reports
第一节　研究报告概述

1. Types of Research Reports(研究报告的类型)

There are several ways to classify research reports. According to the research design, it is divided into two types usually: quantitative research report and qualitative research report; according to the form of research report, it is often divided into four types: journal articles, theses and dissertations, oral reports and poster presentations.

研究报告的分类有多种方法。根据研究设计分类，常分为量性研究报告和质性研究报告两种类型；根据研究报告的形式分类，常分为期刊论文、学位论文、口头报告及海报展示四种类型。

2. Preparation before Reporting the Research Findings(报告研究结果前的准备)

2.1　Choosing a Communication Media and Channel(选择传播媒介和渠道)

The research findings could be presented in oral or written form. Generally, oral presentations are shown in professional meetings, facing the audience to give a formal speech.

Sometimes poster presentations are combined with the formal speech. The main advantages of conference reports are that they can be conducted soon after the research completion (or even in the process of the research stage) and provide opportunities for audiences who are interested in the same topic to communicate with the reporter.

可以通过口头或者书面形式呈现研究结果。口头报告通常是在专业会议中面对观众进行正式的演讲，有时海报展示与口头汇报相结合。口头报告的主要优点是它们可以在研究完成后不久(甚至在研究阶段中)进行，并为对相同主题感兴趣的人提供交流机会。

Except for oral reports, a written report is also a common form. It could take the form of journal articles published in traditional or open-access professional journals. The significant advantage of journal articles is that they can be accessed easily, especially the open-access ones.

除此之外，书面报告也是一种常见的形式。书面报告的呈现形式为在传统或开放获取的专业期刊上发表的期刊文章。期刊文章(尤其是开发获取的期刊文章)的主要优势在于它容易获及。

2.2 Knowing the Audience(了解受众)

Good research communication depends on providing information that can be understood. Therefore, researchers should consider the primary audience for their study. The following are some problems that need to be considered：

良好的研究交流取决于提供可以理解的信息，因此研究人员应该考虑他们的研究的主要受众。以下列举需要考虑到的问题：

(1)Will the audience include professionals in other disciplines except for nurses (e. g., doctors, psychologists, physical therapists)？

受众中除了护士以外是否还包括其他学科的专业人员(例如，医生、心理学研究者、物理治疗师)？

(2)Will the audience be researchers or other professionals (e. g., clinic practitioners, health care policymakers)？

受众是研究人员，还是其他专业人员(例如，临床实践者、卫生保健政策制定者)？

(3)Are there any laymen in the audience？

受众中是否有外行人？

(4)Will the audience understand the language used in the research report？

受众是否可以理解研究报告中所用的语言？

(5)Are the reviewers, editors and readers experts in the field？

审稿人、编辑和读者是该领域的专家吗？

Generally, writing reports should be clear and avoid using academic terms as much as possible when facing multiple and broad audiences.

通常情况下，当面对多样化和广泛的受众时，研究人员在撰写报告时应保证清晰，并且尽量避免使用学术术语。

2.3　Making a Plan(制订计划)

2.3.1　Determining Authorship(确定作者)

Authorship confers credit and has important academic, social, and financial implications. Authorship also implies responsibility and accountability for published work. The International Committee of Medical Journal Editors (ICMJE, 2019) recommends that authorship should be based on the following 4 criteria:

作者身份授予信誉，并具有重要的学术、社会和经济影响，同时还意味着对已发表作品的责任和义务。国际医学期刊编辑委员会 (ICMJE, 2019) 建议作者身份根据以下 4 条标准确定作者资格：

(1) Substantial contributions to the conception or design of the work; or the acquisition, analysis, or interpretation of data for the work;

对文章的构思或设计做出重要贡献；或为研究资料的获取、分析或数据解释做出重要贡献；

(2) Drafting the work or revising it critically for important intellectual content;

起草文章或对文章的重要知识内容做出批判性修改；

(3) Final approval of the version to be published;

对于要发表的文章版本给予最终的同意；

(4) Agreement to be accountable for all aspects of the work in ensuring that questions related to the accuracy or integrity of any part of the work are appropriately investigated and resolved.

同意对文章的所有方面负责，以确保与文章任何部分的准确性或完整性相关的问题得到适当的调查和解决。

2.3.2　Determining the Content(确定内容)

It's important to determine what parts of the research findings will be presented in the paper. If there were multiple research questions, more than one paper may be required to present research findings. Writing several essays is inappropriate and unethical when one article is enough. It's also unethical to simultaneously submit the same or similar paper to two journals.

确定在论文中展示研究结果的哪部分内容很重要。如果有多个研究问题，可能需要多篇论文来呈现研究结果。在一篇论文就足以展现研究结果时，写多篇论文是不合适的，甚至是不道德的，并且，同时向两个期刊投稿相同或相似的论文也是违反伦理原则的。

2.3.3 Assembling Materials(组织材料)

Before starting to write reports, researchers must clarify the materials used in the writing process and then prepare them. Generally, online journals publish guidelines for authors, which should be retrieved and understood. When you write your articles, please follow the guidelines of the journal.

开始动笔写作之前，研究者需要明确写作过程中有可能使用到的材料并且将其准备好。一般在线期刊会在官网上发布投稿指南，应该检索和了解这些投稿指南，并按照期刊要求进行写作。

Section II Quantitative Research Reports
第二节 量性研究报告

1. Journal Articles(期刊论文)

1.1 Overview of Quantitative Journal Articles(量性期刊论文概述)

After completing the research, nursing researchers should sort out and analyze the research data and information timely and write articles to pass the latest research results to their peers, so as to promote the development of the nursing discipline.

护理科研工作者在完成相关研究后，应及时对研究数据和资料进行整理、分析，并撰写成文，将最新的研究成果传递给同行，从而促进护理学科的发展。

1.2 Classification of Journal Articles for Quantitative Research
(量性研究期刊论文的分类)

1.2.1 According to the source of the articles(根据论文的资料来源分类)

(1) Original articles: It is the primary literature, which means that the data used in the

article comes from the first-hand data collected by the author.

论著：即一次文献，指文章中所使用的资料来源于作者所收集的第一手资料。

（2）Compilottion：It refers to the information used in the article from indirect information provided by the author through literature searching or others（e. g., systematic review or second-hand data analysis articles）.

编著：指文章中所使用的资料来源于作者通过文献检索或他人提供的间接资料（例如，系统综述或二手数据分析文章）。

1.2.2　According to the Research Methods of the Articles （根据论文的研究手段分类）

（1）Experimental research articles.（实验研究类论文）

（2）Investigation research articles.（调查研究类论文）

（3）Data analysis articles.（资料分析类论文）

（4）Experience summary articles.（经验总结类论文）

（5）Others.（其他）

1.2.3　According to the Forms of Journal Articles（根据期刊论文体裁分类）

Chinese nursing journal articles usually include original articles, reviews, experience exchange, nursing technology innovation, etc.; English nursing journals also usually include original articles or research reports, reviews（literature review or systematic review）, clinical methods, etc.

中文护理期刊论文通常包括论著、综述、经验交流、护理技术革新等形式；英文护理期刊也通常包括原著或研究报告、综述（文献综述或系统综述）、临床方法学研究等。

1.3　Writing Quantitative Journal Articles（量性期刊论文的撰写）

1.3.1　Structure of Journal Articles for Quantitative Research（量性期刊论文的结构）

The overall structure of nursing journal articles can be roughly divided into three sections: the front part, the main body part, and the back part.

护理期刊论文整体结构大致可分为三个部分，分别是前置部分、正文部分、后置部分。

（1）Front part: Title, author, Chinese and English abstract and keywords.

前置部分：文题、作者、中英文摘要与关键词。

（2）Main body：Introduction, research methods, results, discussions and conclusions.

正文部分：引言、研究方法、结果、讨论与结论。

（3）Back part：References, acknowledgments（optional section）.

后置部分：参考文献、致谢（为非必备项目）。

1.3.2 **Reporting Format for Quantitative Research**（量性研究报告格式）

Quantitative reports usually follow the IMRAD format, which includes four parts — the Introduction, Methods, Results, and Discussion. Each of these parts explains the following questions：I：Why was this research conducted? M：How was the research conducted? R：What was learned? D：What does it mean?

定量报告通常遵循 IMRAD 格式，包含四个部分——引言、方法、结果和讨论。这些部分分别解决以下问题：I：为什么进行这项研究？M：研究是如何进行的？R：从这项研究了解到什么？D：这项研究的研究结果意味着什么？

（1）The introduction.（引言部分）

The introduction allows readers to understand the research questions, significance and background. The introduction lays the foundation by describing the existing literature, the conceptual framework of the research, the problem, the research questions or hypotheses, and the study rationale. Although the introduction includes several parts, it should be concise. A common criticism from reviewers for research manuscripts is that the introduction is too long. Introductions are usually written in a funnel-shaped structure, starting from a broad sense to establish a framework for understanding the study, and then narrowing down to the specifics that researchers are trying to learn.

引言部分让读者了解研究问题、研究意义和研究背景。引言通过描述现有文献、研究的概念框架、存在的问题、研究问题或假设和进行研究的原因来奠定基础。虽然引言包括多个部分，但它应尽量简洁。杂志审稿人对研究手稿的一个普遍批判是引言部分过于冗余。引言部分通常以漏斗形状结构撰写，先从广泛的视角切入，建立一个帮助理解此项研究的框架，然后缩小到研究者想要去了解的特定部分。

（2）The method section.（方法学部分）

In order to assess the quality of research evidence, readers need to know exactly what methods were used to solve the research questions. In journal articles, the method section is usually condensed due to word limitation or layout limitation, but the degree of details should allow readers to conclude the integrity of the results. The defective method section is the main reason for the rejection of papers by research journals. The method section may contain the following subsections：research design, sample and setting, data collection, procedures, and data analysis.

为了评估研究证据的质量，读者需要确切地知道使用了什么研究方法以解决研究问题。在期刊文章中，由于字数或版面限制，方法学部分通常要求精练，但仍需提供足够的细节使读者能够得到真实及完整的结论。方法学部分存在问题是研究期刊拒绝稿件的主要原因。方法部分可包含以下子部分：研究设计、样本和研究场所、资料收集、研究步骤和数据分析。

①Research design.（研究设计）

The method section usually starts by describing the research design and its rationale. Clinical trials usually describe the design in detail, including information about which specific design was used, how subjects were allocated to each group, and whether blinding was used. In all types of quantitative research, it is important to control the research steps and confounding variables.

方法部分通常从研究设计及其基本原理的描述开始。临床试验中通常会详细陈述研究设计内容，其中包含采用了何种特定设计、受试者如何分配到各组，以及是否使用了盲法。在所有类型的定量研究中，重要的是对研究步骤及混杂变量进行控制。

②Sample and setting.（样本与研究地点）

This subsection usually includes a list of eligible criteria to clarify the population to whom results can be generalized, which may be labeled *Research Sample*, *Subjects*, *or Study Participants* in the journal articles. The sample selecting method, recruitment techniques, and sample size should be explained so that readers can determine the representativeness of the subjects in the target population. It should be described if a power analysis was performed to estimate the sample size. Information on response rates and response bias should also be provided.

这一部分在期刊文章中可被命名为研究样本、受试者或是研究参与者，其通常包括一系列纳入标准，从而确定可以将结果推广到的人群。应说明样本选择方法、招募技术和样本量大小，以便读者可以确定研究对象在目标人群中的代表性。如果使用了效能分析来估计样本量，则应予以说明。还应提供有关应答率和应答偏倚的信息。

③Data collection.（资料收集）

Data collection is a critical component of the method section, which may be labeled *Instruments*, *Measures*, *or Data Collection* in the journal articles. A description of the research instruments and the rationale for their use should be provided. If the instrument was constructed specifically for the project, the report should describe its development. Any special equipment used (e. g., to collect bio-physiological or observational data) should be described, including the manufacturer's information. The report should also explain who collected the data (e. g., the authors, research assistants, nurses) and how they received the training. Information related to the data quality and the procedures used to evaluate the quality should be described.

资料收集是方法学部分的重要内容，在期刊文章中可被命名为研究工具、测量方法或资料收集。应提供对研究工具的描述及其使用方法。如果研究工具是特定为某个研究项目进行构建，应报告其开发过程。应描述使用的任何特殊设备(例如，用以收集生物及生理学数据或观察数据)的信息，其中包括有关制造商的信息。报告还应说明由谁收集了资料(例如，作者、研究助理、护士)，以及他们是如何接受培训的。任何与资料质量相关的信息，以及用于评价资料质量的程序都应予以描述。

④Procedures. (研究步骤)

In the intervention study, there is usually a procedures subsection that includes intervening information. What was the specific content of the intervention? How was the intervention theory transformed into components? How and by whom was the intervention performed, and how were they trained? What was the control group condition? How long elapsed between the intervention and the measurement of the dependent variable? How was intervention fidelity monitored?

在干预研究中，通常包含一个研究步骤部分，其涵盖与干预相关的信息。干预的具体内容是什么？干预理论是如何转化为干预组成部分？干预如何实施，由谁实施，实施干预人员是如何进行培训的？对照组的情况如何？干预实施及因变量的测量之间间隔了多长时间？如何对干预的真实性进行监测？

⑤Data analysis. (数据分析)

After data collection is completed, data analysis procedures are required to describe in the method section. It is usually sufficient to determine the statistical test used, and it is not necessary to indicate the statistical formulas or references commonly used.

资料收集完成后，方法学部分需要描述数据分析步骤。通常确定使用的统计学检验就足够了，不需要标明常用的统计公式或参考文献。

⑥Reporting guidelines. (报告规范)

The guidelines for reporting methodological information for various types of studies are being updated or expanded regularly. The EQUATOR Network is a useful website that provides information on reporting guidelines for various types of studies (http://www.equator-network.

org). For example, the CONSORT (Consolidated Standards of Reporting Trials) guidelines focus on reporting information about RCTs, and the PRISMA (Preferred Reporting Items for Systematic reviews and Meta-Analysis) guidelines are for reporting systematic reviews.

报告各类研究方法学信息的指南正在定期更新或扩展。EQUATOR Network 是一个有用的网站，提供有关各类研究报告指南的信息（http://www. equator-network. org）。例如，CONSORT 指南是随机对照试验研究的报告规范，PRISMA 指南是关于系统评价的报告规范。

（3）The result section. （结果部分）

The results section is the core of the report. In quantitative research, the results of statistical analysis should be summarized in an authentic way. Descriptive statistics are provided firstly to give an overview of the research variables, and research results are usually ordered by overall importance. When reporting the results of a statistical hypothesis test, three parts are typically presented: the value of the calculated statistic, the degree of freedom, and the exact probability level. Confidence intervals combine location and precision information and can often be used directly to infer significance levels. Therefore, data of the report need to include it. When reporting the results of multiple statistical analyses, they should be summarized in one table. Good tables with concise titles and notes are essential to avoid repetitious statements. In addition, when using a table, the text should refer to the table by number (e. g., "A shown in Table 1...).

结果部分是研究报告的核心。在量性研究中，统计分析的结果应以事实陈述的方式进行总结。通常首先呈现描述性统计以对研究变量进行概述，且研究结果通常按整体重要性排序进行呈现。在报告假设检验的结果时，通常会报告三部分信息：计算统计量的值、自由度和确切的概率水平。置信区间结合了位置和精度的信息，并且通常可以直接用于推断显著性水平，因此论文数据中最好包含置信区间。当报告多个统计分析的结果时，应将它们汇总在一个表格中。具有简明标题和注释的好表格是避免重复陈述的重要方法。另外，当使用表格时，文本应按编号引用表格（例如，如表 1 所示……）。

（4）The discussion section. （讨论部分）

The meaning assigned to the results by the researchers plays a key role in the report. The discussion is dedicated to a thoughtful analysis of the result and then discussing its clinical and theoretical utility. The typical discussion part addresses the following questions: What are the main findings? What does the research result mean? Is there any evidence that the results and explanations are valid? Which restrictions may threaten validity? How does the result compare to the prior knowledge of the subject? What impact will these findings have on future research?

What is the effect on nursing practice?

研究人员赋予结果的含义在报告中起着重要作用。讨论部分致力于对研究结果进行深度的分析，从而讨论其临床和理论效用。典型的讨论部分解决以下问题：主要发现是什么？研究结果意味着什么？有什么证据表明结果和解释是有效的？哪些研究不足之处可能影响有效性？结果与该主题的先验知识相比如何？这些发现对未来的研究有什么影响？对护理实践有何影响？

Generally, the discussion section starts with a summary of the main findings. However, the summary should be short, because the important point of the discussion is understanding the results. The interpretation of results is a significant process, including research results, methodological advantages and limitations, sample characteristics, relevant research results, clinical aspects and theoretical issues. Researchers should justify their explanations and clearly state why other explanations were excluded. The unsupported conclusion is one of the most common issues in the discussion section. A tentative explanation should be provided if it conflicts with the earlier research. A discussion of the generality of the research results should also be included. It should be noted that the meaning of the research results is speculative. Therefore, it should be expressed in a tentative way. Finally, and importantly, the impact of research findings on nursing practice should be discussed. For example, which aspects of the evidence have clinical significance, and how do nurses use the evidence?

通常，讨论部分以主要发现的总结开始，然而，总结应该简短，因为讨论的重点是解释结果。结果的解释是一个重要的过程，包括研究结果、方法学优点和局限性、样本特征、相关研究结果、临床方面和理论问题。研究人员应该证明他们的解释是合理的，并明确说明为什么排除了其他解释。不受支持的结论是讨论部分中最常见的问题之一，如果发现与早期研究的结果相冲突，应尝试提供解释。讨论部分还应包括对研究结果的普遍性的讨论。需要注意的是，研究结果的含义是推测性的，因此应该以试探性的方式进行表述。最后，也是重要的，需要讨论研究结果对护理实践的影响。例如，证据的哪些方面具有临床意义，以及护士如何使用这些证据？

2. Theses and Dissertations(学位论文)

2.1 Overview of Theses and Dissertations(学位论文概述)

The dissertation is an important part of the nursing science and technology thesis. Writing a dissertation is a significant part of the training process of college students. Writing a dissertation provides students with an opportunity to systematically summarize, analyze and apply the knowledge they have learned. It can not only cultivate students' research skills and improve their comprehensive quality but also test the quality of university education.

学位论文是护理科技论文的重要组成部分。撰写学位论文是高等院校学生科研训练的一个重要环节。通过撰写学位论文，为学生提供一个对所学知识进行系统总结、归纳、分析、应用的机会，不仅可以培养学生的研究技能，提高学生的综合素质，还能检验学校的教学质量。

Strictly speaking, a dissertation refers to an academic dissertation written by degree applicants for professional review in order to obtain a degree certification. It is a standardized record of students' research under the guidance of their tutor. The dissertation is a graduation thesis of the students. It is the basis for judging the academic level of degree applicants, and it is also a necessary condition for students to obtain a certification.

学位论文严格地说是指学位申请者为获取学位证书而撰写的供评审和答辩用的专业性学术论文。它是学生在导师指导下对所完成科研活动的规范性的文字记录。学位论文通常是学生的毕业论文，它是判断学位申请者学术水平的重要依据，也是学位申请者获得学位的必要条件。

2.2　Classification of Dissertations(学位论文的分类)

Generally, dissertations are classified into bachelor's thesis, master's thesis, and doctoral thesis.

一般来说，学位论文通常分为学士学位论文、硕士学位论文和博士学位论文。

（1）Bachelor's thesis: It refers to a professional academic paper submitted by undergraduate students to apply for a bachelor's degree, measuring the graduate's professional knowledge, skills and work ability, with a word length of about 10,000 words.

学士学位论文：指大学本科毕业生为申请学士学位而提交的专业性学术论文，考察本科毕业生专业的知识、技能和工作能力，字数在1万字左右。

（2）Master's thesis: It refers to the thesis submitted by master students to apply for a master's degree. The word length of the thesis is usually about 30,000 words.

硕士学位论文：指硕士研究生为申请硕士学位而提交的论文，论文字数通常在3万字左右。

（3）Doctoral thesis: The dissertations are usually about 50,000 words long.

博士学位论文：论文字数通常要求在 5 万字左右。

2.3 Writing Quantitative Theses and Dissertations(量性学位论文的撰写)

The dissertation should have those characteristics：scientism, innovation, practicality, standardization, authenticity and fullness.

学位论文应该具备科学性、创新性、实用性、规范性、真实性和翔实性的特点。

2.3.1 Overall structure of nursing degree thesis(护理学位论文的整体结构)

The overall structure of the nursing degree thesis can be roughly summarized into three parts：the front part, the main text part, and the back part. The specific content is shown in Table 25.2.1.

护理学位论文的整体结构大致可分为三个部分：前置部分、正文部分、后置部分。具体内容见表 25.2.1。

Table 25.2.1　　　　**Overall structure of nursing degree thesis**
(护理学位论文的整体结构)

Front part (前置部分)	Cover, original statement, title, author, contents, Chinese and English abstract and keywords (封面，原创声明，文题，作者，目录，中英文摘要与关键词)
Main part (正文部分)	Introduction, research methods, results, discussion, conclusion (引言，研究方法，结果，讨论，结论)
Back part (后置部分)	References, appendix, summaries, acknowledgment, research results during the degree study (参考文献，附录，综述，致谢，攻读学位期间研究成果)

2.3.2 The Writing Requirements of Each Part of the Dissertation
(学位论文各部分的撰写要求)

（1）Cover：The cover is the outer surface of the dissertation. According to the national standard, it should provide readers with relevant information, such as the title, the name of the responsible people, the level of the applied degree, the name of the major, the completion date and so on.

封面：封面是学位论文的外表，根据国家标准论文封面应为读者提供相关信息，如题名、责任者姓名、申请学位级别、专业名称、完成日期等。

(2) The original statement of thesis and the consent about using copyright: a document in which the student solemnly declares the originality of the submitted dissertation and assumes the corresponding legal responsibility. The consent of using copyright is students and the tutor authorizing the school to use the dissertation.

论文原创声明及版权使用同意：学生对所提交学位论文的原创性进行郑重声明并承担相应法律责任的文书。版权使用同意书是学生和导师授权学校使用其论文的文本。

(3) Title: The title is a high-level summary of the main content about the dissertation. The standard for a good title is accurately describing the content with the least necessary terms. Therefore, the basic requirements for writing are accuracy, conciseness, standardization, novelty and eye-catching.

题目：论文的题目或题名是学位论文主要内容的高度概括，好标题的标准是用最少的必要术语去准确描述学位论文的内容，因此写作的基本要求是准确、简明、规范、新颖和醒目。

(4) Author: The author's signature of the dissertation is mainly to maintain the labor achievements and to show that he/she is responsible. It is also convenient for readers to communicate with the author. Generally, a dissertation is completed by the student under the guidance of the tutor. Therefore, the paper needs to have their name and identity information.

作者：学位论文作者的署名主要是为了维护作者的劳动成果，同时也表明文责自负，也便于读者与作者的联系。通常是学生在导师指导下完成的成果，因此，论文需要学生和导师的姓名身份信息。

(5) Contents: The catalog displays the content about each part in the dissertation and its page number, making it convenient for readers to gain the structure information and search for the required content.

目录：目录是学位论文各部分内容及其页码的展示，方便读者了解论文构成及查找所需的内容。

(6) Abstract: The abstract is a condensing of the main points in the dissertation. It is the main viewpoint and the essence of this article, and thus it plays a key role in searching and reporting. The abstract consists of two parts: Chinese and English abstract. Chinese abstract writing mainly adopts an inherent structural format.

摘要：摘要是学位论文要点的浓缩，它是文章的主要观点和精华所在，起到检索和报道文献的作用。学位论文的摘要包括中文和英文两部分，中文摘要写作多采用结构式的固定格式。

（7）Keywords：Keywords are usually selected from the paper. Keywords have substantive meaning and reflect the content of the paper without standardization.

关键词：关键词通常是从论文中选取出来的，具有实质性意义的反映论文主题内容的未经过规范化的词汇。

（8）Introduction：The introduction is the prelude to the main body of the dissertation. The purpose is to provide readers with background information related to the thesis. And explain the importance of the research question and clearly state the purpose of the research.

引言：引言是学位论文正文的前导，目的是让读者提供理解论文所需的背景资料，说明研究问题的重要性并清楚地陈述研究的目的。

（9）Research method：The research method is a detailed introduction of the methodology used in the dissertation, which usually includes the research design plan, sampling method, detailed intervention plan, the process of collecting experimental materials or research tools, data analysis methods, the technical route of research, research quality control and so on.

研究方法：研究方法是本研究所采用的研究方法学的详细介绍，通常包括研究设计方案，抽样方法，详细的干预方案，收集实验材料的过程或研究工具，资料分析方法，研究技术路线及研究质量控制等。

（10）Results：The results are the data and facts used to answer the research questions obtained by the researcher through the review of the original material and data, analysis, induction, and statistical processing.

结果：研究结果是研究者通过对原始资料及数据进行审查核对、分析、归纳和统计处理后得出的用于回答研究问题的数据与事实。

（11）Discussion：The discussion is mainly the in-depth analysis of the results. The scientific explanation and evaluation discussion are part of the academic thinking of authors. It focuses on clarifying the internal connections and laws between things, the meaning of the research results in theory and practice, and providing a scientific basis for the conclusion.

讨论：研究讨论主要是对研究结果进行深入分析，科学解释和评价讨论是作者学术思想展开的部分，重在阐明事物间的内在联系与规律，以及研究结果在理论与实践中的意义为结论提供科学依据。

（12）Conclusion：The conclusion is the summary of the full dissertation. The writing of the summary conclusion should be objective, accurate, concise, precise and should not be repeated with the results or the discussion part.

结论：研究结论是学位论文全文的概括。总结结论的书写要客观准确简洁、精练严谨，不要与结果或讨论部分重复。

（13）References：References are the basis of the dissertation. The basic principles of citing documents include authority, accuracy, timeliness, avoiding indirect use and using standardized document citing formats.

参考文献：参考文献是学位论文的基础。引用文献的基本原则包括权威性、准确性、时效性、避免间接引用，以及采用规范的文献引用格式。

（14）Acknowledgement：Acknowledgement is a way for the author to express gratitude to the units and individuals who have substantively helped the completion of the dissertation.

致谢：致谢是作者对完成本学位论文有帮助的单位和个人表达感谢的方式。

（15）Appendix：The appendix is a supplement or reference item. The author usually puts diagrams in the appendix that are related to the main text but hard to put into the main text so that readers can better understand the viewpoint.

附录：附录是正文主体部分的补充或参考内容。作者通常将与正文相关，但又不便于放入正文的图表等放入附录中，以便读者能更好理解作者的观点。

Section Ⅲ　Qualitative Research Reports
第三节　质性研究报告

1. Overview of Qualitative Research Reports(质性研究报告概述)

The definition of qualitative research comes from Denzin and Lincoln（Denzin NK & Lincoln YS，2009）："Qualitative research is a situated activity that locates the observer in the world. Qualitative research consists of a set of interpretive, material practices that make the world visible." These practices tranform the world into a series of representations, including field notes, interviews, conversations, photographs, recordings, and memos to oneself. At this level, qualitative research involves an interpretive, naturalistic approach to the world. This means that qualitative researchers study phenomena in their natural settings, attempting to make sense of or interpret phenomena in terms of the meanings people bring to them.

质性研究被 Denzin 和 Lincoln 定义为（Denzin NK 和 Lincoln YS，2009）："质性研究是一种定位于世界观察者的活动。质性研究由一套使世界可见的解释性的、物质的实践组成."这些实践把世界变成一系列的表征，包括实地笔记、采访、对话、照片、录音和自我备忘录。在这个层面上，质性研究涉及对世界的解释和自然主义的方法。这意味着质性研究人员在自然环境中研究事物，试图从人们带给现象的意义上理解或解释现象。

2. Writing Qualitative Research Reports(质性研究报告的撰写)

Compared with quantitative research，qualitative research requires more ability to dig out useful information and seek people's understanding of this phenomenon，so as to explain this phenomenon better. Therefore，we follow a series of practical guidelines for qualitative research to guide the writing of qualitative research reports.

相比于量性研究来说，质性研究开展起来更加需要一定的能力，更能发掘出有用的信息，寻求人们对这种现象的理解，从而更好地解释这种现象。因此我们依据一系列质性研究的实用指南进行质性研究报告撰写的指导。

2.1 The components of Qualitative Research(质性研究的组成部分)

Research Component	Example
Refine the study question	Given the desire for faculty guidance of the SDL process during residency training, the purpose of the study was to explore residents' perceptions of the role that faculty members play in the promotion and support of resident SDL, to better characterize the SDL process in the clinical learning environment.
Identify the methodology	We previously developed a comprehensive, theoretical model of SDL among internal medicine residents, including the domains of person, process, and context; this theoretical model informed our constructivist grounded theory approach to explore faculty support for SDL among internal medicine residents and further characterize the relationship between context and process.
Choose data-collection methods	To facilitate discussion among residents regarding contextual elements and SDL, we used focus groups to collect data. Focus groups fit within a constructivist paradigm and are well suited for exploring the circumstances through which participants construct meaning, making this an appropriate tool for exploring the context surrounding resident experiences with SDL.
Select a sampling strategy	We purposively sampled internal medicine residents but were limited in our ability to perform theoretical sampling. Theoretical saturation was determined through group consensus, and data collection stopped after seven focus groups.
Plan and outline a strategy for data processing	After the first two focus groups were open-coded, we discussed the dominant themes and the relationships between themes to create a book of axial codes. We applied the axial codes to all transcripts using a qualitative software program that aids in the organization of qualitative research data.
Conduct the data analysis	We analyzed data as it was being collected and processed data through open-coding, axial coding, and writing analytic memos. We continued to analyze the data through group discussion, engaging in constant comparison between themes, and examination of relationships between themes, theoretical models of SDL, and new data as it was collected. Through consensus-building discussions, we developed models to explain the relationships between the emerging themes.
Consider the trustworthiness of your study findings	All the coders were core faculty in the residency program, and to provide additional perspective, we reviewed the coding with the focus group moderator. To establish the trustworthiness of our findings, we invited all participants to two member-check sessions, presented results of the analysis to study participants, and provided time for comments. This process did not identify any need for further analysis or data revision.
Synthesize and interpret data	We identified three explanatory models for categorizing themes describing faculty support for SDL: faculty guidance for the process of SDL, SDL *versus* other-directed learning, and faculty archetypes for supporting SDL. One example of a faculty archetype for supporting SDL was "collaborative SDL," in which the faculty member and the learner work together to answer a question, allowing the faculty member to explicitly model their approach for SDL.

Note: Please see reference 25: Sawatsky AP, Ratelle JT, Bonnes SL, Egginton JS, Beckman TJ. Faculty support for self-directed learning in internal medicine residency: A qualitative study using grounded theory. Acad Med 2018; 93:943–51.
SDL, self-directed learning.

Figure 25.3.1 Components of Qualitative Research：Examples from a Single Research Study（Sawatsky AP et al.，2019）

（质性研究的组成部分：来自单一研究研究的例子（Sawatsky AP 等，2019））

2.2　The Content of Qualitative Research Report(质性研究报告的内容)

Qualitative research can help researchers solve some problems in nursing. Different types of qualitative research require different types of reports to be written. Researchers who are exposed to qualitative research report writing for the first time can refer to the following overall structure and writing requirements for each part.

质性研究可以帮助研究人员解决护理方面的一些问题。不同类型的定性研究需要撰写不同类型的报告，对于初次接触定性研究报告撰写的研究人员，可以参照以下整体结构和各部分的撰写要求进行撰写。

The content and writing requirements of each part of the qualitative research report are as follows (Burnard P, 2004):

质性研究报告各部分的内容和撰写要求如下 (Burnard P, 2004):

2.2.1　Abstract(摘要)

Although the abstract needs to be written before it can be summarized and written, it is the first part of the article so that readers can understand the general content of the article in a short time. A good abstract should contain details of the background to the study, the aim, the sample, the data collection and analysis methods and a summary of the findings.

虽然摘要需要在写完全文才可以进行总结和撰写，但是它是文章的第一个部分，可以让读者短时间内了解文章的大致内容。一个好的摘要应该包含研究的背景、目的、样本、数据收集和分析方法的细节，以及研究结果的总结。

2.2.2　Introduction(引言)

The author should briefly explain what the research is, why it is needed, and the current status of relevant research.

作者需要简要说明这项研究是什么，为什么需要做这项研究，相关研究的现状如何等。

2.2.3　Aims of the study(研究目的)

2.2.4　Review of the literature(文献回顾)

2.2.5　Sample(抽样)

Convenience sampling is probably the most commonly used case in qualitative research. This part needs to clarify the sample size and sample type used in the study. If an unusual variant of sampling is used, it is useful to acknowledge the nature of it. Other comments about the sampling process may be helpful.

便利抽样可能是质性研究中最常用的情况。这部分需要明确研究中使用的样本量和样本类型。如果使用了一种不寻常的抽样方法，需要了解它的性质。关于抽样过程的其他评论可能会有所帮助。

2.2.6　Data collection methods(数据收集方法)

In many qualitative studies (but not all), the data collection method is usually the interview method. How the interviews were carried out should be noted, but this is not the place for a detailed critique of the interview process.

在许多质性研究(但不是全部)中，数据收集方法通常是访谈法。应该注意采访是如何进行的，但这里不需要写对采访过程中的详细批判。

2.2.7　Data analysis methods(数据分析方法)

A variation is to be found in the amount of detail of reporting in this section. It is possible to describe, in full, how the researcher handled the data, or it is possible to write that the interviews were recorded and transcribed. The researcher then sorted those data into a range of categories and made a report.

本节中报告的详细程度有所不同。可以完整地描述研究人员如何处理数据，或者可以写下"采访被记录和转录"。然后，研究人员将这些数据分类为一系列类别进行报告。

2.2.8　Findings(结果)

It should be noted that what is found in a qualitative study are always "findings" and/ "results". The findings of qualitative research are usually based on the analysis of the language and attitude of the research object.

需要注意的是，在质性研究中发现的总是"发现"而不是"结果"。质性研究的发现通常是对研究对象的语言和态度进行分析而得出的。

2.2.9 Discussion(讨论)

2.2.10 Conclusion(结论)

2.2.11 References(参考文献)

The writing method is the same as that of quantitative research.

与量性研究的文章书写方法相同。

2.2.12 Appendix(附录)

Ethical approval, funding sources and division of labor may be added to the appendix according to the requirements of different journals.

附录中根据不同杂志的要求，可能还需要补充伦理批准、资金来源和分工等。

Other notes written for such reports are also agreed to be available (e. g. Hollaway and Wheeler, 1996 & Holliday, 2001). Researchers are required to make appropriate choices based on research types and research results.

此类报告撰写的其他说明也是同意可用的(如 Hollaway 和 Wheeler, 1996; Holliday, 2001)。需要研究人员自行结合研究类型和研究结果做出适当的选择。

2.3 The Key Features of Qualitative Research Reports(质性研究报告的主要特征)

According to practical guidance for qualitative research, qualitative research reports have the following four main characteristics (Moser A & Korstjens I, 2017):

据质性研究的实用指南指出，质性研究报告有以下四个主要特征(Moser A 和 Korstjens I, 2017):

(1)Qualitative research studies phenomena in the natural contexts of individuals or groups.

质性研究研究个体或群体自然环境中的现象。

(2)Qualitative researchers try to gain a deeper understanding of people's experiences, perceptions, behavior and processes and the meanings they attach to them.

质性研究者试图更深入地理解人们的经历、感知、行为和过程，以及他们赋予它们的意义。

(3)During the research process, researchers use "emerging design" to be flexible in adjusting to the context.

在研究过程中，研究人员使用"新兴设计"来灵活地适应环境。

（4）Data collection and analysis are iterative processes that happen simultaneously as the research progresses.

数据收集和分析是随着研究进展而同时发生的迭代过程。

Section Ⅳ　Critiquing Research Reports
第四节　评判研究报告

The evaluation of research reports can improve their application in clinical practice. The evaluation content mainly includes：

对研究报告的评判，可以提高其在临床实践中的运用。评价内容主要包括：

（1）Does the report describe the purpose of the research，the overall structural framework，experimental design and methods，ethical issues，data analysis and discussion in detail so that readers can make a comprehensive judgment？

报告中是否对研究的目的、整体框架、实验设计和方法、伦理问题、数据分析和讨论都进行了细致的描写以便读者进行全面的评判？

（2）Is the language of the report concise and appropriate？

报告的语言是否精练贴切？

（3）Is the report written orderly and logically？Can the report convey the author's thoughts and continuity of expressions？

报告的书写是否有序、合乎逻辑？报告能传递出作者思想和表达的连续性吗？

（4）Can the tables or graphics in the report be effectively combined with the text description？

报告中的表格或图形是否与文字描述能够有效结合起来？

（5）Does the report contain obvious prejudice，exaggeration or distortion？

报告中是否包含明显的偏见、夸大或歪曲内容？

（6）Is gender-discriminatory language avoided in the report？

报告中是否避免使用性别歧视的语言？

（7）Is the report written using appropriately tentative language？

报告是否使用适当的试探性语言？

（8）Does the title of the report fully reflect the key concepts and population？

报告的标题是否充分体现了关键概念和人群？

📖 Studies Cited in Chapter 25(第二十五章参考文献)

[1] ICMJE. The Recommendations for the Conduct, Reporting, Editing, and Publication of Scholarly work[J]. Medical Journals, 2019.

[2] Denzin, N. K., Lincoln, Y. S. Introduction: The Discipline and Practice of Qualitative Research, The SAGE Handbook of Qualitative Research[M]. 5th ed. London: Sage, 2009: 10.

[3] Sawatsky, A. P., Ratelle, J. T., Beckman, T. J. Qualitative research methods in medical education[J]. Anesthesiology, 2019, 131(1): 14-22.

[4] Burnard P. Writing a qualitative research report[J]. Nurse Education Today, 2004, 24 (3): 174-179.

[5] Hollaway, I., Wheeler, S., Qualitative Research for Nurses[M]. Oxford: Blackwell, 1996.

[6] Holliday, A., Doing and Writing Qualitative Research[M]. London: Sage, 2001.

[7] Moser, A., Korstjens, I. Series: Practical guidance to qualitative research[J]. The European Journal of General Practice, 2017, 23(1): 271-273.

Appendix

附　录

Appendix 15. 3. 1　Critical Values for the t Distribution

(附录 15. 3. 1　t 界值表)

TABLE A. 1　∗　Critical Values for the *t* Distribution

df	α, 2-tailed test α, 1-tailed test	0. 10 0. 05	0. 05 0. 025	0. 02 0. 01	0. 01 0. 005	0. 001 0. 0005
1		6.314	12.706	31.821	63.657	636.619
2		2.920	4.303	6.965	9.925	31.598
3		2.353	3.182	4.541	5.841	12.941
4		2.132	2.776	3.747	4.604	8.610
5		2.015	2.571	3.376	4.032	6.859
6		1.953	2.447	3.143	3.707	5.959
7		1.895	2.365	2.998	3.449	5.405
8		1.860	2.306	2.896	3.355	5.041
9		1.833	2.262	2.821	3.250	4.781
10		1.812	2.228	2.765	3.169	4.587
11		1.796	2.202	2.718	3.106	4.437
12		1.782	2.179	2.681	3.055	4.318
13		1.771	2.160	2.650	3.012	4.221
14		1.761	2.145	2.624	2.977	4.140
15		1.753	2.131	2.602	2.947	4.073
16		1.746	2.120	2.583	2.921	4.015
17		1.740	2.110	2.567	2.898	3.965
18		1.734	2.101	2.552	2.878	3.922
19		1.729	2.093	2.539	2.861	3.883

续表

df	α,2-tailed test α,1-tailed test	0.10 0.05	0.05 0.025	0.02 0.01	0.01 0.005	0.001 0.0005
20		1.725	2.086	2.528	2.845	3.850
21		1.721	2.080	2.518	2.831	3.819
22		1.717	2.074	2.508	2.819	3.792
23		1.714	2.069	2.500	2.807	3.767
24		1.711	2.064	2.492	2.797	3.745
25		1.708	2.060	2.485	2.787	3.725
26		1.706	2.056	2.479	2.779	3.707
27		1.703	2.052	2.473	2.771	3.690
28		1.701	2.048	2.467	2.763	3.374
29		1.699	2.045	2.462	2.756	3.759
30		1.697	2.042	2.457	2.750	3.646
40		1.684	2.021	2.423	2.704	3.551
60		1.671	2.000	2.390	2.660	3.450
120		1.658	1.980	2.358	2.617	3.373
∞		1.645	1.960	2.326	2.576	3.291

Appendix 15.4.1 Critical Values for the F Distribution
(附录 15.4.1 F 界值表)

TABLE A.2 * Critical Values for the F Distribution

$\alpha = 0.05$ (Two-Tailed) $\qquad\qquad$ $\alpha = 0.025$ (One-Tailed)

$\dfrac{df_s}{df_w}$	1	2	3	4	5	6	8	12	24	∞
1	161.4	199.5	215.7	224.6	230.2	234.0	238.9	243.9	249.0	254.3
2	18.51	19.00	19.16	19.25	19.30	19.33	19.37	19.41	19.45	19.50
3	10.13	9.55	9.28	9.12	9.01	8.94	8.84	8.74	8.64	8.53
4	7.71	6.94	6.59	6.39	6.26	6.16	6.04	5.91	5.77	5.63
5	6.61	5.79	5.41	5.19	5.05	4.95	4.82	4.68	4.53	4.36
6	5.99	5.14	4.76	4.53	4.39	4.28	4.15	4.00	3.84	3.67
7	5.59	4.74	4.35	4.12	3.97	3.87	3.73	3.57	3.41	3.23

$\dfrac{df_s}{df_w}$	1	2	3	4	5	6	8	12	24	∞
8	5.32	4.45	4.07	3.84	3.69	3.58	3.44	3.28	3.12	2.93
9	5.12	4.26	3.86	3.63	3.48	3.37	3.23	3.07	2.90	2.71
10	4.96	4.10	3.71	3.48	3.33	3.22	3.07	2.91	2.74	2.54
11	4.84	3.98	3.59	3.36	3.20	3.09	2.95	2.79	2.61	2.40
12	4.75	3.88	3.49	3.26	3.11	3.00	2.85	2.69	2.50	2.30
13	4.67	3.80	3.41	3.18	3.02	2.92	2.77	2.60	2.42	2.21
14	4.60	3.74	3.34	3.11	2.96	2.85	2.70	2.53	2.35	2.13
15	4.54	3.68	3.29	3.06	2.90	2.79	2.64	2.48	2.29	2.07
16	4.49	3.63	3.24	3.01	2.85	2.74	2.59	2.42	2.24	2.01
17	4.45	3.59	3.20	2.96	2.81	2.70	2.55	2.38	2.19	1.96
18	4.41	3.55	3.16	2.93	2.77	2.66	2.51	2.34	2.15	1.92
19	4.38	3.52	3.13	2.90	2.74	2.63	2.48	2.31	2.11	1.88
20	4.35	3.49	3.10	2.87	2.71	2.60	2.45	2.28	2.08	1.84
21	4.32	3.47	3.07	2.84	2.68	2.57	2.42	2.25	2.05	1.81
22	4.30	3.44	3.05	2.82	2.66	2.55	2.40	2.23	2.03	1.78
23	4.28	3.42	3.03	2.80	2.64	2.53	2.38	2.20	2.00	1.76
24	4.26	3.40	3.01	2.78	2.62	2.51	2.36	2.18	1.98	1.73
25	4.24	3.38	2.99	2.76	2.60	2.49	2.34	2.16	1.96	1.71
26	4.22	3.37	2.98	2.74	2.59	2.47	2.32	2.15	1.95	1.69
27	4.21	3.35	2.96	2.73	2.57	2.46	2.30	2.13	1.93	1.67
28	4.20	3.34	2.95	2.71	2.56	2.44	2.29	2.12	1.91	1.65
29	4.18	3.33	2.93	2.70	2.54	2.43	2.28	2.10	1.90	1.64
30	4.17	3.32	2.92	2.69	2.53	2.42	2.27	2.09	1.80	1.62
40	4.08	3.23	2.84	2.61	2.45	2.34	2.18	2.00	1.79	1.51
60	4.00	3.15	2.76	2.52	2.37	2.25	2.10	1.92	1.70	1.39
120	3.92	3.07	2.68	2.45	2.29	2.17	2.02	1.83	1.61	1.25
∞	3.84	2.99	2.60	2.37	2.21	2.09	1.94	1.75	1.52	1.00

TABLE A. 2 ＊ Critical Values for the F Distribution(continued)

$\alpha=0.01$ [Two-Tailed]　　　　　　　　　　　　　　　　　　　　　$\alpha=0.005$ (One-Tailed)

$\dfrac{df_s}{df_w}$	1	2	3	4	5	6	8	12	24	∞
1	4052	4999	5403	5625	5764	5859	5981	6106	6234	6366
2	98.49	99.00	99.17	99.25	99.30	99.33	99.36	99.42	99.46	99.50
3	34.12	30.81	29.46	28.71	28.24	27.91	27.49	27.05	26.60	26.12
4	21.20	18.00	16.69	15.98	15.52	15.21	14.80	14.37	13.93	13.46
5	16.26	13.27	12.06	11.39	10.97	10.67	10.29	9.89	9.47	9.02
6	13.74	10.92	9.78	9.15	8.75	8.47	8.10	7.72	7.31	6.88
7	12.25	9.55	8.45	7.85	7.46	7.19	6.84	6.47	6.07	5.65
8	11.26	8.65	7.59	7.01	6.63	6.37	6.03	5.67	5.28	4.86
9	10.56	8.02	6.99	6.42	6.06	5.80	5.47	5.11	4.73	4.31
10	10.04	7.56	6.55	5.99	5.64	5.39	5.06	4.71	4.33	3.91
11	9.65	7.20	6.22	5.67	5.32	5.07	4.74	4.40	4.02	3.60
12	9.33	6.93	5.95	5.41	5.06	4.82	4.50	4.16	3.78	3.36
13	9.07	6.70	5.74	5.20	4.86	4.62	4.30	3.96	3.59	3.16
14	8.86	6.51	5.56	5.03	4.69	4.46	4.14	3.80	3.43	3.00
15	8.68	6.36	5.42	4.89	4.56	4.32	4.00	3.67	3.29	2.87
16	8.53	6.23	5.29	4.77	4.44	4.20	3.89	3.55	3.18	2.75
17	8.40	6.11	5.18	4.67	4.34	4.10	3.78	3.45	3.08	2.65
18	8.28	6.01	5.09	4.58	4.29	4.01	3.71	3.37	3.00	2.57
19	8.18	5.93	5.01	4.50	4.17	3.94	3.63	3.30	2.92	2.49
20	8.10	5.85	4.94	4.43	4.10	3.87	3.56	3.23	2.86	2.42
21	8.02	5.78	4.87	4.37	4.04	3.81	3.51	3.17	2.80	2.36
22	7.94	5.72	4.82	4.31	3.99	3.76	3.45	3.12	2.75	2.31
23	7.88	5.66	4.76	4.26	3.94	3.71	3.41	3.07	2.70	2.26
24	7.82	5.61	4.72	4.22	3.90	3.67	3.36	3.03	2.66	2.21
25	7.77	5.57	4.68	4.18	3.86	3.63	3.32	2.99	2.62	2.17
26	7.72	5.53	4.64	4.14	3.82	3.59	3.29	2.96	2.58	2.13
27	7.68	5.49	4.60	4.11	3.78	3.56	3.26	2.93	2.55	2.10
28	7.64	5.45	4.57	4.07	3.75	3.53	3.23	2.90	2.52	2.06
29	7.60	5.42	4.54	4.04	3.73	3.50	3.20	2.87	2.49	2.03
30	7.56	5.39	4.51	4.02	3.70	3.47	3.17	2.84	2.47	2.01
40	7.31	5.18	4.31	3.83	3.51	3.29	2.99	2.66	2.29	1.80
60	7.08	4.98	4.13	3.65	3.34	3.12	2.82	2.50	2.12	1.60
120	6.85	4.79	3.95	3.48	3.17	2.96	2.66	2.34	1.95	1.38
∞	6.64	4.60	3.78	3.32	3.02	2.80	2.51	2.18	1.79	1.00

TABLE A. 2　*　Critical Values for the F Distribution(continued)

α = 0. 001　[Two-Tailed]　　　　　　　　　　　　　　　　　　　　　　α = 0. 0005　(One-Tailed)

$\dfrac{df_s}{df_w}$	1	2	3	4	5	6	8	12	24	∞
1	405284	500000	540379	562500	576405	585937	598144	610667	623497	636619
2	998.5	999.0	999.2	999.2	999.3	999.3	999.4	999.4	999.5	999.5
3	167.5	148.5	141.1	137.1	134.6	132.8	130.6	128.3	125.9	123.5
4	74.14	61.25	56.18	53.44	51.71	50.53	49.00	47.41	45.77	44.05
5	47.04	36.61	33.20	31.09	29.75	28.84	27.64	26.42	25.14	23.78
6	35.51	27.00	23.70	21.90	20.81	20.03	19.03	17.99	16.89	15.75
7	29.22	21.69	18.77	17.19	16.21	15.52	14.63	13.71	12.73	11.69
8	25.42	18.49	15.83	14.39	13.49	12.86	17.04	11.19	10.30	9.34
9	22.86	16.39	13.90	12.56	11.71	11.13	10.37	9.57	8.72	7.81
10	21.04	14.91	12.55	11.28	10.48	9.92	9.20	8.45	7.64	6.76
11	19.69	13.81	11.56	10.35	9.58	9.05	8.35	7.63	6.85	6.00
12	18.64	12.97	10.80	9.63	8.89	8.38	7.71	7.00	6.25	5.42
13	17.81	12.31	10.21	9.07	8.35	7.86	7.21	6.52	5.78	4.97
14	17.14	11.78	9.73	8.62	7.92	7.43	6.80	6.13	5.41	4.60
15	16.59	11.34	9.34	8.25	7.57	7.09	6.47	5.81	5.10	4.31
16	16.12	10.97	9.00	7.94	7.27	6.81	6.19	5.55	4.85	4.06
17	15.72	10.66	8.73	7.68	7.02	6.56	5.96	5.32	4.63	3.85
18	15.38	10.39	8.49	7.46	6.81	6.35	5.76	5.13	4.45	3.67
19	15.08	10.16	8.28	7.26	6.61	6.18	5.59	4.97	4.29	3.52
20	14.82	9.95	8.10	7.10	6.46	6.02	5.44	4.82	4.15	3.38
21	14.59	9.77	7.94	6.95	6.32	5.88	5.31	4.70	4.03	3.26
22	14.38	9.61	7.80	6.81	6.19	5.76	5.19	4.58	3.92	3.15
23	14.19	9.47	7.67	6.69	6.08	5.65	5.09	4.48	3.82	3.05
24	14.03	9.34	7.55	6.59	5.98	5.55	4.99	4.39	3.74	2.97
25	13.88	9.22	7.45	6.49	5.88	5.46	4.91	4.31	3.66	2.89
26	13.74	9.12	7.36	6.41	5.80	5.38	4.83	4.24	3.59	2.82
27	13.61	9.02	7.27	6.33	5.73	5.31	4.76	4.17	3.52	2.75
28	13.50	8.93	7.19	6.25	5.66	5.24	4.69	4.11	3.46	2.70
29	13.39	8.85	7.12	6.19	5.59	5.18	4.64	4.05	3.41	2.64
30	13.29	8.77	7.05	6.12	5.53	5.12	4.58	4.00	3.36	2.59
40	12.61	8.25	6.60	5.70	5.13	4.73	4.21	3.64	3.01	2.23
60	11.97	7.76	6.17	5.31	4.76	4.37	3.87	3.31	2.69	1.90
120	11.38	7.31	5.79	4.95	4.42	4.04	3.55	3.02	2.40	1.56
∞	10.83	6.91	5.42	4.62	4.10	3.74	3.27	2.74	2.13	1.00

Appendix 15.5.1 Critical Values for the χ^2 Distribution

附录 15.5.1 χ^2 界值表

TABLE A.3 ∗ Critical Values for the χ^2 Distribution

df	LEVEL OF SIGNIFICANCE				
	0.10	0.05	0.02	0.01	0.001
1	2.71	3.84	5.41	6.63	10.83
2	4.61	5.99	7.82	9.21	13.82
3	6.25	7.82	9.84	11.34	16.27
4	7.78	9.49	11.67	13.28	18.46
5	9.24	11.07	13.39	15.09	20.52
6	10.64	12.59	15.03	16.81	22.46
7	12.02	14.07	16.62	18.48	24.32
8	13.36	15.51	18.17	20.09	26.12
9	14.68	16.92	19.68	21.67	27.88
10	15.99	18.31	21.16	23.21	29.59
11	17.28	19.68	22.62	24.72	31.26
12	18.55	21.03	24.05	26.22	32.91
13	19.81	22.36	25.47	27.69	34.53
14	21.06	23.68	26.87	29.14	36.12
15	22.31	25.00	28.26	30.58	37.70
16	23.54	26.30	29.63	32.00	39.25
17	24.77	27.59	31.00	33.41	40.79
18	25.99	28.87	32.35	34.81	42.31
19	27.20	30.14	33.69	36.19	43.82
20	28.41	31.41	35.02	37.57	45.32
21	29.62	32.67	36.34	38.93	46.80
22	30.81	33.92	37.66	40.29	48.27
23	32.01	35.17	38.97	41.64	49.73
24	33.20	36.42	40.27	42.98	51.18
25	34.38	37.65	41.57	44.31	52.62
26	35.56	38.89	42.86	45.64	54.05
27	36.74	40.11	44.14	46.96	55.48
28	37.92	41.34	45.42	48.28	56.89
29	39.09	42.56	46.69	49.59	58.30
30	40.26	43.77	47.96	50.89	59.70

（扫一扫，获得更多学习资料）